Managing Instability of the Wrist, Forearm and Elbow

Editor

JULIE E. ADAMS

HAND CLINICS

www.hand.theclinics.com

Consulting Editor
KEVIN C. CHUNG

November 2020 • Volume 36 • Number 4

ELSEVIER

1600 John F. Kennedy Boulevard ● Suite 1800 ● Philadelphia, Pennsylvania, 19103-2899

http://www.theclinics.com

HAND CLINICS Volume 36, Number 4
November 2020 ISSN 0749-0712, ISBN-13: 978-0-323-75994-6

Editor: Lauren Boyle
Developmental Editor: Kristen Helm

Hand Clinics (ISSN 0749-0712) is published quarterly by Elsevier Inc., 360 Park Avenue South, New York, NY 10010-1710. Months of publication are February, May, August, and November. Business and Editorial Offices: 1600 John F. Kennedy Blvd., Ste. 1800, Philadelphia, PA 19103-2899. Customer Service Office: 3251 Riverport Lane, Maryland Heights, MO 63043. Periodicals postage paid at New York, NY and at additional mailing offices. Subscription price is $439.00 per year (domestic individuals), $854.00 per year (domestic institutions), $100.00 per year (domestic students/residents), $501.00 per year (Canadian individuals), $994.00 per year (Canadian institutions), $562.00 per year (international individuals), $994.00 per year (international institutions), $256.00 (international students/residents), and $100.00 (Canadian students/residents). Foreign air speed delivery is included in all *Clinics* subscription prices. All prices are subject to change without notice. **POSTMASTER:** Send address changes to *Hand Clinics*, Elsevier Health Sciences Division, Subscription Customer Service, 3251 Riverport Lane, Maryland Heights, MO 63043. Customer Service (orders, claims, online, change of address): Elsevier Health Sciences Division, Subscription **Customer Service, 3251 Riverport Lane, Maryland Heights, MO 63043. Tel: 1-800-654-2452 (U.S. and Canada); 314-447-8871 (outside U.S. and Canada). Fax: 314-447-8029. E-mail: journalscustomerservice-usa@elsevier.com (for print support); journalsonlinesupport-usa@elsevier.com (for online support).**

Reprints. For copies of 100 or more of articles in this publication, please contact the Commercial Reprints Department, Elsevier Inc., 360 Park Avenue South, New York, New York 10010-1710. Tel.: 212-633-3874; Fax: 212-633-3820; E-mail: reprints@elsevier.com.

Hand Clinics is covered in *MEDLINE/PubMed (Index Medicus)*, *Current Contents/Clinical Medicine*, *EMBASE/Excerpta Medica*, and *ISI/BIOMED*.

Contributors

CONSULTING EDITOR

KEVIN C. CHUNG, MD, MS
Charles B. G. de Nancrede Professor of
Surgery, Professor of Plastic Surgery and
Orthopaedic Surgery, Chief of Hand Surgery,
Michigan Medicine, Assistant Dean for Faculty
Affairs, Associate Director of Global REACH,
University of Michigan Medical School, Ann
Arbor, Michigan, USA

EDITOR

JULIE E. ADAMS, MD
Professor of Orthopaedic Surgery, University
of Tennessee College of Medicine–
Chattanooga, Erlanger Orthopaedic Institute,
Chattanooga, Tennessee, USA

AUTHORS

EMILY E. ABBOTT, DO
Fellow, Orthopaedic Surgery, UPMC,
Pittsburgh, Pennsylvania, USA

BRIAN ADAMS, MD
Professor, Department of Orthopedic Surgery,
Baylor College of Medicine, Houston, Texas,
USA

JULIE E. ADAMS, MD
Professor of Orthopaedic Surgery, University
of Tennessee College of Medicine–
Chattanooga, Erlanger Orthopaedic Institute,
Chattanooga, Tennessee, USA

MARK E. BARATZ, MD
Program Director, Orthopaedic Surgery,
UPMC, Pittsburgh, Pennsylvania, USA

JUAN MANUEL BREYER, MD
Hand Surgeon, Orthopedic Department,
Hospital del Trabajador, Santiago,
Providencia, Chile; Hand Surgeon, Orthopedic
Department, Clinica Alemana-Universidad del
Desarrollo, Santiago, Chile

RICHARD A. CAMBO, MA
Research Associate, Research Department,
Miami Hand & Upper Extremity Institute,
Miami, Florida, USA

LOGAN W. CARR, MD
Fellow, Department of Orthopedic Surgery,
Baylor College of Medicine, Houston, Texas,
USA

KEVIN C. CHUNG, MD, MS
Charles B. G. de Nancrede Professor of
Surgery, Professor of Plastic Surgery and
Orthopaedic Surgery, Chief of Hand Surgery,
Michigan Medicine, Assistant Dean for Faculty
Affairs, Associate Director of Global REACH,
University of Michigan Medical School, Ann
Arbor, Michigan, USA

NILOOFAR DEHGHAN, MD, FRCS
The CORE Institute, Phoenix, Arizona, USA

FELICITY G. FISHMAN, MD
Assistant Professor, Department of
Orthopaedic Surgery & Rehabilitation, Loyola

University Medical Center, Maywood, Illinois, USA; Staff Hand Surgeon, Shriners Hospital for Children, Chicago, Illinois, USA

ROHIT GARG, MD
Hand and Upper Extremity Surgery, Department of Orthopaedics, Massachusetts General Hospital, Boston, Massachusetts, USA

DOUGLAS HANEL, MD
Professor, Department of Orthopaedics and Sports Medicine, University of Washington, Seattle, Washington, USA

MICHAEL R. HAUSMAN, MD
Lippmann Professor of Orthopaedics, Chief of Upper Extremity Surgery, Department of Orthopaedic Surgery, Mount Sinai Hospital, New York, New York, USA

GRAHAM J.W. KING, MD, MSc, FRSC
Roth | McFarlane Hand & Upper Limb Centre, Professor of Surgery, Division of Orthopaedics, Western University, St. Joseph's Health Care, London, Ontario, Canada

ANTHONY L. LOGLI, MD
Orthopedic Surgery Resident, Department of Orthopedic Surgery, Mayo Clinic, Rochester, Minnesota, USA

TIMOTHY J. LUCHETTI, MD
Fellow, Orthopaedic Surgery, UPMC, Pittsburgh, Pennsylvania, USA

TYLER C. MILLER, MD
Hand Fellow, Department of Orthopaedic Surgery & Rehabilitation, Loyola University Medical Center, Maywood, Illinois, USA

STEVEN L. MORAN, MD
Professor, Departments of Plastic & Reconstructive Surgery, and Orthopedic Surgery, Mayo Clinic, Rochester, Minnesota, USA

CHAITANYA MUDGAL, MD
Hand and Upper Extremity Surgery, Department of Orthopaedics, Massachusetts General Hospital, Boston, Massachusetts, USA

JORGE L. ORBAY, MD
Medical Director, Orthopaedic Surgery Department, Miami Hand & Upper Extremity

Institute, Clinical Associate Professor of Orthopaedic Surgery, The Herbert Wertheim School of Medicine, Florida International University, Miami, Florida, USA

A. LEE OSTERMAN, MD
Professor of Orthopedic Surgery, Thomas Jefferson University, Philadelphia Hand to Shoulder Center, Philadelphia, Pennsylvania, USA

MIDHAT PATEL, MD
Department of Orthopedic Surgery, University of Arizona College of Medicine–Phoenix, Phoenix, Arizona, USA

JOEY G. PIPICELLI, MScOT, CHT
Roth | McFarlane Hand and Upper Limb Centre, Division of Hand Therapy, St. Joseph's Health Care, Lecturer, Faculty of Health Sciences, School of Occupational Therapy, Western University, London, Ontario, Canada

LOUIS H. POPPLER, MD, MSCI
Consultant, Department of Plastic & Reconstructive Surgery, St. Luke's Health System, Boise, Idaho, USA

NICHOLAS PULOS, MD
Assistant Professor, Department of Orthopedic Surgery, Mayo Clinic, Rochester, Minnesota, USA

PHILLIP R. ROSS, MD
Assistant Professor, Department of Orthopaedic Surgery, University of Cincinnati Medical Center, Cincinnati, Ohio, USA

DANIL A. RYBALKO, MD
Hand Surgery Fellow, Department of Orthopaedic Surgery, Mount Sinai Hospital, New York, New York, USA

BRETT SCHIFFMAN, MD
Resident, Department of Orthopaedics and Sports Medicine, University of Washington, Seattle, Washington, USA

PAMELA VERGARA, MD
Hand Surgeon, Orthopedic Department, Hospital del Trabajador, Santiago, Providencia, Chile; Hand Surgeon, Orthopedic Department, Clinica Las Condes, Santiago, Chile

Contents

> Three predictable patterns of forearm fracture-dislocation—Essex-Lopresti, Monteg-gia, and Galeazzi—can occur and are eponymously labeled for the investigators who appreciated their unique characteristics and offered a framework by which to under-stand them. Subsequent investigation has resulted in an improved understanding of forearm anatomy and stability. Management of the instability component differs based on the type of fracture-dislocation, timing of intervention, and surgeon preference. Despite advances in both understanding and treating these injuries, several nuances continue to make them challenging entities for the modern day surgeon to handle.

> In the forearm, ligaments and joints act in unison to facilitate placement of the hand in 3-dimensional space and transmit loads across the upper extremity. Intricate, effective forearm stabilizers facilitate physiologic motions and restrict abnormal ones. The proximal radioulnar joint, interosseous ligament complex, and distal radio-ulnar joint work together to ensure the forearm is stable. Each ligament and joint is designed to leverage its biomechanical advantages. Damage destabilizes the syn-ergy of the forearm and results in debilitating injury patterns. Physicians need to un-derstand how all these structures work together to be able to quickly diagnose and treat these forearm injuries.

> Distal radius fractures with severe displacement or concomitant triangular fibrocar-tilage complex tears may be accompanied by distal radioulnar joint instability. Clini-cians should examine the distal radioulnar joint closely when managing wrist fractures and treat coexisting instability appropriately. Chronic instability from distal radius malunion may require osteotomy or radioulnar ligament reconstruction. With proper management, most patients recover forearm stability and rotational motion after distal radius fracture.

> This article reviews the anatomy and mechanics of pronation and supination (axial rotation) of the forearm through the distal radioulnar joint (DRUJ), and the proximal

radioulnar joint (PRUJ). Injuries to the bones and/or ligaments of the forearm, wrist, or elbow can result in instability, pain, and limited rotation. Acute dislocations of the DRUJ commonly occur along with a fracture to the distal radius, radial metadiaphysis, or radial head. These injuries are all caused by high-energy trauma. Outcomes are predicated on anatomic reduction and restoration of stability to the DRUJ and PRUJ with or without ligamentous repair or reconstruction.

The distal radioulnar joint is inherently unstable, relying primarily on ligaments for stability. Disruption of the joint-stabilizing structures can occur in isolation or concomitantly with osseous trauma. Instability can result from dislocations, fractures, ligament injuries, or malunions. Untreated instability alters wrist and forearm kinematics, leading to pain, weakness, and possibly arthritis. In chronic instability, the native ligaments may not be reparable, necessitating a reconstructive procedure.

Fractures of the radial shaft associated with disruption of the distal radioulnar joint (DRUJ) are termed Galeazzi fractures. These fractures are unstable injuries requiring open reduction and internal fixation of the fracture to achieve optimal outcomes. DRUJ stability should be carefully assessed intraoperatively and addressed accordingly.

This article describes evaluation and treatment considerations for Essex-Lopresti injuries. Specific information about pattern recognition and treatment options is provided.

Monteggia fracture-dislocations in the pediatric population have unique patterns of injury that require distinct considerations in diagnosis and management. When appropriately diagnosed and treated early, acute pediatric Monteggia injuries have favorable outcomes. Missed or inadequately treated injuries result in chronic Monteggia lesions that require more complex surgical reconstructions and are associated with less predictable outcomes. This article reviews the classification, diagnosis, and treatment of acute and chronic pediatric Monteggia injuries as well as the controversies there in.

Monteggia fracture-dislocation of the elbow is a fracture of the proximal ulna with associated dislocation of the radial head or radial neck fracture. In adults, this injury is managed with open reduction and internal fixation of the ulna fracture. Care should be taken to ensure anatomic reduction of the proximal ulna. If radial head dislocation or subluxation persists, reduction of the ulna should be reassessed. Rarely, interposed soft tissue may block radial head reduction, and requires removal. Complications include hardware prominence, stiffness, infection, heterotopic ossification, nerve injury, malunion or nonunion of the ulna, radioulnar synostosis, and persistent radial head instability.

Acute elbow dislocations are commonly seen in clinical practice, and attention to management principles and strategies can help facilitate improved outcomes. Patients may present with simple elbow dislocation, in which nonoperative treatment is highly successful. Alternatively, fracture dislocations can be sometimes easily managed but frequently are associated with the need for surgical intervention and operative and postoperative challenges.

Elbow dislocations represent common injuries. A quarter of these injuries involve at least 1 fracture. The sequel of elbow fracture-dislocations can be fraught with complications, including recurrent instability, posttraumatic arthritis, elbow contracture, and poor functional results. The 3 main patterns of injury are valgus posterolateral rotatory instability, varus posteromedial rotatory instability, and transolecranon fracture-dislocation. This article discusses each pattern individually, including the anatomy, the typical injury pattern, and treatment strategies. It also discusses common complications that can occur.

The elbow is the second most commonly dislocated major joint in adults with estimated incidence of 5 dislocations per 100,000 persons per year. A comprehensive understanding of elbow anatomy and biomechanics is essential to optimize rehabilitation of elbow injuries. This allows for implementation of a systematic therapy program that encourages early mobilization within a safe arc of motion while maintaining joint stability. To optimize outcomes, close communication between surgeon and therapist is necessary to allow for implementation of an individualized rehabilitation program. This article reviews key concepts that enable the clinician to apply an evidence-informed approach when managing elbow instability.

An unstable and osteoarthritic distal radioulnar joint presents with considerable functional impairment, pain, and weakness in gripping manipulation of objects. A wide variety of surgical alternatives have been described to address these concerns. Resection arthroplasties include different types of distal ulna resection and soft tissue procedures; good overall results have been described for these types of procedures, although they have shown limitations in achieving and maintaining pain relief and stability, especially in more active patients. Since the late 1980s, partial and total joint arthroplasties have emerged as good alternatives for treatment in young and more active patients.

The One Bone Forearm

Brett Schiffman and Douglas Hanel

The one bone forearm is a salvage procedure for treatment of painful, instability of the forearm that results from trauma, congenital deformity, tumor, infection, and failed reconstructive efforts. By creating a stable osseous bridge between the ulno-humeral and radiocarpal joints, one bone forearm addresses defects in the bony architecture of the radius and ulna, their articulations, and their associated ligamentous complexes. Global instability of the forearm is a complex clinical pathology with few other answers. Choice of technique should be dictated by adjacent bone loss. This article presents experience with creating a one bone forearm in patients using synostosis procedures.

Solutions for the Unstable and Arthritic Elbow Joint

Danil A. Rybalko and Michael R. Hausman

An unstable, arthritic elbow presents a therapeutic challenge. Patients may have painful, limited range of motion, often due to trauma or progressive joint destruction from rheumatologic disease. The options for management may be particularly challenging when treating young, active patients. While elbow arthroplasty usually provides predictable pain relief and joint range of motion, concerns exist regarding postoperative activity limitations and implant survival. Therefore, these procedures are limited to select subsets of patients, typically low-demand, elderly patients. Interposition arthroplasty is an option for the young, active patient with a painful arthritic elbow.

HAND CLINICS

SERIES OF RELATED INTEREST:

Clinics in Plastic Surgery
https://www.plasticsurgery.theclinics.com/

Orthopedic Clinics of North America
https://www.orthopedic.theclinics.com/

Physical Medicine and Rehabilitation Clinics of North America
https://www.pmr.theclinics.com/

THE CLINICS ARE AVAILABLE ONLINE!
Access your subscription at:
www.theclinics.com

Introduction

In this issue, experienced and expert authors share their insights on the problems of instability of the forearm.

A review of the history of our recognition of these problems with a nod to the owners of the eponyms by which many of these conditions are known, is presented by Dr Anthony Logli and Dr Nick Pulos. It is especially remarkable to read this article in light of the knowledge that Dr Pulos, at the time his article is written, is serving his country in the US Navy in Afghanistan. Thank you, Dr Pulos, for your service.

An understanding of the biomechanical factors contributing to stability of the forearm in the normal state and the pathologic factors associated with instability is beautifully and pictorially described by Dr Jorge Orbay and Mr Richard Campo in their article.

Distal radius fractures are common and may be associated with distal radioulnar joint instability. An understanding of the factors associated with instability, the treatment options, and alternatives is described in the article by Dr Phillip Ross and Dr Kevin Chung.

The optimal evaluation and treatment options in the setting of acute distal radioulnar joint injuries are discussed by Dr Louis Poppler and Dr Steve Moran and in the setting of chronic distal radioulnar joint injuries are discussed by Dr Logan Carr and Dr Brian Adams.

The fracture dislocations and injuries that bear eponyms are also covered: Galeazzi fractures (by Dr Rohit Garg and Dr Chai Mudgal), Essex Lopresti (by Dr Julie Adams and Dr A. Lee Osterman), and Monteggia fractures in both children (by Dr Tyler and Dr Felicity Fishman) and adults (by Dr Midhat Patel and Dr Niloofar Dehghan).

The elbow is discussed next, including evaluation and treatment of the unstable elbow (Dr Julie Adams) and elbow fracture dislocations (Dr Timothy Luchetti, Dr Emily Abbott, and Dr Mark Baratz). Important rehabilitation principles are outlined by Mr Joey Pipicelli and Dr Graham King.

Salvage options for end stage arthrosis or instability are discussed, including solutions for the unstable and arthritic distal radioulnar joint (Dr. Juan Manual Breyer); the one-bone forearm (Dr Doug Hanel and Dr Brett Alan Schiffman); and the unstable and arthritic elbow joint (Dr Danil Rybalko and Dr Michael Hausman).

All in total, this issue looks closely at evaluation and treatment for instability of the forearm axis from the distal radioulnar joint to the elbow and in between, and the authors provide a valuable resource to understand and treat these conditions.

Julie E. Adams, MD
University of Tennessee College of Medicine–Chattanooga
Erlanger Orthopaedic Institute
975 E 3rd Street Suite C 225
Chattanooga, TN 37403, USA

E-mail address:
adams.julie.e@gmail.com

Hand Clin 36 (2020) xi
https://doi.org/10.1016/j.hcl.2020.08.002
0749-0712/20/© 2020 Published by Elsevier Inc.

Preface

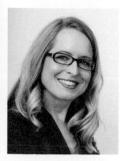

Julie E. Adams MD
Editor

In the year 2020, the year of this issue's publication, we have faced unprecedented challenges to our society, to our patients, and to us as surgeons and health care workers providing musculoskeletal health. The pandemic of COVID-19 has altered all our lives, perhaps for a few months or perhaps permanently.

We have changed the way we provide care and the way we educate ourselves and others. We have canceled in-person meetings and have experienced disruption of the way in which we interact and provide surgical and nonsurgical care for patients, and even in ways we live our lives, with social distancing being the norm. Some of us have practiced "outside of the scope" of our training, rising to challenges of which previously we never dreamed. Nevertheless, the challenges of forearm injuries continue to present and will remain problems, even after COVID-19 is a memory. It is for that reason I am especially grateful to the authors of this *Hand Clinics*, and the Elsevier staff, who even in the midst of this situation, have created an issue focusing upon instability of the forearm. This reference serves as a guide to aid in evaluation and management of these often challenging conditions. Likewise, I am indebted to my family, including my husband, Scott Steinmann, and our children, Sarah and Hannah, for their patience and support.

Julie E. Adams, MD
University of Tennessee College of Medicine–
Chattanooga
Erlanger Orthopaedic Institute
975 E 3rd Street Suite C 225
Chattanooga, TN 37403, USA

E-mail address:
adams.julie.e@gmail.com

Hand Clin 36 (2020) xiii
https://doi.org/10.1016/j.hcl.2020.08.001

Problems of Eponymous Proportions
The History Behind Recognizing Forearm Instability Issues

Anthony L. Logli, MD, Nicholas Pulos, MD*

KEYWORDS

- Forearm instability • Essex-Lopresti • Monteggia • Galeazzi • "Fracture of necessity"
- Piedmont fracture • Interosseous membrane • Longitudinal radioulnar dissociation

KEY POINTS

- Eponymous forearm injuries include Essex-Lopresti, Monteggia, and Galeazzi fracture-dislocations.
- Lessons learned from successes and failures in treating these injuries have fostered a greater understanding of forearm anatomy and stability.
- Conceptually, the forearm's bony and soft tissue structures are understood to function together as a single unit, consisting of the radius, ulna, distal radioulnar joint, proximal radioulnar joint, and interosseous membrane, where disruption of more than any one of these results in forearm instability.
- Although knowledge and experience with these injuries continue to grow, the foundation set forth by early investigators, who provided the descriptions and shared their namesakes, continues to be of relevance when treating these challenging injuries.

INTRODUCTION

Early surgeon investigators recognized that certain forearm fractures occurred with predictable patterns of instability. They were descriptive in their evaluation and established a foundation for understanding these injuries. Although relatively rare, when a forearm fracture-dislocation does occur, the fracture component often is simpler to appreciate and address. In these cases, it is important to have a high index of suspicion to avoid missing the component of instability. When missed, patients unfortunately may face the consequences of pain, poor motion, loss of function, and further instability. Although contemporaries may call for a more descriptive designation of these injuries, oponyms persist within the orthopedic vernacular, partly due to familiarity and tradition, but also to commemorate the early leaders in the field who

have contributed to understanding of these complex problems. This article discusses the history behind recognizing the 3 most common types of forearm instability—Essex Lopresti, Monteggia, and Galeazzi—starting first with insights gained from these injuries as related to forearm function, anatomy, and stability.

THE FOREARM—ANATOMIC CONSIDERATIONS OF FOREARM STABILITY

The forearm may be thought of as having 3 primary functions, to (1) permit pronosupination to position the hand in space, (2) transfer axial loads from the wrist to the elbow, and (3) serve as a site of attachment for muscles of the hand and wrist.[1] Stability of the forearm is conferred by the intricate interplay of bony and soft tissue structures and articulations within the forearm's proximal radioulnar

Department of Orthopedic Surgery, Mayo Clinic, 200 1st Street Southwest, Rochester, MN 55905, USA
* Corresponding author.
E-mail address: pulos.nicholas@mayo.edu
Twitter: @AnthonyLogliMD (A.L.L.); @NickPulosMD (N.P.)

Hand Clin 36 (2020) 397–406
https://doi.org/10.1016/j.hcl.2020.07.010

joint (PRUJ) and distal radioulnar joint (DRUJ) as well as from the humerus and carpus. The individual contributions to stability are outlined.

Bony

Radius
Proximally, the radial head has a slight elliptical shape that is offset from the radial shaft by approximately 15°. It is the primary contributor to longitudinal forearm stability, protects against posterior forearm displacement, and acts as a secondary stabilizer to valgus stress of the elbow in conjunction with the anterior bundle of the medial collateral ligament.

Ulna
Proximally, the ulna conforms to the trochlea of the distal humerus by means of a 190° bony arc known as the greater sigmoid notch. The coronoid process is a triangular, bony projection at the anterior, terminal extent of the greater sigmoid notch that serves as a key stabilizer to varus stress and to elbow extension by preventing posterior displacement of the forearm.[2]

Soft Tissue

Annular ligament
Also known as the orbicular ligament[3], this thick and strong band of fibrocartilage tissue both originates and insert on the lesser sigmoid notch of the ulnar after encircling the radial head-neck junction. It may be ruptured, ruptured and interposed, or intact in a Monteggia injury.[4]

Quadrate ligament
This thin ligamentous band of tissue covers the joint capsule inferior to the annular ligament and extends from just below the lesser sigmoid notch to the radial neck.[5] It is often disrupted in Monteggia injuries.

Interosseous membrane
This complex ligamentous structure, sometimes referred to as the middle radioulnar joint (MRUJ)[6,7] links radial and ulnar diaphyses and consists of 5 discrete parts. From proximal to distal these are the proximal oblique cord, dorsal oblique accessory cord, accessory band, central band (CB), additional accessory band, the distal oblique bundle (DOB). The CB is by far the strongest component of the IOM and runs obliquely from the proximal one third of the radius to the distal one-fourth of the ulna at a 21o angle.[8,9] Absence of CB restraint at the distal one-third of the radius is thought to contribute to the higher risk of radial shortening when this area is fractured.[10] The DOB is the other structure thought

to confer stability to the DRUJ in all positions of forearm rotation.[11,12] This structure is injured in Essex-Lopresti injuries.

Triangular fibrocartilage complex
This structure consists of palmar and dorsal components each having superficial and deep attachments sharing a common origin at the ulnar aspect of the radius in between the lunate fossa and sigmoid notch. The superficial TFCC attachments insert on the ulnar styloid whereas the deep attachments insert within the fovea.[13] The TFCC serves as a soft tissue stabilizer of the DRUJ. Thus, injury can lead to DRUJ instability and radial shortening. Radial shortening for another reason, e.g. IOM injury, may also stress and injure the TFCC.[14] The TFCC is injured in Galeazzi and Essex-Lopresti injuries.

Forearm Articulations

PRUJ
The PRUJ is a bony and soft tissue articulation between the radius and ulna at the level of the elbow. It is primarily stabilized by the annular ligament and CB of the IOM in pronation and the CB of the IOM in supination.[15] Instability of the PRUJ is seen in Monteggia injuries.

DRUJ
The DRUJ is a bony and soft tissue articulation between the radius and ulna at the level of the wrist. It receives primary stability from the TFCC and secondary bony stability from the sigmoid notch. The DRUJ is at greatest risk of injury with middle and distal one-third fractures of the radius. Instability of the DRUJ is seen in Essex-Lopresti and Galeazzi injuries.

ESSEX-LOPRESTI INJURIES

In a 1946 publication of the *British Journal of Surgery*, Curr and Coe[16] describe a single case report of a young coal miner who sustained a "vertical dislocation of the inferior radio-ulnar joint associated with posterior dislocation and fracture of the upper end of the radius" when his arm was caught between 2 mining hutches. This mechanism was very different from the forced abduction moment that typically causes radial head fractures. The patient presented with severe pain and swelling and limited mobility of the forearm that was attributed to disruption of the IOM. After an open reduction and period of immobilization in full supination for 6 weeks, these investigators reported satisfactory results with 1-year follow-up in the first confirmed case of this unusual injury.

Five years later, a posthumously published account provided a detailed description of Peter Essex-Lopresti's experience with 2 similar cases of the condition that now bears his name.[17] In this description, he talks of the importance of always suspecting DRUJ instability with a radial head fracture (**Fig 1.**). Despite being relatively uncommon, the consequences of a missed injury often are further surgery and morbidity Additionally, he observed that excision of the radial head in this injury was a mistake, because the radial head is an important restraint to proximal migration of the radius.

Essex-Lopresti advocated for repair of the radial head whenever possible or excision and prosthetic replacement if not. The first developed prosthetic radial head is attributed to Kellogg Speed in 1941, but they were not commonly implanted at the time of Essex-Lopresti's publication.[18,19] The first reported case of radial head replacement for severe radial head comminution in an Essex-Lopresti injury was not until more than 20 years later.[20] Use of metallic radial head implants occurred in the early 1990s and represents the standard treatment of any unreconstructable radial head fracture today. In comparison to silicone, these implants have demonstrated improved valgus stability, greater durability, and better restoration of forearm rotation.[21] Potential complications largely include loosening in the setting of press fit or cemented stems, overstuffing of the joint, and the development of capitellar arthritis.[22]

An Essex-Lopresti injury is characterized as much by its mechanism (a violent longitudinal and compressive force) as it is the anatomy involved (radial head fracture, disruption of the IOM, and instability of the DRUJ). Motor vehicle accidents or falls from a great height are the most common mechanisms.[23] It is far less

common than an isolated radial head fracture (accounting for only 1% of all radial head fractures) but also far easier to miss on initial assessment.[24] As Essex-Lopresti warned, a high index of suspicion is imperative when assessing for this injury because wrist and forearm pain can be mild, elbow pain can act as a distractor, and even radiographs of the wrist may be normal or show only a subtle loss of radial height[7] (**Fig. 2**).

Since Essex-Lopresti's early work, interest and investigation into understanding this specific injury pattern have led to an increased appreciation of the intricacies of IOM anatomy and biomechanics of the forearm. The complex interplay between the forearm, wrist, and elbow is now better understood to function as a forearm unit, ring, or joint.[25] This can be thought of as consisting of 5 composite parts—the radius, the ulna, the PRUJ, the DRUJ, and the IOM—with an injury to any 2 of these structures making the ring unstable.[26]

Conceptual understanding of this injury is aided further by considering the forearm to have 3 primary stabilizers against an axial loading force. In order of their contribution to conferring forearm stability, these are (1) the radial head, (2) the IOM, and (3) the DRUJ. Since the original description of an Essex-Lopresti injury, the TFCC has been shown to be the primary stabilizer of the DRUJ and, thus, often is included in contemporary descriptions of Essex-Lopresti injuries.[27]

In 1988, Edwards and Jupiter[23] formulated a descriptive, treatment-based classification system for Essex-Lopresti injuries based on injury patterns presenting to their practice (**Table 1**). Although this classification schema is widely used today and is helpful in considering both the status of the radial head and timing of the injury relative to surgical intervention, it suggests that forearm stability will be re-established after achieving a united and reduced radial head.

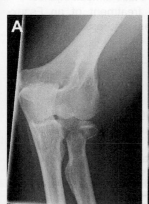 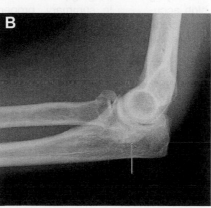

Fig. 1. (A) Anteroposterior radiograph of an Essex-Lopresti injury demonstrating a comminuted radial head fracture. (B) On the lateral view, an arrow points out a malrotated and displaced articular fragment. This patient presented with elbow, forearm, and wrist pain. (From Dodds SD, Yeh PC, Slade JF. Essex-lopresti injuries. Hand Clin 2008;24(1):130; with permission.)

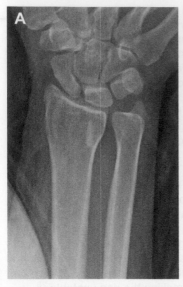

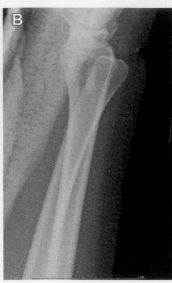

Fig. 2. (*A*) The same patient's posteroanterior radiograph of the wrist revealed subtle widening at the DRUJ. (*B*) The lateral wrist radiograph confirmed dorsal subluxation of the distal ulna. (*From* Dodds SD, Yeh PC, Slade JF. Essex-lopresti injuries. Hand Clin 2008;24(1):131; with permission.)

However, stability at the wrist also is critical. Surgical treatment of the DRUJ, therefore, has been aimed not only at re-establishing radio-ulnar variance and reducing the ulnar head but also restoring DRUJ stability.[28] Often, this is accomplished through repair or reconstruction of the TFCC whenever possible.[2,28,29]

Furthermore, although some investigators believe a reduced PRUJ and DRUJ is enough to stabilize the forearm and restore longitudinal stability,[28,30] ie, reconstitute the forearm ring to establish enough relative stability for IOM healing, others believe there may be a role for directly addressing the IOM. More recently, there has been growing interest in either directly repairing the IOM or augmenting or reconstructing the IOM in acute or chronic situations, respectively.[31,32]

In the acute setting, preoperative ultrasonography or magnetic resonance imaging both have been shown to be capable of reliably identifying tears or a disruption in the IOM with high accuracy.[33–35] Furthermore, intraoperative maneuvers,

such as the radial pull test, can be performed to assess the status of the IOM and TFCC when the radial head is irreparable and resection or arthroplasty is planned.[36]

Strategies for the augmentation or reconstruction of the ever more challenging chronic Essex-Lopresti injury have included various autograft (eg, palmaris longus, flexor carpi radialis, and bone-patellar-bone), allograft (eg, Achilles tendon), and synthetic materials (eg, suture button), all intending to replicate the position, orientation, and function of the CB component of the IOM.[7]

Although results of early efforts to surgically address an incompetent IOM have been promising, further research with comparative cohorts and long-term follow-up is needed to determine the value of repair or reconstruction of the IOM as well as to develop a standard algorithm for managing patients with these difficult injuries.

In summary, proper treatment of an Essex-Lopresti injury involves addressing both the

Table 1
Edwards and Jupiter classification of Essex-Lopresti injuries

Type I	Radial head fracture with fragments amenable to ORIF
Type II	Comminuted radial head fractures requiring excision and prosthetic replacement
Type III	Chronic injuries with a proximally migrated, irreducible radial head requiring ulnar shortening osteotomy and radial head excision with prosthetic replacement

Data from Edwards JG, Jupiter JB. Radial head fractures with acute distal radioulnar dislocation. Essex-Lopresti revisited. *Clinical orthopaedics and related research.* 1988(234):61-69.

fracture and instability to restore the forearm ring and confer pain-free forearm rotation and function. Although some investigators may advocate for the adoption of a more descriptive term for this unique injury pattern, such as longitudinal radioulnar dissociation, it is important not to forget the impact Essex-Lopresti had on understanding of this injury, as his insights made some 70 years ago continue to guide treatment today.

MONTEGGIA INJURIES

In 1814, Giovanni Battista Monteggia[37] described 2 cases of fractures at the upper end of the ulna with concomitant radial head dislocations. In his initial description, it was noted that radial head reduction was imperative but also difficult to achieve in a closed manner. In a 1909 publication it was Perrin[38] who referred to the injury pattern eponymously as a Monteggia fracture and it has been cataloged in the literature as such ever since. Although the energy incurred is of a magnitude great enough to cause fractures of both the ulnar and radial shafts, the transmitted force is thought to instead disrupt the annular ligament, thereby preventing containment of the radial head.[39] Furthermore, interposition of the ruptured annular ligament and deforming forces of muscular attachments often lead to unsuccessful results with closed reduction maneuvers even if fracture realignment is achieved (**Fig. 3**).

Speed and Boyd[39] reported on one of the largest early series of Monteggia fractures in the English literature and stressed how critical open reduction and internal fixation (ORIF) of the ulna and reduction of the radial head were to treating this injury in order to avoid future restrictions of function and motion. Even with anatomic realignment of the fracture, they comment that failure to maintain a reduced radial head, may lead to an increased carrying angle, muscle atrophy, weakness, and radial head arthrosis. This thinking represented a paradigm shift in the treatment of Monteggia injuries, because, prior to this, treating the ulnar fracture and radial head dislocation in a closed fashion was standard practice, reserving open treatment for chronic cases.[40]

Speed and Boyd[39] also distinguished between pediatric Monteggia injuries and those occurring in adults. In their experience with pediatric patients, closed reduction was more successful in both realigning the ulna and maintaining a reduced radial head. Furthermore, the growth potential of children permitted some degree of residual angulation without compromising outcomes. They caution, however, that if there is any difficulty in obtaining near-anatomical alignment or any question of radial head instability after closed reduction, ORIF is warranted. Finally, resection of the radial head was performed only if deemed necessary to reduce the ulna or PRUJ, such as in a chronic Monteggia injury with a nonunited or malunited ulna and a dislocated radial head.[39]

Until the cadaveric report of E.M. Evans[41], Monteggia injuries were thought to occur only secondary to a direct and violent impact. In 1949, Evans showed that anterior dislocation of the radial head more likely was a result of extreme pronation of the forearm beyond its inherent limit and around a fixed hand (often fixed to the ground). (often to the ground). This caused the ulna to fracture while at the same time levering the radial head out of its

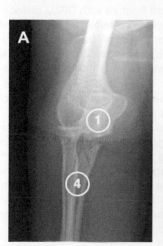
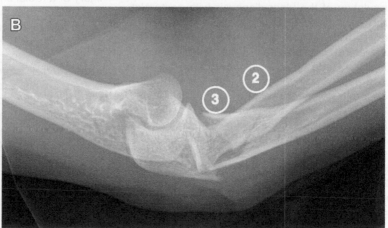

Fig. 3. Right elbow radiographs showcasing deforming forces of the Monteggia injury. 1. Supinator—directs proximal ulnar fragment radially. 2. Biceps—directs radius anteriorly. 3. Brachialis—directs ulna anteriorly. 4. IOM—prevents radio-ulnar diastasis and proximal migration of the radius.

anatomic location. More than 20 years later, D.G Tompkins[42] proposed an alternative mechanism of injury related less to forearm position and more to the synchronized soft tissue forces occurring during a fall. He suggested that the inciting event is a sudden and violent contraction of the biceps muscle that causes the radial head to dislocate anteriorly during a fall onto an outstretched hand. Tension from the attached IOM and the force of the contracting brachialis muscle subsequently causes the ulna to fracture.

Both of these mechanisms, however, only describe the anterior Monteggia fracture variety. In 1951, J.H Penrose[30] devised a cadaveric experiment to illustrate and reproduce the mechanism of posterior radial head dislocation, which was much less appreciated than the anterior dislocations at the time. Based on the radial head shear fracture commonly associated with this Monteggia type, Penrose reasoned that the forearm is often in a 30° pronated position with the elbow flexed to 120° before receiving a direct blow to the elbow. When the bone is stronger than the surrounding elbow ligaments, an elbow dislocation is seen; when the ligamentous structures are stronger than the bone, an ulnar fracture and Monteggia injury are seen.

In 1962, José Luis Bado[43] reported on 3200 forearm fractures and found the Monteggia injury to account for only 1.7%. Furthermore, he proposed a classification system for Monteggia injuries consisting of 4 types based on mechanism, treatment, and prognosis. The injury Evans and Tompkins attempted to explain was the most common Monteggia injury and labeled a type I (ie, anterior angulation of the ulnar diaphysis with anterior dislocation of the radial head).[41,42] A Bado type II injury was characterized by posterior angulation of the ulnar diaphysis with posterolateral radial head dislocation and a type III by a very proximal ulna shaft fracture (ie, metaphyseal) with lateral or anterolateral radial head dislocation. Finally, a Bado type IV was considered the same as a type I injury, except the radial shaft is concomitantly fractured at the same level as the ulna. In 1991, Jupiter and colleagues[44] later subclassified the Bado type II injuries into 4 subtypes based on the ulnar fracture type and location. In 1998, Ring and colleagues[45] proposed 1 of 2 different mechanisms of injury thought to produce Bado type II injuries based on the differing patient populations and levels of energy observed most commonly.

Investigation into each Monteggia type has elucidated unique characteristics associated with each.[46] Bado type I injuries occur with comparable frequency in children and young adults whereas type II injuries are found primarily in middle-aged and elderly adults and commonly are associated with a radial head shear fracture as it strikes the capitellum during posterior dislocation.[30,46] Type III injuries also occur in both children and adults but are more common in children and often are associated with radial nerve injuries.[30,46] In general, children do better both with closed reduction and immobilization and operative intervention regardless of Bado type.[44,45] Results of types I and III injuries are more favorable than type II injuries.[46,47]

Today, the most widely accepted approach to acute Monteggia fracture-dislocations is similar to that proposed by Speed and Boyd in 1940. In adults, ORIF of the ulna is performed first, which, if anatomically realigned, often permits a closed reduction of the radial head. If a reduced and stable radial head is not achieved, then interposed tissue is the most likely culprit and an open reduction of the radial head is warranted.[48,49] In 1 large series of 121 Monteggia injuries, open reduction of the PRUJ was most common in Bado type I injuries and was necessary in approximately 1 in every 5 injuries.[49] In children, a closed reduction of the ulna should initially be attempted and is usually sufficient in simultaneously reducing the radial head. ORIF is reserved for instances when this is not the case and, in those instances, can be accomplished with flexible intramedullary nails or plates and screws.[45,48,50]

GALEAZZI INJURIES

Eight years after Monteggia described the fracture-dislocation injury that bears his name, Astley Cooper,[51] reported on a similarly unique injury of a radial shaft fracture with DRUJ dislocation. Although sometimes referred to as a reverse Monteggia, Piedmont fracture, fracture of necessity, or Darrach-Hughston-Milch fracture, it is most widely recognized as a Galeazzi fracture-dislocation,[26] after Riccardo Galeazzi, who reported on his experience treating 18 cases of this unique injury in 1934.[52]

Galeazzi fractures occur at a slightly higher incidence than Monteggia injuries, both of which are uncommon among all forearm fractures.[10,26,52] Similar to Monteggia injuries, instability is the fundamental feature of this injury, albeit instability of the DRUJ. As translated by Sebastin and Chung[26] from Galeazzi's 1935 German-language publication, Galeazzi writes[52]:

   ...when a person falls on his hand and fractures the radius, the weight acts longitudinally on the ulna because of the sudden

superposition of the radius fragments. The ulna in proportion to the radius becomes too long and bends inevitably. If the bone does not resist the force of longitudinal energy, it breaks. However when the bone resists the force, it is forced to luxate at the lower end, as the upper end is connected very strongly to the humerus.

Closed reduction and immobilization of both the radial shaft fracture and DRUJ dislocation were the initial management strategy, separately attempted by Cooper and Galeazzi in the early treatment of this injury.[51,52] Unfortunately, these cases often were fraught with persistent DRUJ instability; in part, this is due to the many deforming forces present in the forearm (**Fig. 4**). Other early surgeons attempted performing an open reduction of the ulna,[53] open reduction of the radius with immobilization of the DRUJ,[54] reconstruction of the DRUJ,[55,56] and pinning of the DRUJ.[57] Unfortunately, despite these various attempts and trials, none seemed to be a safeguard against the poor motion, poor function, and poor outcomes associated with the recurrent DRUJ instability that often developed.

The first attempt at ORIF of the radial shaft fracture in a Galeazzi injury was by Valande[58] in 1929. He attempted fixation with a series of wire loops and published this report in the French literature.[26,58] Despite this early attempt, the true effectiveness of ORIF was not demonstrated until the advent of early plate and screw constructs, developed and subsequently studied by Hughston[59,60] and the Piedmont Orthopedic Society. In his 1957 publication, Hughston reports on a series of 41 isolated, distal one-third radial shaft fractures.[59] Because a high percentage of these fractures were treated on referral, the exact number of patients presenting with concomitant DRUJ

subluxation or dislocation was recognized and appreciated by Hughston but not reported. Initial closed treatment in 35 of 38 of these fractures resulted in failure and a transition to either early (21 patients) or delayed (>4 weeks; 7 patients) ORIF, depending on timing of return follow-up. Fixation methods included plates and screws, screws, or the more traditional Kirschner wires or intramedullary pins with or without autologous bone grafting. Results of early ORIF were deemed satisfactory in 67% of cases whereas delayed intervention yielded a satisfactory result in only 33% of cases. Nonunion and malunions were a large part of the failures. Ultimately, the investigators suggested testing DRUJ stability relative to the contralateral side once "anatomic reduction with rigid and secure internal fixation" of the radius is achieved. If any instability is appreciated or if the fracture presents for delayed treatment, they then advocate for acute distal ulna resection—the so-called Darrach procedure[53]—to prevent any malunion or nonunion of the fracture site. Another method of assessing DRUJ instability in Galeazzi injuries is based on cadaveric work.[61] Moore and colleagues[61] demonstrated that radial shortening at the DRUJ of 5 mm or more was associated with DRUJ instability, with 5 mm to 10 mm of migration representing disruption of either the TFCC or IOM and greater than 10 mm representing concomitant disruption of both structures.

Subsequent investigators agreed with ORIF of the radius but thought routine use of the Darrach procedure to be unnecessary. Instead, opinions on how to manage DRUJ instability ranged from doing nothing,[62] to immobilization in some degree of supination,[14,61,63] or to temporary pin fixation,[64–67] each supported by reasonably good results.

Efforts have been made to classify Galeazzi injuries. This would both ensure appropriate

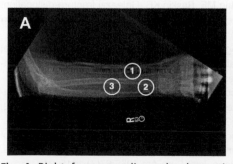
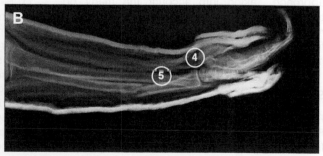

Fig. 4. Right forearm radiographs showcasing deforming forces of the Galeazzi injury. 1. Brachioradialis—shortens the distal radial fragment. 2. Pronator quadratus—rotates distal radial fragment toward the ulna. 3. IOM—prevents radio-ulnar diastasis and proximal migration of the radius. 4. Gravity—directs distal radial fragment volarly. 5. Thumb abductors and extensors—shortens distal radius fragment.

comparisons were made across study populations and to see determine if the level of intervention necessary for DRUJ instability could be predicted by the characteristics of the fracture-dislocation. Accordingly, classifications were developed based on radial shaft fracture obliquity and on distance of the fracture to the distal-most aspect of the radius.[9,68–70] In the former, type A fractures were those with obliquity mirroring radial inclination, considered more unstable and, therefore, amenable to pin fixation; type B fractures were those with reverse obliquity.[69] Three groups independently looked at the latter and found that radial shaft fractures in closer proximity to the DRUJ tended to be more unstable, specifically those within 7.5 cm to 10 cm of the distal end of the radius or distal one-third.[9,68,70] One plausible explanation for this finding is that the TFCC and distal portion of the IOM, including the DOB, are more likely affected, whereas the CB remains intact and prohibitive of proximal radial migration. These investigators advocate for empirical pinning of distal Galeazzi variants, followed by immobilization in supination, where DRUJ instability is a concern as well as when it is clinically unstable. Although the location of the radial shaft fracture can be helpful in providing some guidance on how to manage the DRUJ injury, Tsismenakis and Tornetta[71] recently challenged the clinical relevance of this radiographic cue, as well as the one proposed by Moore and colleagues,[61] finding them to only be moderately accurate predictors of DRUJ instability. Furthermore, they found a concomitant ulnar styloid fracture to have a similar, if not better, predictive value for DRUJ instability.[71]

Today, the current treatment of the Galeazzi fracture-dislocation involves ORIF of the radius and intraoperative assessment of the DRUJ. Although algorithms have been proposed for when and how to stabilize an unstable DRUJ, no standard exists. Instead a selective, case-based approach, taking into account the many options—temporary DRUJ pinning, TFCC repair or reconstruction, immobilization, and ulnar styloid fracture fixation—is reasonable and adhered to most often in everyday practice.

SUMMARY

Peter Essex-Lopresti, Giovanni Monteggia, and Riccardo Galeazzi identified specific forearm fracture-dislocation injuries that continue to bear significance today. Of utmost importance is to recognize these injuries when present. Management of the component of instability differs based on the type of fracture-dislocation, the timing of

intervention, and surgeon preference. Finally, although eponymous designations may not serve as descriptive labels for these unique injuries, they are a reminder that what is known and learned now is deeply rooted in the work of others.

DISCLOSURE

The authors have nothing to disclose.

REFERENCES

1. Kapandji A. 5th édition. Physiologie Articulaire, vol. II. Paris: Maloine; 1996.
2. Tashjian RZ, Katarincic JA. Complex elbow instability. J Am Acad Orthop Surg 2006;14(5):278–86.
3. Martin BF. The annular ligament of the superior radio-ulnar joint. J Anat 1958;92(3):473–82.
4. Smith FM. Monteggia fractures; an analysis of 25 consecutive fresh injuries. Surg Gynecol Obstet 1947;85(5):630–40.
5. Spinner M, Kaplan EB. The quadrate ligament of the elbow—its relationship to the stability of the proximal radio-ulnar joint. Acta Orthop Scand 1970;41(6):632–47.
6. Soubeyrand M, Wassermann V, Hirsch C, et al. The middle radioulnar joint and triarticular forearm complex. J Hand Surg Eur Vol 2011;36(6):447–54.
7. Dumontier C, Soubeyrand M. The forearm joint. In: Bentley G, editor. European surgical orthopaedics and traumatology: the EFORT textbook. Berlin: Springer Berlin Heidelberg; 2014. p. 1509–24.
8. LaStayo PC, Lee MJ. The forearm complex: anatomy, biomechanics and clinical considerations. J Hand Ther 2006;19(2):137–45.
9. Adams JE. Forearm instability: anatomy, biomechanics, and treatment options. J Hand Surg Am 2017;42(1):47–52.
10. McGinley JC, Hopgood BC, Gaughan JP, et al. Forearm and elbow injury: the influence of rotational position. J Bone Joint Surg Am 2003;85(12):2403–9.
11. Rettig ME, Raskin KB. Galeazzi fracture-dislocation: a new treatment-oriented classification. J Hand Surg Am 2001;26(2):228–35.
12. Ring D, Rhim R, Carpenter C, et al. Isolated radial shaft fractures are more common than Galeazzi fractures. J Hand Surg 2006;31(1):17–21.
13. Nicolaidis SC, Hildreth DH, Lichtman DM. Acute injuries of the distal radioulnar joint. Hand Clin 2000;16(3):449–59.
14. Moore TM, Klein J, Patzakis M, et al. Results of compression-plating of closed Galeazzi fractures. J Bone Joint Surg Am 1985;67(7):1015–21.
15. Weiss A-PC, Hastings H. The anatomy of the proximal radioulnar joint. J Shoulder Elbow Surg 1992;1(4):193–9.

16. Curr J, Coe W. Dislocation of the inferior radio-ulnar joint. Br J Surg 1946;34(133):74–7.

17. Essex-Lopresti P. Fractures of the radial head with distal radio-ulnar dislocation. Orthop Trauma Dir 2008;6(03):29–32.

18. McGlinn EP, Sebastin SJ, Chung KC. A historical perspective on the Essex-Lopresti injury. J Hand Surg Am 2013;38(8):1599–606.

19. van Riet RP, Van Glabbeek F. History of radial head prosthesis in traumatology. Acta Orthop Belg 2007; 73(1):12.

20. Levin PD. Fracture of the radial head with dislocation of the distal radio-ulnar joint: case report: Treatment by prosthetic replacement of the radial head. J Bone Joint Surg Am 1973;55(4):837–40.

21. Hotchkiss RN, Weiland AJ. Valgus stability of the elbow. J Orthop Res 1987;5(3):372–7.

22. Knight D, Rymaszewski L, Amis A, et al. Primary replacement of the fractured radial head with a metal prosthesis. J Bone Joint Surg Br 1993;75(4): 572–6.

23. Edwards JG, Jupiter JB. Radial head fractures with acute distal radioulnar dislocation. Essex-Lopresti revisited. Clin Orthop Relat Res 1988;(234):61–9.

24. Wegmann K, Dargel J, Burkhart K, et al. The Essex-Lopresti lesion. Strategies Trauma Limb Reconstr 2012;7(3):131–9.

25. Dodds SD, Yeh PC, Slade JF. Essex-lopresti injuries. Hand Clin 2008;24(1):125–37.

26. Sebastin SJ, Chung KC. A historical report on Riccardo Galeazzi and the management of Galeazzi fractures. J Hand Surg Am 2010;35(11):1870–7.

27. Palmer AK, Werner FW. The triangular fibrocartilage complex of the wrist—anatomy and function. J Hand Surg 1981;6(2):153–62.

28. O'driscoll S, Bell D, Morrey B. Posterolateral rotatory instability of the elbow. J Bone Joint Surg Am 1991; 73(3):440–6.

29. O'Driscoll SW, Jupiter JB, Cohen MS, et al. Difficult elbow fractures: pearls and pitfalls. Instructional Course Lectures 2003;52:113–34.

30. Penrose JH. The Monteggia fracture with posterior dislocation of the radial head. J Bone Joint Surg Br 1951;33 B(1):65–73.

31. Adams JE, Culp RW, Osterman AL. Central band interosseous membrane reconstruction for forearm longitudinal instability. J Wrist Surg 2016;5(3):184–7.

32. Gaspar MP, Adams JE, Zohn RC, et al. Late reconstruction of the interosseous membrane with bone-patellar tendon-bone graft for chronic essex-lopresti injuries: outcomes with a mean follow-up of over 10 years. J Bone Joint Surg Am 2018;100(5): 416–27.

33. Failla JM, Jacobson J, van Holsbeeck M. Ultrasound diagnosis and surgical pathology of the torn interosseous membrane in forearm fractures/dislocations. J Hand Surg 1999;24(2):257–66.

34. Jaakkola JI, Riggans DH, Lourie GM, et al. Ultrasonography for the evaluation of forearm interosseous membrane disruption in a cadaver model. J Hand Surg 2001;26(6):1053–7.

35. Fester EW, Murray PM, Sanders TG, et al. The efficacy of magnetic resonance imaging and ultrasound in detecting disruptions of the forearm interosseous membrane: a cadaver study. J Hand Surg 2002;27(3):418–24.

36. Smith AM, Urbanosky LR, Castle JA, et al. Radius pull test: predictor of longitudinal forearm instability. J Bone Joint Surg Am 2002;84(11):1970–6.

37. Monteggia G. Lussazioni delle ossa delle estremita superiori. Instituzioni chirurgiches 1814;5:131–3.

38. Perrin J. Les fractures du cubitus accompagnées d'une luxation de l'extrémité supérieure du radius 1909.

39. Speed JS, Boyd HB. Treatment of fractures of ulna with dislocation of head of radius: (monteggia fracture). J Am Med Assoc 1940;115(20):1699–705.

40. Cunningham SR. Fractures of the ulna with dislocations of the head of the radius. J Bone Joint Surg Am 1934;16(2):351–4.

41. Evans EM. Pronation injuries of the forearm, with special reference to the anterior Monteggia fracture. J Bone Joint Surg Br 1949;31 B(4):578–88. illust.

42. Tompkins DG. The anterior Monteggia fracture: observations on etiology and treatment. J Bone Joint Surg Am 1971;53(6):1109–14.

43. Bado J. The Monteggia lesion. Springfield (IL): Charles C Thomas; 1962. translated by IV Ponseti.

44. Jupiter JB, Leibovic SJ, Ribbans W, et al. The posterior Monteggia lesion. J Orthop Trauma 1991;5(4): 395–402.

45. Ring D, Jupiter JB, Waters PM. Monteggia fractures in children and adults. J Am Acad Orthop Surg 1998;6(4):215–24.

46. Bryan RS. Monteggia fracture of the forearm. J Trauma 1971;11(12):992–8.

47. Pavel A, Pitman JM, Lance EM, et al. The posterior Monteggia fracture: a clinical study. J Trauma Acute Care Surg 1965;5(2):185–99.

48. Ring D. Monteggia fractures. Orthop Clin 2013; 44(1):59–66.

49. Hamaker M, Zheng A, Eglseder WA, et al. The adult monteggia fracture: patterns and incidence of annular ligament incarceration among 121 cases at a single institution over 19 years. J Hand Surg Am 2018;43(1):85.e1-6.

50. Bae DS, Waters PM. Surgical treatment of acute and chronic monteggia fracture-dislocations. Oper Tech Orthop 2005;15(4):308–14.

51. Cooper A. Simple fracture of the radius and dislocation of the ulna. A treatise on dislocations, and on fractures of the joints. London: Longman; 1825. p. 470–6.

52. Galeazzi R. Über ein besonderes Syndrom bei Verletzungen im Bereich der Unterarmknochen. Archiv für orthopädische und Unfall-Chirurgie, mit besonderer Berücksichtigung der Frakturenlehre und der orthopädisch-chirurgischen Technik 1934;35(1):557–62.

53. Darrach W. Forward dislocation at the inferior radioulnar joint with fracture of the lower third of the shaft of the radius. Ann Surg 1912;56:801–3.

54. Homans J, Smith JA. Fracture of the lower end of the radius associated with fracture or dislocation of the lower end of the ulna. Boston Med Surg J 1922;187(11):401–7.

55. Milch H. Dislocation of the inferior end of the ulna: suggestion for a new operative procedure. Am J Surg 1926;1(3):141–6.

56. Wilson PD, Cochrane WA. Fractures and dislocations: immediate management, aftercare, and convalescent treatment with special reference to the conservation and restoration of function. Philadelphia: JB Lippincott Company; 1925.

57. Bohler L. The treatment of fractures. 4th English edition. Bristol (England): John Wright and Sons; 1935.

58. Valande M. Luxation en arrière du cubitus avec fracture de la diaphyse radiale. Bull Mem Soc Mat Chir 1929;55:435–7.

59. Hughston JC. Fracture of the distal radial shaft: mistakes in management. J Bone Joint Surg Am 1957;39(2):249–402.

60. Hughston JC. Fractures of the forearm: anatomical considerations. J Bone Joint Surg Am 1962;44(8):1664–7.

61. Moore TM, Lester DK, Sarmiento A. The stabilizing effect of soft-tissue constraints in artificial Galeazzi fractures. Clin Orthop Relat Res 1985;(194):189–94.

62. Kraus B, Horne G. Galeazzi fractures. J Trauma 1985;25:1093–5.

63. Mestdagh H, Duquennoy A, Letendart J, et al. Long-term results in the treatment of fracture-dislocations of Galeazzi in adults. Report on twenty-nine cases. Ann Chir Main 1983;2(2):125–33.

64. Reckling FW, Peltier LF. Riccardo Galeazzi and Galeazzi's fracture. Surgery 1965;58(2):453–9.

65. Mikić ZD. Galeazzi fracture-dislocations. J Bone Joint Surg Am 1975;57(8):1071–80.

66. Reckling FW. Unstable fracture-dislocations of the forearm (Monteggia and Galeazzi lesions). J Bone Joint Surg Am 1982;64(6):857–63.

67. Reckling FW, Cordell LD. Unstable fracture-dislocations of the forearm. The Monteggia and Galeazzi lesions. Arch Surg 1968;96(6):999–1007.

68. Maculé Beneyto F, Arandes Renú JM, Ferreres Claramunt A, et al. Treatment of Galeazzi fracture-dislocations. J Trauma 1994;36(3):352–5.

69. Chattopadhyay A, Chatterjee ML. Recognition of two types of Galeazzi fracture-dislocation and their management. J Indian Med Assoc 1986;84(10):307–8.

70. Korompilias AV, Lykissas MG, Kostas-Agnantis IP, et al. Distal radioulnar joint instability (galeazzi type injury) after internal fixation in relation to the radius fracture pattern. J Hand Surg 2011;36(5):847–52.

71. Tsismenakis T, Tornetta P. Galeazzi fractures: Is DRUJ instability predicted by current guidelines? Injury 2016;47(7):1472–7.

Biomechanical Factors in Stability of the Forearm

Jorge L. Orbay, MD[a,b,*], Richard A. Cambo, MA[c]

KEYWORDS

• Forearm • Biomechanics • IOM • PRUJ • DRUJ • Stability

KEY POINTS

- The forearm operates as a series of interconnected parts where damage to one can affect stability in multiple areas.
- The proximal radioulnar joint, interosseous ligament complex, and distal radioulnar joint are key biomechanical components of forearm stability.
- The proximal radioulnar joint, interosseous ligament complex, and distal radioulnar joint are important for facilitating force transmission and forearm rotation.
- Physicians need a holistic understanding of these components to quickly diagnose the proper injury patterns before the condition worsens.

The forearm has evolved into a highly complex and versatile part of human anatomy. Ligaments and joints act in unison to facilitate placement of the hand in 3-dimensional space and transmit loads across the upper extremity. Intricate but effective forearm stabilizers facilitate physiologic motions and restrict abnormal ones. This article is intended to integrate current knowledge of forearm biomechanics into a cohesive and practical picture.

BASIC STRUCTURE AND FUNCTION

The forearm connects the carpus to the humerus and is the site for forearm rotation or pronosupinatory motion. The forearm is also responsible for transmitting force in longitudinal and transverse directions. Two bones, the radius and ulna, form its basic structure. These articulate by means of a single forearm joint having 2 condyles, the proximal radioulnar joint (PRUJ) and distal radioulnar joint (DRUJ). As a pivot joint, the axis of forearm rotation is aligned longitudinally and slightly obliquely

through the center of the radial head and ulnar fovea.[1] The interosseous ligament complex (IOLC) is the main forearm stabilizer. The annular ligament contributes to proximal stability, and the triangular fibrocartilage complex (TFCC) also contributes to distal stability (**Fig. 1**).

The DRUJ and PRUJ share anatomic and biomechanical similarities. During forearm rotation at the DRUJ, the seat of the ulnar head serves as the articular surface for the sigmoid notch, the surface around which the radius rotates.[2] The radius of curvature of the sigmoid notch is twice the radius of curvature of the ulnar head; this incongruity allows for rotational motion and translational motion.

The force transmission profiles at the DRUJ and PRUJ are similar, although not identical. Peak force transmission at the PRUJ is slightly higher; therefore, there is a larger surface area at the radial notch compared with the sigmoid notch.[3] The 2 joints also have a connected pathology, because some studies have shown that, when 1 joint is

[a] Orthopaedic Surgery Department, Miami Hand & Upper Extremity Institute, 8905 Southwest 87th Avenue, Suite 100, Miami, FL 33176, USA; [b] The Herbert Wertheim School of Medicine, Florida International University, 11200 SW 8th Street, Miami, Florida, 33199, USA; [c] Research Department, Miami Hand & Upper Extremity Institute, 8905 Southwest 87th Avenue, Suite 100, Miami, FL 33176, USA
* Corresponding author. The Miami Hand & Upper Extremity Institute, 8905 SW 87th Ave, Suite 100, Miami, FL 33176.
E-mail address: jlorbay@gmail.com

Hand Clin 36 (2020) 407–415
https://doi.org/10.1016/j.hcl.2020.06.001
0749-0712/20/© 2020 Elsevier Inc. All rights reserved.

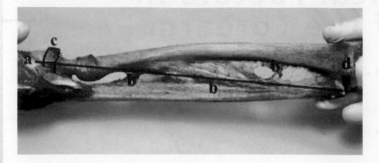

Fig. 1. (a) The forearm is a pivot joint and its axis of rotation courses through the center of the radial head (PRUJ) and ulnar fovea (DRUJ). (b) The IOLC with its 3 components is the main forearm stabilizer. (c) The annular ligament is a proximal stabilizer. (d) The TFCC is a distal stabilizer.

damaged, axial loads place added stress on the other, leading to clinical problems.[4]

The IOLC presents proximal, central, and distal components that are generally arranged in a zigzag configuration.[5] These are distinguished by their location and fiber direction. The most proximal component (proximal interosseous ligament [PIOL]) presents fibers that originate most proximally on the ulna and insert more distally on the radius, restricting distal radial translation. The proximal component contains the proximal oblique cord found on the volar side, and a dorsal oblique accessory cord ligament than can only be seen dorsally.[5] The most substantial central component also known as the central band (CB) has fibers that roughly originate on the distal half of the ulnar shaft and insert on the proximal half of the radial shaft, restricting proximal radial translation.[5] The most variable distal component (distal interosseous ligament [DIOL]) presents fibers that originate proximally on the distal ulnar shaft, insert most distally on the radius or course in a transverse direction, and is roughly homologous to the proximal component.[6] This component can present itself in different ways. The fibers can arrange themselves into a thickly defined "bundle" that appear as a linear section, or they can display as a spread-out membrane the span the entire portion of the distal interosseous membrane (DIOM).[7] The DIOL is taut in all positions of forearm

rotation and acts as an isometric stabilizer[8] (**Fig. 2**).

These 3 components, acting together and in the presence of intact distal and proximal articular structures, stabilize the radius to the ulna restricting motion in all directions, except that of rotation around the axis of pronosupination. During the non-physiologic motion of hypersupination, the ligaments of the PIOL (proximal oblique cord and dorsal oblique accessory cord) get taut upon over-rotation.[1] These ligaments create a biomechanical stop that helps to restrict any increased supination that can lead to dislocation. Distal or proximal displacement of the radius with respect to the ulna is prevented by the zigzag configuration of the IOLC. Diastasis and anteroposterior or sagittal radial translation at the PRUJ and the DRUJ articulations is also restricted by the IOLC (**Fig. 3**).

Muscular function affects forearm stability in multiple ways. The biceps muscle inserting into the bicipital tuberosity, the pronator quadratus, the supinator, and most muscles located along the forearm axis act to power forearm rotational motion. The biceps action is very powerful and generates an anteriorly directed force, not normal to the radioulnar articular surfaces, which is restricted by the IOLC and the annular ligament.[9] The supinator and pronator muscles are

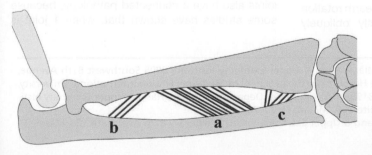

Fig. 2. The IOLC has a zigzag architecture and consists of 3 components. (a) The most substantial CB, its fibers are arranged in a distal ulnar to proximal radial direction. (b) The proximal component of the interosseous ligament has fibers arranged in an opposite proximal ulnar to distal radial direction. (c) The distal component of the interosseous ligament has fibers arranged proximal ulnar to distal radial or in a more transverse direction and

is the most variable.

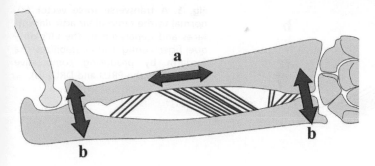

Fig. 3. (a) The zigzag arrangement of the IOLC prevents longitudinal displacement of the radius against the ulna. (b) The IOLC also prevents diastasis and subluxation of the PRUJ and DRUJ.

generally stabilizing, because their line of pull is normal to the radioulnar articular surfaces.

Most forearm muscles, including all that power the wrist and all extrinsic hand muscles, are arranged in a longitudinal manner. Therefore, they generate significant axial loads along the forearm during function. At the level of the wrist, the radius sustains the major part of these loads (80%–90%).[10] Because the forearm carries the radial load proximally, the CB of the IOLC transfers a large portion of this load to the ulna. This occurs to the degree that the radial head and coronoid process of the ulna sustain similar loads at the elbow (**Fig. 4**).

This effect, known as the forearm load transfer mechanism, occurs because the CB is arranged from distal on the ulna to more proximally on the radius at an average angle of 21° to the forearm axis.[11] This arrangement suspends the radius from the ulna while generating a vector force that approximates the radius to the ulna. This transverse force component is normal to the radioulnar articular surfaces and further stabilizes the forearm during function (**Fig. 5**).

Disruption of the ligamentous and bony structures of the forearm can cause great disability. A thorough understanding of their function and normal biomechanics is necessary for optimal treatment. We analyze patterns of disruption to the PRUJ, CB, and DRUJ to discuss the principles of their treatment.

PROXIMAL RADIOULNAR JOINT INJURY

Injuries to the PRUJ can involve bony, ligamentous, or combined structures. Radial head fractures are most common. The surgeon must understand the direction and magnitude of the forces that the radial head experiences. Besides an obvious axial load, the radial head is subject to a convergent transverse force of great magnitude generated by the function of the CB and a proximally directed or divergent force induced by the pull of the biceps tendon. The convergent PRUJ transverse force is the cause of proximal radioulnar convergence after radial head excision and of loosening of poorly fixed radial head replacements. Bipolar radial heads often collapse into a valgus alignment because of this force. To resist transverse forces, radial head implants must have sufficiently long stems to provide 3-point fixation for initial stability (**Fig. 6**).

Proximal dislocation of the radial head is a rare but disabling problem that may be difficult to treat. It is caused by the divergent pull of the biceps tendon after disruption of the annular ligament and IOLC. Simple disruption of the annular ligament is insufficient to allow radial head dislocation. Studies have shown that PRUJ divergence is minimal upon damage to the annular ligament when compared with damage to the IOLC[12] (**Fig. 7**).

The treatment of PRUJ dislocation may require tendon graft reconstruction of the IOLC (**Fig. 8**).

CENTRAL BAND INJURY

The CB is the most important component of the IOLC and responsible for maintaining forearm longitudinal alignment. Loss of this structure affects all other components of the IOLC, significantly disrupting forearm rotation, carrying angle, and load-bearing capacity. Injury to the CB is usually

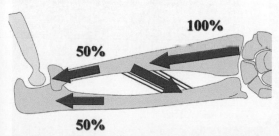

Fig. 4. The CB's oblique fiber configuration transfers load from the radius to the ulna leveling loads at coronoid and radial head levels. This is known as the forearm load transfer mechanism.

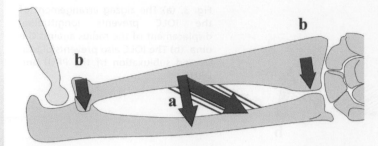

Fig. 5. A transverse force vector (a), normal to the radio-ulnar articular surfaces and generated by the CB's oblique fiber configuration stabilizes the forearm by producing compressive loads across the PRUJ and DRUJ (b).

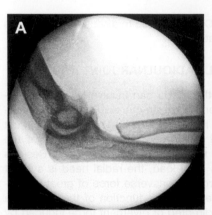

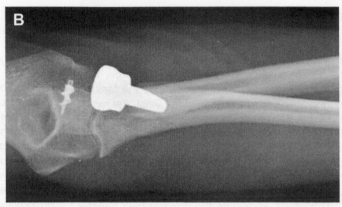

Fig. 6. (A) Distal radioulnar convergence after radial head resection and (B) loosening of poorly fixed radial head replacement is due to the convergent transverse forearm force generated by the function of the CB of the IOLC.

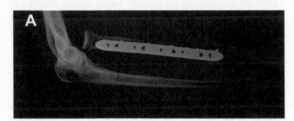

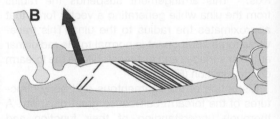

Fig. 7. (A) PRUJ dislocation after high-energy injury of the proximal radius. (B) Disruption of the annular ligament and IOLC will allow the pull of the biceps tendon to dislocate the radial head in a proximal direction.

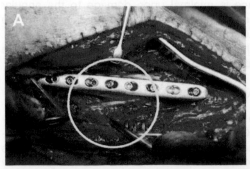

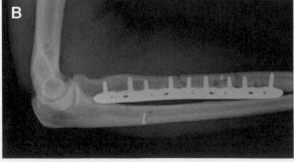

Fig. 8. (A) Tendon graft reconstruction of the proximal component of the IOLC and PIOL. (B) Restoration of PRUJ alignment.

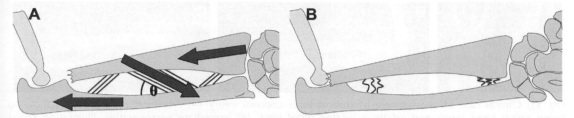

Fig. 9. The mechanism of the Essex–Lopresti injury. (*A*) First, the radial head fractures and all remaining loads are then resisted by the CB. (*B*) After the CB fails, the radius displaces proximally. The proximal and distal components of the CB remain intact but foreshortened (PIOL and DIOL).

associated with a radial head fracture and disruption of the TFCC.[13] It is a well-known clinical problem that is very difficult to treat and is caused by a high energy axial load.[14] The impact initially fractures the radial head, which is the most rigid link in the chain of loaded structures. After the radial head fractures, the CB receives the remaining energy in its attempt to transfer the load to the ulna. The CB has limited strength, having been measured to average 250 lbs.[15] Once the radial head is damaged, the CB becomes responsible for 71% of the longitudinal stiffness of the forearm.[11] This added load can result in eventual CB failure.[11] After its rupture, the radius translates proximally, often abutting the capitellum. The PIOL and DIOL remain intact as their fiber direction is opposite that of the CB and not loaded (**Fig. 9**).

Treatment of this injury has proven a challenge because simple repair or replacement of the radial head fails to restore radial longitudinal alignment and forearm function. One important study outlines that the problem with using metal head arthroplasties for radial head fractures, while CB damage is present, Is that long-term clinical outcomes are still unsatisfactory owing to excessive radiocapitellar load and leading to pain.[16] To reestablish forearm stability and alignment, it is necessary to reconstruct the CB at its native length. This process will reestablish the longitudinal alignment and stability of the radius and ulna. It is also necessary to repair or replace the radial head at its original anatomic dimensions to avoid overstuffing the radiocapitellar joint while simultaneously supporting the CB reconstruction. Restoring longitudinal alignment of the radius and ulna with a reconstructed CB and repaired radial head will recreate proper tension in the intact PIOL and DIOL and therefore reestablish stability of the PRUJ and DRUJ (**Figs. 10 and 11**).

With the Essex–Lopresti injury, optimal treatment requires not only the technical components of radial head and CB treatment, but also depends on quick recognition of the scale of the injury.

Adams and colleagues[17] evaluated a series of 106 referral cases, and the correct Essex–Lopresti diagnoses made before referral only occurred in 38% of them. Quick recognition is necessary to correct the CB and radial head damage properly, or else risk long-term forearm instability. The common orthopedic caveat to "examine a joint above and below" the obvious injury is important to remember.[14]

CENTRAL BAND ATTRITION

Idiopathic ulnocarpal impaction syndrome is a cause for wrist pain in middle-aged patients. During the patient's lifetime, the CB is loaded every time the hand is used in grasp or pinching activities. Degenerative or attritional lengthening of the CB can allow proximal translation of the radius with respect to the ulna. Because bony length does not change, slight angular realignment of these bones will result in relative prominence of the ulna distally and increased contact with the carpus resulting overloading and clinical symptoms. This has been called the parallelogram effect[18] (**Fig. 12**). Treatment of this condition consists of shortening the ulna to correct ulnar variance. The shortening osteotomy should be made distal to the origin of the CB to avoid inducing more laxity in this structure.

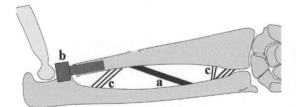

Fig. 10. Restoring the forearm after the Essex–Lopresti injury. (a) Reconstructing the CB under its native tension to restore radial alignment. (b) Anatomic radial head replacement or reconstruction. (c) Reestablishment of physiologic tension in proximal and distal components of the IOLC (PIOL and DIOL).

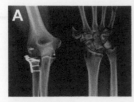
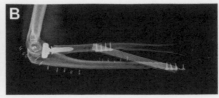
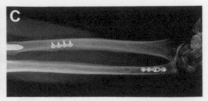

Fig. 11. Clinical case of management of chronic Essex–Lopresti injury. (*A*) Preoperative radiographs showing failed radial head repair and axially dislocated distal ulna. (*B*) Immediate postoperative, illustrating radial head replacement and CB allograft reconstruction. (*C*) One year follow-up showing restoration of longitudinal alignment.

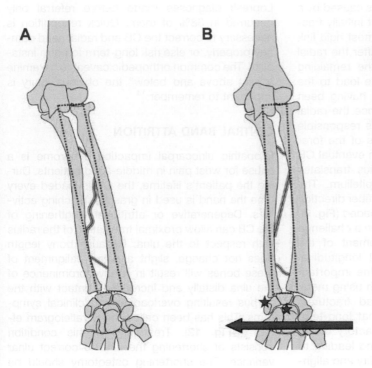

Fig. 12. Attritional failure of the CB can produce idiopathic ulnocarpal impaction syndrome via the parallelogram effect: (*A*) degenerative elongation of the CB (*B*) allows slight angular forearm bony realignment resulting in a distally prominent ulna and positive ulnar variance. The *red arrow* shows the direction of the forearm realignment. The *red stars* indicate pain.

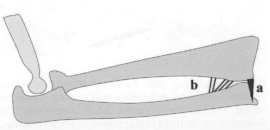

Fig. 13. The 2 static stabilizers of the DRUJ: the TFCC (a) and the distal component of the IOLC (b).

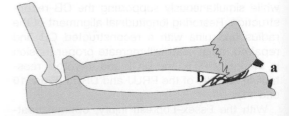

Fig. 14. DRUJ instability after a distal radius fracture: a ruptured TFCC (a) and incompetent distal component of the IOLC (b).

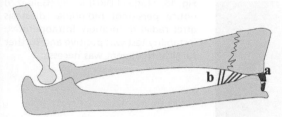

Fig. 15. Restoration of DRUJ stability after anatomic restoration of distal radius fracture: approximation of TFCC rupture (a) with restoration of tension at the distal component of the IOLC (b).

	TFCC	DIOL
Type I	+	+
Type II	–	+
Type III	–	–

Fig. 16. The 3 stages of DRUJ injury concomitant to distal radius fracture. Type I: Intact DIOL and TFCC, no need to treat instability. Type II: Incompetent TFCC, intact DIOL instability treated by anatomic radial restoration. Type III: Incompetent DIOL and TFCC, DRUJ instability requires specific treatment.

DISTAL RADIOULNAR JOINT INJURY

Injuries to the DRUJ can also involve bony, ligamentous, or a combination of these structures. Injuries associated with distal radius fractures are the most common, but those that occur in isolation are also well-known. The surgeon must understand the direction and magnitude of the physiologic forces sustained by this structure. Like the radial head, the distal ulna is subject to an axial force, but of lesser magnitude and depends on ulnar variance.[19] There is as a significant transverse force at the distal ulna of comparable magnitude as that seen by the radial head. The forearm load transfer mechanism and the pull of the brachialis during resisted elbow flexion generates this transverse force.[20] An absence of the distal ulna often results in radioulnar impingement, which can be very debilitating, particularly for physically demanding individuals.[21] The particular transverse force component produced by the brachialis can have a shearing or destabilizing direction depending on the position of forearm rotation during this muscle's activity. The principal static stabilizers at the DRUJ are the TFCC and DIOL[22] (**Fig. 13**).

The loss of both structures results in significant instability and clinical dysfunction. The presence or reconstruction of only 1 of these 2 structures often provides sufficient stability to allow satisfactory function. Even with a disrupted TFCC, an intact DIOL can still provide enough stability to

minimize DRUJ translation. In 2017, Omokawa and colleagues[23] in a cadaveric investigation determined that, upon TFCC sectioning, DRUJ translation increases minimally, but it is not until DIOL sectioning where the translation maximizes (increasing from 10 mm of dorsal translation to 23 mm of dorsal translation).

Commonly, distal radius fractures disrupt the TFCC but not the DIOL. Recent studies have shown that TFCC injury in distal radius fractures occur in 30% to 70% of cases.[24] The injury plane courses through the distal radial metaphysis distal to the insertion of the DIOL and continues between the TFCC and the ulna disrupting its foveal insertion and often avulsing the styloid process. With displacement of the distal radial fragment, the DIOL becomes foreshortened and incompetent allowing for DRUJ instability[25] (**Fig. 14**).

Anatomic restoration of the distal radius fracture restores tension on the DIOL therefore stabilizing the DRUJ. Correcting the radial deformity also

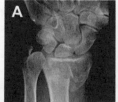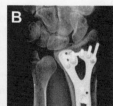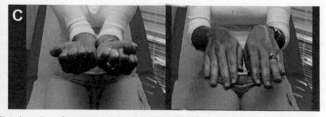

Fig. 17. Stage II DRUJ injury concomitant to distal radius fracture. (*A*) Severe radial displacement, dislocation DRUJ and large displaced ulnar styloid. (*B*) DRUJ and ulnar styloid reduction after anatomic radial restoration. (*C*) DRUJ stability and forearm rotation restored without additional intervention.

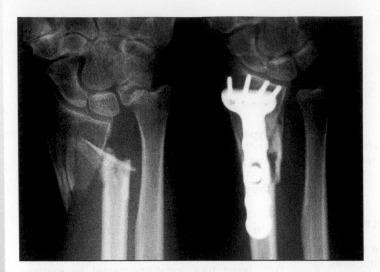

Fig. 18. Stage III DRUJ injury (Galeazzi) notice persistent radioulnar diastasis after radial restoration. Intraoperative instability test was positive and further surgical treatment was necessary.

approximates the ruptured TFCC and further healing usually results in an asymptomatic DRUJ. Surgeons documented this experience after the introduction of contemporary stable distal radius fracture fixation implants[26] (**Fig. 15**).

Categorizing the stages of DRUJ injury concomitant to a distal radius fracture in light of this mechanism leads to a clinically useful classification based on the remaining stabilizers.[27] Three combinations are possible: both the TFCC and DIOL stabilizers are intact, only the DIOL is intact, or both stabilizers are absent. The first type are usually minimally displaced, the second type are the common distal radius fractures with intact DIOL, and the third type are usually Galeazzi fractures or high-energy injuries with DIOL tears, which may need intraoperative clinical instability testing after radial restoration to identify. Only the third type would require the surgeon to address DRUJ instability after restoring the radius anatomically. Stability can be reestablished by either immobilizing the forearm in a reduced and stable rotational position or by actually repairing the torn TFCC (**Figs. 16–18**). Reconstruction of the distal oblique ligament is possible,[28] but infrequently done.

SUMMARY

The forearm is a mechanical structure consisting of 2 long bones that articulate by means of 1 joint having 2 condyles and whose motion is determined by an intricate set of ligaments, the IOLC. Injuries to the forearm often involve several of its components and understanding how the forearm works is crucial to selecting best therapeutic options. Several well known injury patterns combine

bone fractures with joint instability and surgeons often do not agree on their proper treatment. A knowledge of biomechanical factors is needed to understand how seemingly 1 isolated injury, such as a radial head fracture, can affect the stability of the entire forearm. The same principle applies to the common distal radius fracture and its concurrent TFCC disruption that may or may not lead to DRUJ instability. Ligaments and bony structures work together like complementary parts in a machine. A disruption to 1 component can affect others, and understanding the entire construct is necessary for the surgical community to improve and standardize current treatment methods.

DISCLOSURE

The authors have nothing to disclose.

REFERENCES

1. Hollister AM, Gellman H, Waters RL. The relationship of the interosseous membrane to the axis of rotation of the forearm. Clin Orthop Relat Res 1994;298: 272–6.
2. Huang JI, Hanel DP. Anatomy and biomechanics of the distal radioulnar joint. Hand Clin 2012;28: 157–63.
3. Malone PS, Shaw OG, Lees VC. Anatomic relationships of the distal and proximal radioulnar joints articulating surface areas and of the radius and ulna bone volumes – implications for biomechanical studies of the distal and proximal radioulnar joints and forearm bones. Front Bioeng Biotechnol 2016; 4:61.

4. Leung YF, Shirley PS, Wong A, et al. Isolated dislocation of the radial head, with simultaneous dislocation of proximal and distal radio-ulnar joints without fracture in an adult patient: case report and review of the literature. Injury. Int J Care Injured 2002;33: 271–3.

5. Noda K, Goto A, Murase T, et al. Interosseous membrane of the forearm: an anatomical study of ligament attachment locations. J Hand Surg Am 2009; 34A:415–22.

6. Kitamura T, Moritomo H, Arimitsu S, et al. The biomechanical effect of the distal interosseous membrane on distal radioulnar joint stability: a preliminary anatomic study. J Hand Surg Am 2011;36A: 1626–30.

7. Moritomo H. The distal interosseous membrane: current concepts in wrist anatomy and biomechanics. J Hand Surg Am 2012;37A:1501–7.

8. Moritomo H, Noda K, Goto A, et al. Interosseous membrane of the forearm: length change of ligaments during forearm rotation. J Hand Surg Am 2009;34A:685–91.

9. Anderson A, Werner FW, Tucci ER, et al. Role of the Interosseous membrane and annular ligament in stabilizing the proximal radial head. J Shoulder Elbow Surg 2015;24(12):1926–33.

10. Jupiter JB. Current concepts review: fractures of the distal end of the radius. J Bone Joint Surg 1991; 73A(3):461–9.

11. Skahen JR, Palmer AK, Werner FW, et al. The interosseous membrane of the forearm: anatomy and function. J Hand Surg Am 1997;22A:981–5.

12. Weiss AP, Hastings H 2nd. The anatomy of the proximal radioulnar joint. J Shoulder Elbow Surg 1992; 1(4):193–9.

13. Loeffler BJ, Green JB, Zelouf DS. Forearm Instability. J Hand Surg Am 2014;39(1):156–67.

14. Adams JE. Forearm instability: anatomy, biomechanics, and treatment options. J Hand Surg Am 2017;42(1):47–52.

15. Wallace AL, Walsh WR, van Rooijen M, et al. The interosseous membrane in radio-ulnar dissociation. J Bone Joint Surg Br 1997;79B:422–7.

16. Tomaino MM, Pfaeffle J, Stabile K, et al. Reconstruction of the interosseous ligament of the forearm reduces load on the radial head in cadavers. J Hand Surg Br 2003;28(3):267–70.

17. Adams JE, Culp RW, Osterman AL. Interosseous membrane reconstruction for the Essex-Lopresti injury. J Hand Surg Am 2010;35A:129–36.

18. Orbay JL, Levaro-Pano F, Vernon LJ, et al. The parallelogram effect: the association between central band and positive ulnar variance. J Hand Surg Am 2018;43(9):827–32.

19. Faucer GK, Zimmerman RM, Zimmerman NB. Instability and arthritis of the distal radioulnar joint: a critical analysis review. JBJS Rev 2016;4(12):e3.

20. Johnson RK, Shrewsbury MM. The pronator quadratus in motions and in stabilization of the radius and ulna at the distal radioulnar joint. J Hand Surg 1976;1(3):205–9.

21. Van Schoonhoven J, Fernandez DL, Bowers WH, et al. Salvage of failed resection arthroplasties of the distal radioulnar joint using a new ulnar head prosthesis. J Hand Surg 2000;25(3):438–46.

22. Watanabe H, Berger RA, Berglund LJ, et al. Contribution of the interosseous membrane to distal radioulnar joint constraint. J Hand Surg Am 2005;30(6): 1164–71.

23. Omokawa S, Iida A, Kawamura K, et al. A Biomechanical Perspective on Distal Radioulnar Joint Instability. J Wrist Surg 2017;6:88–96.

24. Kazemian GH, Bakhshi H, Lilley M, et al. DRUJ instability after distal radius fracture: a comparison between cases with and without ulnar styloid fracture. Int J Surg 2011;9(8):648–51.

25. Matthias R, Wright TW. Interosseous membrane of the forearm. J Wrist Surg 2016;5:188–93.

26. Atesok KI, Jupiter JB, Weiss AP. Galeazzi fracture. J Am Acad Orthop Surg 2011;19:623–33.

27. Orbay JL, Mijares MR. Wrist injuries. In: Cheema TA, editor. Complex injuries of the hand. London: Jaypee Brothers Medical Pub; 2014. p. 101–14.

28. Riggenbach MD, Wright TW, Dell PC. Reconstruction of the distal oblique bundle of the interosseous membrane: a technique to restore distal radioulnar joint stability. J Hand Surg Am 2015;40(11): 2279–82.

Instability in the Setting of Distal Radius Fractures
Diagnosis, Evaluation, and Treatment

Phillip R. Ross, MD[a],*, Kevin C. Chung, MD, MS[b]

KEYWORDS

- Instability • Distal radius fracture • DRUJ • TFCC • Malunion • Osteotomy
- Distal radioulnar joint instability

KEY POINTS

- Displaced distal radius fractures can cause osseous deformities and soft tissue injuries of the triangular fibrocartilage complex (TFCC) and interosseous membrane, which can lead to rotational forearm instability.
- The TFCC is the primary stabilizer of the distal radioulnar joint (DRUJ) and is a major component of forearm rotational stability.
- Anatomic fracture alignment restores proper soft tissue tensions and DRUJ stability in a majority of patients.
- The DRUJ should be evaluated for acute instability after radius fixation and treated with immobilization, styloid fracture reduction, or TFCC repair.
- Chronic instability after distal radius fracture may require radius or ulna osteotomy or TFCC reconstruction in persistently symptomatic patients.

OVERVIEW

Distal radius fractures are one of the most common fractures of the upper extremity,[1] frequently occurring with a bimodal distribution; they typically occur in the elderly after low-energy trauma, such as a fall on an outstretched hand, whereas in younger patients they are associated with high-energy trauma.[2,3] Distal radius malunions occur in approximately 23% of nonoperatively treated and 11% of operatively treated distal radius fractures.[4] Axial forearm instability manifested at the distal radioulnar joint (DRUJ) commonly is unnoticed initially but, if untreated, can lead to substantial disability.[5]

NORMAL DISTAL RADIOULNAR JOINT MOTION AND ANATOMY

The DRUJ is a complex diarthrodial joint which, along with the proximal radioulnar joint, facilitates forearm rotation along a longitudinal axis from the center of the radial head to the foveal sulcus of the ulna. Motion at the DRUJ includes rotation as well as translation. Normal range of motion ranges from 150° to 180° of pronation and supination through the DRUJ, with additional rotational motion (up to 30° in some) through the carpal joints.[6] During pronation, the distal radius moves proximally and palmarly with respect to the distal ulna and appears to shorten on posteroanterior (PA) radiographs. In supination, the converse occurs (distal and dorsal translation) and the radius is relatively longer than the ulna.[7]

Numerous structures contribute to the rotatory motion and axial stability of the forearm, including the osseous anatomy of the radius and ulna, the triangular fibrocartilage complex (TFCC), the extensor retinaculum, pronator quadratus, the interosseous membrane (IOM), and the annular ligament in the elbow.[6]

[a] Department of Orthopaedic Surgery, University of Cincinnati Medical Center, 231 Albert Sabin Way, Cincinnati, OH 45267-0212, USA; [b] Section of Plastic Surgery, Department of Surgery, University of Michigan Medical School, 2130 Taubman Center, SPC 5340, 1500 East Medical Center Drive, Ann Arbor, MI 48109-5340, USA
* Corresponding author.
E-mail address: phillip.ross@uc.edu

Hand Clin 36 (2020) 417–427
https://doi.org/10.1016/j.hcl.2020.06.002

At the DRUJ, the concave sigmoid notch on the distal medial radius rotates around the fixed, round ulna head, of which move to after "circumference" over 220° of its circumference is covered in articular cartilage.[8] The radius of curvature of the ulna head (8–10 mm) is much smaller than that of the sigmoid notch (15–19 mm), leading to incongruity between the articular surfaces and translational movement in addition to rotation.[6] In neutral forearm rotation, only 60% of the sigmoid notch and ulna head may be opposed; this contact area decreases to 10% in full pronation or supination.[8] Furthermore, the shape of the sigmoid notch has been found to vary, with a flat surface most common (42%), followed by C-shaped (30%), S-shaped (14%), and ski slope–shaped (14%) notches (**Fig. 1**).[9] Bony architecture accounts for only 20% of DRUJ stability; rather, stability of this poorly constrained joint relies largely on associated soft tissues.[6] An extra-articular volar osteocartilaginous lip is present in many wrists, which confers additional stability.[9]

The TFCC provides the most robust soft tissue constraint of the DRUJ and a large component of rotational forearm stability. It is a constellation of soft tissue structures comprising the dorsal radioulnar ligament (DRUL) and palmar radioulnar ligament (PRUL), the articular disk, the ulnocarpal ligaments, the extensor carpi ulnaris (ECU) subsheath, and the meniscal homologue. Of these, the DRUL and PRUL have the most substantial impact on DRUJ stability. Both ligaments have superficial and deep fibers,[7] originating from the sigmoid notch of the radius. The superficial fibers insert on the ulnar styloid, whereas the deep fibers (also called the ligamentum subcruentum) attach to the fovea on the ulna head (**Fig. 2**).[6,7] The superficial DRUL becomes taut in pronation to prevent dorsal ulna subluxation, whereas in supination the PRUL tightens and pulls the ulna palmarly.[2,6,10] The deep fibers act as checkreins in opposite directions of their superficial counterparts: the deep DRUL resists subluxation in supination and the deep PRUL is taut in pronation.[6,11]

The remaining components of the TFCC provide auxiliary support to the wrist and forearm. The articular disk provides a smooth surface for the ulnocarpal joint and undergoes significant deformation with forearm rotation. As long as the peripheral 2 mm are left intact, central portions of the disk can be removed without causing DRUJ instability.[6] The ulnocarpal ligaments originate on the volar ulna by the styloid and insert on the lunate and triquetrum[12]; they provide resistance to wrist extension and alternatively tighten in radial and ulnar deviation.[13] The ECU tendon resides in a groove dorsoradial to the ulnar styloid, and its subsheath attaches to the dorsal ulna and triquetrum.[14] The tendon serves as a dynamic stabilizer to keep the ulna head depressed during pronation.[6]

The IOM transfers axial loads from the radius to the ulna. Its central band provides the strongest contribution to this function,[6] whereas the inconsistently present distal oblique bundle (DOB) helps resist dorsal and volar DRUJ laxity. When present,

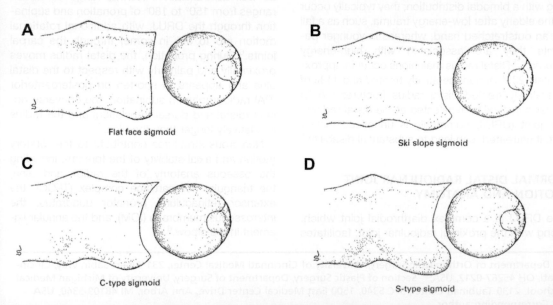

Fig. 1. Sigmoid notch shape variations. (*A*) Flat face; (*B*) Ski slope; (*C*) C-type; (*D*) S-type. (*From* Tolat AR, Stanley JK, Trail IA. A cadaveric study of the anatomy and stability of the distal radioulnar joint in the coronal and transverse planes. J Hand Surg Br. 1996 Oct;21(5):587-94; with permission.)

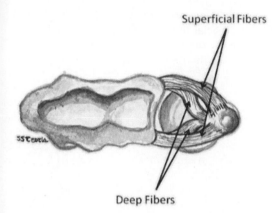

Superficial Fibers

Deep Fibers

Fig. 2. The superficial and deep dorsal and palmar radioulnar ligaments arise from the sigmoid notch to insert on the ulnar styloid and fovea, respectively. (*From* Sammer DM & Chung KC. Management of the Distal Radioulnar Joint and Ulnar Styloid Fracture. Hand Clin 28 (2012) 199–206; with permission.)

the DOB serves as an isometric stabilizer, which is under tension throughout forearm rotation.[15,16]

PATHOLOGY

Fractures of the distal radius may disrupt any number of structures that can result in DRUJ instability. Radius or ulna malalignment, TFCC injury, ulnar styloid fractures, and DRUJ articular incongruity may need to be treated to ensure smooth and stable forearm rotation after injury.

A significant degree of extra-articular distal radius malposition can be tolerated before instability or loss in forearm motion develops,[17] but large derangements in tilt, translation, inclination, and height have been shown to alter the biomechanics at the DRUJ.

Distal radial tilt, which normally averages 11° volar,[18] results in significant DRUJ incongruity after 20° of dorsal angulation.[19] Dorsally tilted malunions displace the ulna in volar, ulnar, and distal directions relative to the radius and typically cause a loss of pronation.[17,19,20] Conversely, volar malunions cause limitations in supination and dorsal translation of the ulna.[21] With other supporting structures intact, malunion alone rarely results in instability, but, if there are simultaneous disruptions of the TFCC and IOM, significant radioulnar diastasis occurs.[19]

Radial translation of the distal radius, or coronal shift, results in the proximal radius being closer to the ulna and effectively changes the radial bow. This deformity loosens the tension of the IOM, contributing to DRUJ instability. Dy and colleagues[22] noted increased DRUJ laxity with coronal shifts as small as 2 mm, and, in a prospective cohort of 163 patients, Fujitani and colleagues[23] found coronal shift to be the most important factor predictive of DRUJ instability in the setting of distal radius fractures.

Pure dorsal translation of the radius has been found to limit forearm pronation, especially after 10 mm.[17] In vitro studies show that changes in radial inclination also lead to stiffness more than instability.[24] Radial height may have the most pronounced effect on rotational kinematics. Shortening of 10 mm can cause loss of both pronation (47% reduction) and supination (29%).[25]

Although most extra-articular malunions cause stiffness, intra-articular fractures of the dorsal lunate facet lead to instability in pronation. Impaction of the lunate into the distal radius often causes a sagittal split in the lunate facet and the resulting free dorsal fragment renders the DRUL incompetent.[26] Typically, facet fractures alone do not cause instability in other positions[2] but may contribute to DRUJ arthrosis.[26]

TFCC injury occurs concomitantly in 40% to 96% of distal radius fractures.[7,27] More severely displaced fractures are more likely to have an accompanying soft tissue injury.[28] Most of these injuries do not confer any instability to the DRUJ and are along for the ride. Many are asymptomatic or may become so after a period of time. Although complete tears are uncommon, they more likely are associated with DRUJ instability.[7] When combined with osseous malalignment, TFCC tears impart a more pronounced effect on instability than when isolated and allow for increased radial shortening.[17] With dorsally angulated radius fractures, volar ulnar displacement increases once the TFCC tears.[20] Nishiwaki and colleagues[21] found the ulna to subluxate dorsally throughout forearm motion with volar radial malalignment and a TFCC tear. In cadavers, Kihara and colleagues[19] found that the DRUJ would not dislocate in the setting of a distal radius fracture without a TFCC tear. After a volar lunate facet fracture, loss of the dorsal TFCC and superficial DRUL restraint causes instability in pronation. Similarly, disruption of the volar TFCC combined with a dorsal lunate facet fracture can cause DRUJ instability.[2]

Distal ulna and styloid fractures also can affect stability in the setting of a distal radius fracture. When the TFCC is injured and the distal ulna is fractured, the distal IOM loses tension and no longer functions as a secondary DRUJ stabilizer. Without a TFCC injury, however, extra-articular distal ulna fractures alone rarely lead to dislocation.[15]

Ulna styloid fractures accompany almost 50% of distal radius fractures and 25% to 66% go on to eventual nonunion.[7,29] Most are asymptomatic but occasionally cause pain, stylocarpal impaction, and ECU tendonitis. Basilar styloid fractures can cause an injury to the radioulnar ligaments; larger fragments with increased displacement may result in instability.[7]

EVALUATION

A proper evaluation begins with a thorough history and physical examination. Patients may report frank episodes of DRUJ dislocation, but more commonly pain and loss of function are presenting complaints. In the acute fracture setting, the mechanism of injury should be elicited, because high-energy injuries are associated with more severe fractures and worse outcomes.[30]

A patient with a healed fracture may report difficulty lifting objects or clicking with forearm rotation. Painful wrist clicking with forearm rotation should raise suspicion for DRUJ instability.

The physical examination in acute injuries generally is limited by pain. Swelling, ecchymosis, and wrist deformity are observed quickly after injury. Immediate evaluation should ensure that the distal hand is neurovascularly intact, with good perfusion and functioning median, radial, and ulnar nerves. Particular attention should be paid to the median nerve sensory distribution, because acute carpal tunnel syndrome may occur and should warrant urgent reduction, and carpal tunnel release, if needed.

For patients with healed fractures, the examination should identify sites of tenderness and gross deformity. Wrist range of motion must be compared with the uninjured site. ECU subluxation and foveal tenderness should be checked for.[31]

DRUJ instability is assessed with the ballottement test, or shuck, test (**Fig. 3**). To perform this test, the examiner holds the distal radius fixed while applying alternating dorsal and volar forces to the mobile distal ulna. The degree of translation is evaluated in neutral, pronation, and supination and then compared with the asymptomatic wrist. Markedly increased displacement, lack of discernible endpoints, and pain with examination all are indicators of instability.[32]

The press test involves asking the patient to push up from a chair. Reproduction of a patient's symptoms or pain over the ulnar aspect of the wrist is highly sensitive for a TFCC tear.[33]

Standard PA and lateral wrist radiographs begin the work-up for instability after a distal radius fracture. Many dorsally angulated fractures have fracture lines extending into the DRUJ.[7] Although radiographic malalignment has been shown unreliable in predicting instability,[34] increased radial

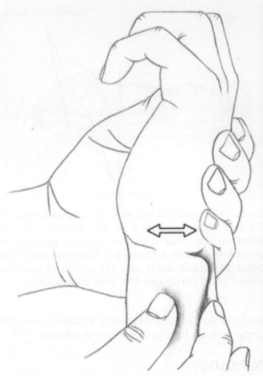

Fig. 3. The DRUJ ballottement, or shuck, test for instability. (*From* Kim JP, Park MJ. Assessment of distal radioulnar joint instability after distal radius fracture: comparison of computed tomography and clinical examination results. J Hand Surg Am 2008; 33 (09) 1486–1492; with permission.)

translation, decreased radial inclination, shortening, and a large radially displaced ulna styloid all are predictors of radioulnar ligament injury.[35] The degree of dorsal or palmar tilt is not always correlated with TFCC injury,[35] and films of the contralateral wrist are useful for comparison.

Computed tomography (CT) is an excellent tool to evaluate the articular integrity and osseous congruity of the DRUJ. Coronal fracture lines invisible on plain radiographs are readily apparent on CT.[7] Although it highlights alterations in static alignment, axial imaging does not always reveal dynamic instability.[32] Several measures have been developed to predict DRUJ instability from CT. Mino and colleagues[36] examined the position of the ulna relative to the dorsal and volar boarders of the sigmoid notch. Nakamura and colleagues[37] defined instability as dorsal ulnar displacement greater than 25% of sigmoid notch diameter. The epicenter method, described by Wechsler and colleagues[38] calculates a displacement ratio of the ulna epicenter between center of the head and the styloid along the length of the sigmoid notch. A similar method, proposed by Lo and

Table 1
Indications for operative treatment

Anatomic Parameter	Deformity
Radius shortening	>5 mm
Radial inclination	<12°
Dorsal angulation	>20°
Articular step-off	>2 mm

colleagues,[39] uses the center of the ulnar head in concentric circles to calculate their radioulnar ratio.

Unfortunately, these calculations often are cumbersome in clinical practice and all have high false-positive rates.[32,40] At best, studies have shown moderate correlation between CT evaluation and clinical instability.[32,41]

Magnetic resonance imaging may be useful as an adjunct in the work-up of instability. It can evaluate the soft tissue supports of the DRUJ and is close to 94% sensitive for a TFCC tear. Clinical correlation is imperative, and, like CT DRUJ evaluation, there is a high false-positive rate.[31]

TREATMENT
Acute Distal Radius Fractures

In the setting of an acute distal radius fracture, treatment options consist of splinting/casting, Kirschner wires, external fixation, open reduction and internal fixation (ORIF), and arthroscopic reduction. The goal of all acute treatment is to achieve healing with nearly anatomic reduction. Closed reduction with splint immobilization should be attempted when a patient initially presents to the emergency department. For fractures that cannot be adequately reduced and maintained with closed methods, operative intervention should be considered (**Table 1**).[7]

Open reduction should attempt to restore anatomic radial height, inclination, and volar tilt.

Correcting the distal radius dorsal tilt to within 10° of normal helps maintain normal DRUJ kinematics, even if the TFCC is torn.[21] Mobilizing the dorsal cortex, with an osteotome through the fracture site, for example, aids in achieving acceptable volar tilt.

Restoring the anatomic radial-ulnar coronal shift to within than 2 mm is recommended to restore the native tension of the distal oblique IOM. Intraoperatively, a Gelpi, Hohmann, or Army-Navy retractor may be placed in the interosseous space to exert a radially directed reduction force on the proximal radial shaft (**Fig. 4**).[42] Ross and colleagues[43] describe a technique using one screw as a fulcrum and the plate as a reduction aid to correct coronal shift.

Articular step-offs in both the radiocarpal joint and DRUJ should be addressed with surgery. Many articular incongruities reduce with traction, ligamentotaxis, and extra-articular fragment manipulation. Occasionally, arthrotomy or arthroscopy is needed to evaluate the scaphoid and lunate fossae and sigmoid notch cartilage surfaces.

After radial fixation, the DRUJ must be tested for stability before leaving the operating room. Forearm rotation and DRUJ ballottement should be similar to the uninjured side. Crepitus, grinding, or clunking may indicate a malreduction or implant malposition and warrant a careful re-evaluation of reduction and fixation.[7]

An unstable DRUJ may benefit from slightly increased radial distraction during ORIF. Overcorrection of the radial height indirectly shortens the ulna and tightens the IOM and radioulnar ligaments.[44] The distal radius can be lengthened slightly through the oblong hole of many plating systems if DRUJ stability is assessed before screws are placed in all the proximal plate holes. Slight increases beyond the native radial length have not been shown to be detrimental.[45]

Even after anatomic radius reduction, the DRUJ may be persistently unstable, likely secondary to

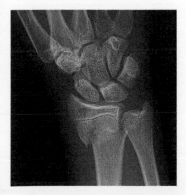
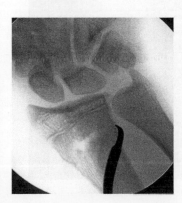

Fig. 4. (*Left*) Distal radius fracture with significant coronal shift. (*Right*) Open reduction of coronal shift using a radially directed Hohmann retractor. (*From* Trehan SK, Orbay JL, Wolfe SW. Coronal shift of distal radius fractures: influence of the distal interosseous membrane on distal radioulnar joint instability. J Hand Surg Am. 2015 Jan;40(1):159-62; with permission.)

TFCC injury.[2,7,17,20,26,28] Frequently it feels unstable in pronation but is stable in supination. For these patients, the forearm should be immobilized in the position of stability for 6 weeks. A sugar-tong splint, long arm cast, or percutaneous pins across the DRUJ all are effective methods to keep the DRUJ reduced while it heals.[7]

When the DRUJ is unstable in all positions, the TFCC may be addressed to restore ligamentous constraints. If there is a fracture through the base of the ulnar styloid, ORIF with a plate or headless compression screw reestablishes the insertions of the radioulnar ligaments, provided that they remain attached to the styloid fragment. Otherwise, acute TFCC repair may be performed open or arthroscopically.[7] Styloid fixation or TFCC repair permit shorter immobilization and can result in good motion and strength.[46]

Ulna Styloid Fractures

Most ulna styloid fractures do not need separate treatment, especially if the radius is fixed and the

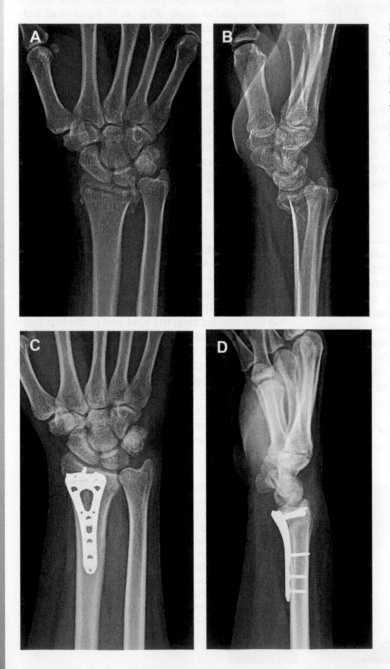

Fig. 5. Distal radius osteotomy for distal radius malunion. (*A*) PA and (*B*) lateral radiographs showing distal radius malunion with loss of radial height and inclination, positive ulnar variance, and significantly increased volar tilt. Postoperative AP (*C*) and lateral (*D*) radiographs after osteotomy.

DRUJ is stable. Distal radius reduction often indirectly reduces the ulna styloid. Although many ulna styloid fractures do not unite, outcomes are comparable between those that heal and nonunions.[4,7] In a meta-analysis by Mulders and colleagues,[4] there was no difference in patient-rated outcome measures, motion, strength, pain scores, or instability between 1196 patients with styloid union and 1047 patients with nonunion. Subset analysis further found no differences between base and nonbase styloid fractures.

If the DRUJ is acutely unstable and there is a concomitant ulna styloid base fracture, however, early repair within 3 months can lead to improved clinical outcomes.[47,48] Thus, the authors consider fixation of an ulna styloid base fracture only if there is persistent multidirection DRUJ instability on intraoperative examination after distal radius fixation.

Chronic Distal Radius Malunion

Conservative management is the first line of treatment of symptomatic instability and pain after a distal radius fracture. Rest, nonsteroidal anti-inflammatory drugs, corticosteroid injections, physical therapy, and splinting all can be effective nonoperative measures that should be exhausted before considering surgery.[31]

For those who remain symptomatic, operative intervention can be considered. Proper preoperative planning requires careful examination to identify all the structures contributing to instability. The surgeon must also consider a patient's pain, activity level, and functional limitations before proceeding.

Distal radius osteotomy is a reliable treatment option for a young, physically active patient with an incongruent and unstable DRUJ.[49,50] Malunion with volar angulation greater than 15°, dorsal angulation greater than 10°, or radial shortening greater than 3 mm all are indications for osteotomy (**Fig. 5**).[49] The procedure is contraindicated if there are marked articular degenerative changes.[50]

The procedure can be performed through either a dorsal or volar approach, with an opening wedge osteotomy based at the apex of deformity.[51] Placing the bone cuts proximal or distal to the IOM insertion has not been found to have an effect on outcome.[42] Kirschner wires placed parallel to the radius articular surface and perpendicular to the diaphysis help visualize angles and manipulate the proximal and distal segments (**Fig. 6**).[50] Kapandji pinning within the osteotomy site can aid with correction as well.[52] If there is residual articular incongruity, an intra-articular osteotomy may be performed simultaneously.[53]

Because an opening wedge osteotomy is needed to help correct lost radial height, the resultant void should be filled with bone graft. Classically, a wedge of iliac crest autograft was inserted in the osteotomy site to provide structure and osteocytes.[50] Some investigators report high union rates with morselized autograft or no graft at all, with comparable healing times.[54,55] Autograft also adds donor site morbidity, a risk of delayed union at the bone-graft interface, potential size mismatches, and additional anesthesia time, all of which must be discussed with the patient.[55]

Once the malunion is corrected, it should be fixed with locking plates. Perpendicular (90–90) plating also is an option for securing the osteotomy.[56] Advances in computer-assisted design and 3-dimensional (3-D) printing have led to new patient-specific guides and implants, which can greatly aid in understanding and correcting multiplanar

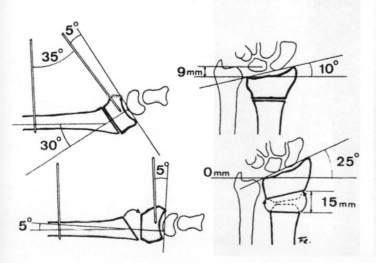

Fig. 6. Kirschner wires inserted perpendicularly to the radial diaphysis and in line with the articular surface (*upper left*) allow simple correction of the dorsal angulation deformity (*lower left*) and radial inclination (*upper right*, pre-correction; *lower right*, post-correction). (*From* Fernandez DL. Correction of post-traumatic wrist deformity in adults by osteotomy, bone-grafting, and internal fixation. J Bone Joint Surg Am. 1982 Oct;64(8):1164-78; with permission.)

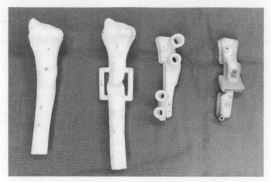

Fig. 7. Patient-specific 3-D printed radius models (left-most, pre-operative deformity; left middle, model of planned correction); drill (right middle) and cutting blocks (rightmost) can facilitate a precise osteotomy according to a CT-based preoperative plan.

deformities. Bilateral preoperative CT scans allow for matched, superimposed 3-D reconstructions.[57,58] Drill and resection guides, titanium plates, and even wedge bone graft models then are custom manufactured with 3-D printing, based on the preoperative reconstruction plan (**Fig. 7**).[57–59]

Outcomes after distal radius osteotomy show improvements in flexion-extension and pronation-supination arcs, pain, grip strength, and functional scores, although final motion often is less than the uninjured side.[57,58,60] Patient-specific guides can achieve corrections to within 1.5° of the preoperative plan, and have shown

near normal motion, pain, and grip strength.[58] Buijze and colleagues,[57] however, found no difference between patient-specific and conventional osteotomies in their randomized trial. In general, radius osteotomies have high complication rates, with revision surgery in up to 38%.[56,60–62] Implant removal is higher with dorsal approaches,[51] and postoperative extensor pollicis longus ruptures reported. Nonunion may occur in up to 12%.[62]

For older patients with instability and radius deformity angulated less than 20°, ulnar shortening osteotomy (USO) is another option.[63] USO can result in a 26% to 44% increase in DRUJ stiffness, as the TFCC tightens (**Fig. 8**).[64] Bone cuts placed more proximally on the ulna lead to more DRUJ stability, as tension in the DOB of the IOM increases.[65] Studies of USO typically show improved range of motion, pain scores, and patient-reported outcomes. Reported nonunion rates are low (4%–6%), but, due to the subcutaneous location of the ulna, hardware removal is frequent (18%–50%).[66,67]

Elderly patients and those with significant medical comorbidities, who require a quick recovery, may benefit from a Darrach ulna head resection. Motion may be initiated quickly and the procedure avoids the need to heal an osteotomy.

Triangular Fibrocartilage Complex Tears

TFCC tears that require intervention should be treated early, with splinting or pinning in the position

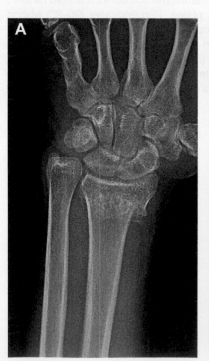
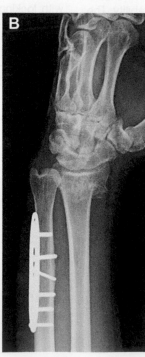

Fig. 8. (*A*) Preoperative and (*B*) postoperative radiographs of ulna shortening osteotomy for an unstable DRUJ after distal radius malunion.

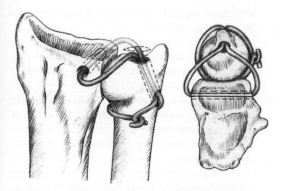

Fig. 9. Coronal (*left*) and axial (*right*) schematic diagramming reconstruction of the dorsal and palmar radioulnar ligaments with a single palmaris longus tendon graft. (*From* Adams BD, Berger RA. An anatomic reconstruction of the distal radioulnar ligaments for posttraumatic distal radioulnar joint instability. J Hand Surg Am. 2002 Mar;27(2):243-51; with permission.)

of stability rather than waiting for chronic instability.[7] Acute TFCC repairs with distal radius fractures generally do well; Johandi and Sechachalam[68] reported 72% returning to work and 91% achieving preinjury function. They noted that the DRUJ remained stable over time in 83%. Open and arthroscopic repair techniques show no difference in long-term recurrence of instability.[69]

Chronic TFCC tears resulting in DRUJ instability after distal radius fracture may not be amenable to primary repair. In cases of DRUJ laxity with minimal osseous deformity, the DRUL and PRUL may require reconstruction with a tendon graft. The technique described by Adams and Berger[70] routes a palmaris longus tendon graft through bone tunnels in the radius and distal ulna to recreate both ligaments at once (**Fig. 9**). Gillis and colleagues[71] reported that 90% achieve a stable DRUJ after this procedure and 75% get adequate pain relief.

SUMMARY

DRUJ instability is an uncommon sequela of distal radius fractures, which is more likely with severely displaced fractures and concomitant TFCC tears. Clinicians should closely examine the DRUJ when treating distal radius fractures and treat instability appropriately. Chronic instability may require osteotomy or radioulnar ligament reconstruction. With proper management, most patients recover forearm stability and motion after distal radius fracture.

DISCLOSURE

Dr P.R. Ross has received travel, education, and food from Skeletal Dynamics, Synthes, and Zimmer. Dr K.C. Chung has nothing to disclose.

REFERENCES

1. Owen RA, Melton LJ III, Johnson KA, et al. Incidence of Colles' fracture in a North American community. Am J Public Health 1982;72:605–7.
2. Cole DW, Elsaidi GA, Kuzma KR, et al. Distal radioulnar joint instability in distal radius fractures: the role of sigmoid notch and triangular fibrocartilage complex revisited. Injury 2006;37(3):252–8.
3. Porrino JA Jr, Maloney E, Scherer K, et al. Fracture of the distal radius: epidemiology and premanagement radiographic characterization. Am J Roentgenol 2014;203(3):551–9.
4. Mulders MAM, Fuhri Snethlage LJ, de Muinck Keizer R, et al. Functional outcomes of distal radius fractures with and without ulnar styloid fractures: a meta-analysis. J Hand Surg Eur Vol 2018;43(2):150–7.
5. Altissimi M, Antenucci R, Fiacca C, et al. Long-term results of conservative treatment of fractures of the distal radius. Clin Orthop Relat Res 1986;206:202–10.
6. Huang JI, Hanel DP. Anatomy and biomechanics of the distal radioulnar joint. Hand Clin 2012;28:157–63.
7. Sammer DM, Chung KC. Management of the distal radioulnar joint and ulnar styloid fracture. Hand Clin 2012;28:199–206.
8. Ekenstam F, Hagert CG. Anatomical studies on the geometry and stability of the distal radio ulnar joint. Scand J Plast Reconstr Surg 1985;19:17–25.
9. Tolat AR, Stanley JK, Trail IA. A cadaveric study of the anatomy and stability of the distal radioulnar joint in the coronal and transverse planes. J Hand Surg Br 1996;21(5):587–94.
10. Schuind F, An KN, Berglund L, et al. The distal radioulnar ligaments: A biomechanical study. J Hand Surg 1991;16A:1106–14.
11. Hagert E, Hagert CG. Understanding stability of the distal radioulnar joint through an understanding of its anatomy. Hand Clin 2010;26(4):459–66.
12. Nakamura T, Takayama S, Horiuchi Y, et al. Origins and insertions of the triangular fibrocartilage complex: a histological study. J Hand Surg Br 2001;26(5):446–54.
13. Moritomo H, Murase T, Arimitsu S, et al. Change in the length of the ulnocarpal ligaments during radiocarpal motion: possible impact on triangular fibrocartilage complex foveal tears. J Hand Surg Am 2008;33(8):1278–86.
14. Pidgeon TS, Waryasz G, Carnevale J, et al. Triangular fibrocartilage complex: an anatomic review. JBJS Rev 2015;3(1). 01874474-201501000-00003.
15. Miyamura S, Shigi A, Kraisarin J, et al. Impact of distal ulnar fracture malunion on distal radioulnar joint instability: a biomechanical study of the distal

interosseous membrane using a cadaver model. J Hand Surg Am 2017;42(3):e185–91.

16. Moritomo H. The distal interosseous membrane: current concepts in wrist anatomy and biomechanics. J Hand Surg Am 2012;37(7):1501–7.

17. Fraser GS, Ferreira LM, Johnson JA, et al. The effect of multiplanar distal radius fractures on forearm rotation: in vitro biomechanical study. J Hand Surg Am 2009;34(5):838–48.

18. Medoff RJ. Essential radiographic evaluation for distal radius fractures. Hand Clin 2005;21(3): 279–88.

19. Kihara H, Palmer AK, Werner FW, et al. The effect of dorsally angulated distal radius fractures on distal radioulnar joint congruency and forearm rotation. J Hand Surg 1996;21A:40–7.

20. Nishiwaki M, Welsh M, Gammon B, et al. Distal radioulnar joint kinematics in simulated dorsally angulated distal radius fractures. J Hand Surg Am 2014; 39(4):656e663.

21. Nishiwaki M, Welsh M, Gammon B, et al. Effect of Volarly Angulated Distal Radius Fractures on Forearm Rotation and Distal Radioulnar Joint Kinematics. J Hand Surg Am 2015;40(11):2236–42.

22. Dy CJ, Jang E, Taylor SA, et al. The impact of coronal alignment on distal radioulnar joint stability following distal radius fracture. J Hand Surg Am 2014;39(7):1264–72.

23. Fujitani R, Omokawa S, Akahane M, et al. Predictors of distal radioulnar joint instability in distal radius fractures. J Hand Surg Am 2011;36(12):1919–25.

24. Bessho Y, Nakamura T, Nagura T, et al. Effect of volar angulation of extra-articular distal radius fractures on distal radioulnar joint stability: a biomechanical study. J Hand Surg Eur Vol 2015;40(8): 775–82.

25. Bronstein AJ, Trumble TE, Tencer AF. The effects of distal radius fracture malalignment on forearm rotation: a cadaveric study. J Hand Surg Am 1997; 22(2):258–62.

26. Melone CP Jr. Articular fractures of the distal radius. Orthop Clin North Am 1984;15(2):217–36.

27. Yan B, Xu Z, Chen Y, et al. Prevalence of triangular fibrocartilage complex injuries in patients with distal radius fractures: a 3.0T magnetic resonance imaging study. J Int Med Res 2019;47(8):3648–55.

28. Richards RS, Bennett JD, Roth JH, et al. Arthroscopic diagnosis of intra-articular soft tissue injuries associated with distal radial fractures. J Hand Surg Am 1997;22(5):772–6.

29. Daneshvar P, Chan R, MacDermid J, et al. The effects of ulnar styloid fractures on patients sustaining distal radius fractures. J Hand Surg Am 2014; 39(10):1915–20.

30. van der Vliet QMJ, Sweet AAR, Bhashyam AR, et al. Polytrauma and high-energy injury mechanisms are associated with worse patient-reported outcomes after distal radius fractures. Clin Orthop Relat Res 2019;477(10):2267–75.

31. Faucher GK, Zimmerman RM, Zimmerman NB. Instability and arthritis of the distal radioulnar joint: a critical analysis review. JBJS Rev 2016;4(12). 01874474-201612000-00001.

32. Kim JP, Park MJ. Assessment of distal radioulnar joint instability after distal radius fracture: comparison of computed tomography and clinical examination results. J Hand Surg Am 2008;33(09):1486–92.

33. Lester B, Halbrecht J, Levy IM, et al. "Press test" for office diagnosis of triangular fibrocartilage complex tears of the wrist. Ann Plast Surg 1995;35(1):41–5.

34. Lindau T, Hagberg L, Adlercreutz C, et al. Distalradioulnar instability is an independent worsening factor in distalradial fractures. Clin Orthop 2000;376: 229–35.

35. Nakamura T, Iwamoto T, Matsumura N, et al. Radiographic and arthroscopic assessment of DRUJ instability due to foveal avulsion of the radioulnar ligament in distal radius fractures. J Wrist Surg 2014; 3(1):12–7.

36. Mino DE, Palmer AK, Levinsohn EM. The role of radiography andcomputerized tomography in the diagnosis of subluxation and dis-location of the distal radioulnar joint. J Hand Surg 1983;8:23–31.

37. Nakamura R, Horii E, Imaeda T, et al. Criteria for diagnosingdistal radioulnar joint subluxation by computed tomography. Skeletal Radiol 1996;25: 649–53.

38. Wechsler RJ, Wehbe MA, Rifkin MD, et al. Computed tomography diagnosis of distal radioulnar subluxation. Skeletal Radiol 1987;16:1–5.

39. Lo IK, MacDermid JC, Bennett JD, et al. The radioulnar ratio: a new method of quantifying distal radioulnar jointsubluxation. J Hand Surg 2001;26A: 236–43.

40. Wijffels M, Stomp W, Krijnen P, et al. Computed tomography for the detection of distal radioulnar joint instability: normal variation and reliability of four CT scoring systems in 46 patients. Skeletal Radiol 2016;45(11):1487–93.

41. van Leerdam RH, Wijffels MME, Reijnierse M, et al. The value of computed tomography in detecting distal radioulnar joint instability after a distal radius fracture. J Hand Surg Eur Vol 2017;42(5):501–6.

42. Trehan SK, Orbay JL, Wolfe SW. Coronal shift of distal radius fractures: influence of the distal interosseous membrane on distal radioulnar joint instability. J Hand Surg Am 2015;40(1):159–62.

43. Ross M, Allen L, Couzens GB. Correction of residual radial translation of the distal fragment in distal radius fracture open reduction. J Hand Surg Am 2015;40(12):2465–70.

44. Wang JP, Huang HK, Fufa D. Radial distraction to stabilize distal radioulnar joint in distal radius fixation. J Hand Surg Am 2018;43(5):493.e1-4.

45. Isa AD, McGregor ME, Padmore CE, et al. Effect of radial lengthening on distal forearm loading following simulated in vitro radial shortening during simulated dynamic wrist motion. J Hand Surg Am 2019;44(7):556–63.e5.

46. Gong HS, Cho HE, Kim J, et al. Surgical treatment of acute distal radioulnar joint instability associated with distal radius fractures. J Hand Surg Eur Vol 2015;40(8):783–9.

47. Chen AC, Chiu CH, Weng CJ, et al. Early and late fixation of ulnar styloid base fractures yields different outcomes. J Orthop Surg Res 2018; 13(1):193.

48. Lee SK, Kim KJ, Cha YH, et al. Conservative treatment is sufficient for acute distal radioulnar joint instability with distal radius fracture. Ann Plast Surg 2016;77(3):297–304.

49. Buijze GA, Prommersberger KJ, González Del Pino J, et al. Corrective osteotomy for combined intra- and extra-articular distal radius malunion. J Hand Surg Am 2012;37(10):2041–9.

50. Fernandez DL. Correction of post-traumatic wrist deformity in adults by osteotomy, bone-grafting, and internal fixation. J Bone Joint Surg Am 1982; 64(8):1164–78.

51. Schurko BM, Lechtig A, Chen NC, et al. Outcomes and complications following volar and dorsal osteotomy for symptomatic distal radius malunions: a comparative study. J Hand Surg Am 2020;45(2): 158.e1-8.

52. Huang HK, Hsu SH, Hsieh FC, et al. Extra-articular corrective osteotomy with bone grafting to achieve lengthening and regain alignment for distal radius fracture malunion. Tech Hand Up Extrem Surg 2019;23(4):186–90.

53. Ring D, Prommersberger KJ, González del Pino J, et al. Corrective osteotomy for intra-articular malunion of the distal part of the radius. J Bone Joint Surg Am 2005;87(7):1503–9.

54. Fok MW, Fernandez DL, Rivera YL. A less invasive distal osteotomy of the radius for malunited dorsally displaced extra-articular fractures. J Hand Surg Eur Vol 2015;40(8):812–8.

55. Disseldorp DJ, Poeze M, Hannemann PF, et al. Is bone grafting necessary in the treatment of malunited distal radius fractures? J Wrist Surg 2015; 4(3):207–13.

56. Gaspar MP, Kho JY, Kane PM, et al. Orthogonal plate fixation with corrective osteotomy for treatment of distal radius fracture malunion. J Hand Surg Am 2017;42(1):e1–10.

57. Buijze GA, Leong NL, Stockmans F, et al. Three-dimensional compared with two-dimensional preoperative planning of corrective osteotomy for extra-articular distal radial malunion: a multicenter randomized controlled trial. J Bone Joint Surg Am 2018;100(14):1191–202.

58. Byrne AM, Impelmans B, Bertrand V, et al. Corrective osteotomy for malunited diaphyseal forearm fractures using preoperative 3-dimensional planning and patient-specific surgical guides and implants. J Hand Surg Am 2017;42(10):836.e1-12.

59. Honigmann P, Thieringer F, Steiger R, et al. A simple 3-dimensional printed aid for a corrective palmar opening wedge osteotomy of the distal radius. J Hand Surg Am 2016;41(3):464–9.

60. Delclaux S, Trang Pham TT, Bonnevialle N, et al. Distal radius fracture malunion: Importance of managing injuries of the distal radio-ulnar joint. Orthop Traumatol Surg Res 2016;102(3):327–32.

61. Mulders MA, d'Ailly PN, Cleffken BI, et al. Corrective osteotomy is an effective method of treating distal radius malunions with good long-term functional results. Injury 2017;48(3):731–7.

62. Haghverdian JC, Hsu JY, Harness NG. Complications of corrective osteotomies for extra-articular distal radius malunion. J Hand Surg Am 2019; 44(11):987.e1-9.

63. Kamal RN, Leversedge FJ. Ulnar shortening osteotomy for distal radius malunion. J Wrist Surg 2014; 3(3):181–6.

64. Nishiwaki M, Nakamura T, Nakao Y, et al. Ulnar shortening effect on distal radioulnar joint stability: a biomechanical study. J Hand Surg Am 2005; 30(4):719–26.

65. Arimitsu S, Moritomo H, Kitamura T, et al. The stabilizing effect of the distal interosseous membrane on the distal radioulnar joint in an ulnar shortening procedure: a biomechanical study. J Bone Joint Surg Am 2011;93(21):2022–30.

66. Owens J, Compton J, Day M, et al. Nonunion rates among ulnar-shortening osteotomy for ulnar impaction syndrome: a systematic review. J Hand Surg Am 2019;44(7):612.e1–12.

67. Chan SK, Singh T, Pinder R, et al. Ulnar shortening osteotomy: are complications under reported? J Hand Microsurg 2015;7(2):276–82.

68. Johandi F, Sechachalam S. Clinical and functional outcome of open primary repair of triangular fibrocartilage complex tears associated with distal radius fractures. J Orthop Surg (Hong Kong) 2017;25(1): 1–5.

69. Andersson JK, Åhlén M, Andernord D. Open versus arthroscopic repair of the triangular fibrocartilage complex: a systematic review. J Exp Orthop 2018; 5(1):6.

70. Adams BD, Berger RA. An anatomic reconstruction of the distal radioulnar ligaments for posttraumatic distal radioulnar joint instability. J Hand Surg Am 2002;27(2):243–51.

71. Gillis JA, Soreide E, Khouri JS, et al. Outcomes of the Adams-Berger ligament reconstruction for the distal radioulnar joint instability in 95 consecutive cases. J Wrist Surg 2019;8(4):268–75.

Acute Distal Radioulnar Joint Instability
Evaluation and Treatment

Louis H. Poppler, MD, MSCI[a], Steven L. Moran, MD[b,c],*

KEYWORDS

- Distal radioulnar joint • DRUJ • DRUJ dislocation • Wrist fracture • TFCC

KEY POINTS

- Pronation and supination (axial rotation) occur through both the proximal radioulnar joint and distal radioulnar joint (DRUJ), which function as 1 unit.
- Injury to the triangular fibrocartilage complex (TFCC) is common and associated with fractures of the distal radius and ulna.
- Injuries to the radial head, the interosseous membrane (IOM), and the TFCC result in dissociation of the radius and ulna, instability, proximal migration of the radius relative to the ulna, and impingement of the distal ulna on the carpus (Essex-Lopresti injury). For this reason, it is important to always examine the elbow along with the wrist.
- Anatomic reduction and fixation of fractures of the radius and ulna is imperative to restoring axial stability to the forearm.
- Understanding the complex anatomy of the TFCC, DRUJ, and IOM allows anatomic reconstruction of these structures at the initial surgery, restoring stability and proper rotation, and avoiding the need for secondary procedures or salvage procedures in future.

INTRODUCTION

Pronation and supination of the forearm occur through the proximal radioulnar joint (PRUJ) and distal radioulnar joint (DRUJ), which function as 1 unit. A combination of bony support and ligamentous constraints are essential for stability and motion. Failure to recognize, anatomically reduce, and stabilize injuries to these joints leads to instability, stiffness, and/or painful arthritis. This article focuses on acute DRUJ instability in the context of triangular fibrocartilage complex (TFCC) injuries, distal radius fractures (DRFs), distal ulnar fractures, Galeazzi fractures, Essex-Lopresti injuries, and DRUJ dislocation. The emphasis is on understanding the primary and secondary stabilizers of the DRUJ and PRUJ so that acute injuries to these stabilizers are recognized and treated before the need for later salvage procedures arises.

Anatomy

The ulna is the fixed unit of the forearm, although by convention the nomenclature implies that the ulna moves. Nevertheless, pronation and supination of the radius occur around the ulna through the DRUJ and PRUJ. Although motion through these joints is primarily rotational, both axial (proximal-distal) and translational (volar-dorsal) motion occur at the DRUJ with load and rotation.[1,2] In pronation, ulnar length at the wrist relative to radial

[a] Department of Plastic & Reconstructive Surgery, St. Luke's Health System, Boise, ID, USA; [b] Department of Plastic & Reconstructive Surgery, Mayo Clinic, Rochester, MN, USA; [c] Department of Orthopedic Surgery, Mayo Clinic, Rochester, MN, USA
* Corresponding author. Department of Orthopedic Surgery, Mayo Clinic, Rochester, MN.
E-mail address: Moran.steven@mayo.edu

Hand Clin 36 (2020) 429–441
https://doi.org/10.1016/j.hcl.2020.07.005
0749-0712/20/© 2020 Elsevier Inc. All rights reserved.

length (ulnar positivity or negativity) may be 2 mm greater than in supination.[3–6]

Stability of the DRUJ arises from a combination of bony architecture and ligamentous constraints. The bony anatomy of the sigmoid notch is variable but accounts for only 20-30% of the joints stability[7,8] (**Fig. 1**A). Deepening of the sigmoid notch has been suggested to improve stability.[9]

The primary stabilizer of the DRUJ is the TFCC.[10,11] The TFCC is composed of several structures that are not readily distinguishable on histologic dissection but are subdivided based on injury patterns and clinical experience. These structures include the dorsal and palmar radioulnar ligaments, the subsheath of the extensor carpi ulnaris (ECU) tendon, triangular fibrocartilage (TFC), the ulnocarpal meniscus, and the ulnar collateral ligament (**Fig. 1**B, C). The dorsal and palmar radioulnar ligaments are subdivided into deep and superficial ligaments.[12] Both the superficial and deep radioulnar ligaments originate from the ulnar side of the radius. The superficial

radioulnar ligaments insert at the base of the styloid, whereas the deep radioulnar ligaments insert at the fovea. Along with normal bony anatomy, the deep dorsal and palmar radioulnar ligaments are thought to be the most important contributors to DRUJ volar-dorsal stability.[7,12–14] The superficial palmar and dorsal radioulnar fibers act to restrain supination and pronation, respectively, and are less important to DRUJ stability. The remainder of the TFCC serves as secondary stabilizers (ECU subsheath, ulnar collateral ligament) or to cushion the distal ulna from the carpus (TFC, ulnocarpal meniscus).

Extensive research has been performed in an attempt to determine whether the palmar or dorsal radioulnar ligament complex is more important to DRUJ stability, and the answer is that the two work together to achieve stability, with neither being more important.[12,15–17] The superficial palmar and deep dorsal radioulnar ligaments tighten in supination, working together to constrain motion. In contrast, the superficial

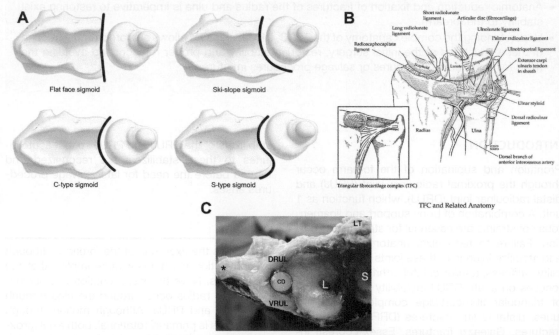

Fig. 1. (*A*) Bony anatomy of the DRUJ. The sigmoid notch has been shown to have 4 anatomic variations as described by Tolat and colleagues.[8] Flat or shallow joints are hypothesized to be more prone to dislocation. (*B*) The primary stabilizer of the DRUJ is the TFCC. The TFCC is composed of the triangular fibrocartilage articular disc, the ulnocarpal meniscus (meniscus homologue), the ulnar collateral ligament, the dorsal radioulnar ligament, the palmar radioulnar ligament, and the subsheath of the extensor carpi ulnaris (ECU). (*C*) Cadaveric dissection of the TFCC showing a distal view of the DRUJ, with the fibrocartilaginous portion of the central disc (CD) shown in light gray. The dorsal radioulnar (DRUL) and volar radioulnar ligaments (VRUL) are seen emanating from the dorsal and volar ulnar corners of the distal radius, inserting onto the distal ulna. Also seen is the lunate facet (L); the scaphoid facet (S); Lister tubercle (LT), and the ulnar styloid (*asterisk*). (*From* [A] Kakar S, Carlsen BT, Moran SL, Berger RA, Hand Clin. 2010, 26: 518; with permission; and [C] *From* Hagert E, Chim H, Moran SL. Anatomy of the distal radioulnar joint. In: JA G, editor. Ulnar sided wrist pain: A master skills publication. Rosemont: American Society for Surgery of the Hand; 2013. p. 11-22; with permission.)

dorsal and deep palmar radioulnar ligaments tighten in pronation. Dorsal displacement of the distal ulna relative to the radius is caused by failure of the palmar radioulnar ligaments, whereas volar displacement is caused by failure of the dorsal radioulnar ligaments.[7,18–20]

Other secondary stabilizers of the DRUJ include the interosseous membrane (IOM), the pronator quadratus (PQ), and the DRUJ joint capsule. The PQ has 2 heads: superficial and deep.[21] The deep head passes between the radius and ulna, inserting on the dorsal ulna. This head may resist dorsal displacement of the ulna relative to the ulna.[22] Of particular importance in fractures of the radius and ulna is the distal oblique bundle (DOB) of the IOM.[17,23–25] This structure is present, or thick, in 29% to 36% of patients.[26–28] This distal thickening of the IOM runs obliquely from the ulna proximally at the proximal end of the PQ to insert on the radius at the capsule of the DRUJ (**Fig. 2**). The DOB is responsible for seating the head of the ulna in the sigmoid notch and is slackened when the radius is shortened because of fracture. Similarly, the IOM is slackened when radial translation of a DRF is not corrected.[29] Tightening of the DOB in addition to the radioulnar ligaments has been shown to improve DRUJ stability following ulnar shortening osteotomy.[30]

Diagnosis of Distal Radioulnar Joint Instability

Diagnosis of DRUJ instability relies on the examiner having a high index of suspicion. DRUJ instability occurs most commonly following high-energy injuries of radius or ulna. DRUJ dislocation or instability may be apparent on physical examination, with inspection revealing a prominent ulnar head suggesting dorsal translation of the ulnar head relative to the radius, or a dimple suggesting volar translation. Clinical diagnosis of DRUJ instability is the gold standard and consists of stabilizing the radius and carpus with 1 hand while "shucking" the ulna volar and dorsal.[31,32] This test can only be done following fixation of any associated fractures. A stable DRUJ should have a firm end point, especially in pronation or supination. Comparison with the contralateral side is essential. Ruch and colleagues[33] suggest greater than 1 cm of dorsal-volar translation is abnormal and instability should be assumed.

There are several radiographic indications of DRUJ instability that should be noted. Radial diaphyseal fractures within 7.5 cm of articular surface (**Fig. 3**A), fractures through the base of the ulnar styloid or with a second foveal fragment (**Fig. 3**B), DRUJ widening or overlap of the radius and ulna on anteroposterior (AP) radiographs, volar or dorsal dislocation of the ulna relative to the radius on a true lateral view, or greater than 5-mm to 7-mm (**Fig. 4**)[34] radial shortening suggest DRUJ injury.[35,36] AP radiographs of the contralateral wrist are helpful in determining changes in radial or ulnar length, and ulnar positivity. If there is significant shortening of the radius without DRF, obtaining forearm and elbow radiographs may help diagnose an Essex-Lopresti injury. Large ulnar styloid fragments, ulnar styloid fragments displaced more than 2 mm, or displacement of the styloid volar to the axis of the ulnar shaft also suggest DRUJ instability.[33,37–39]

Computed tomography (CT) protocols for diagnosing instability of the DRUJ have been

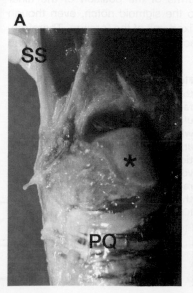
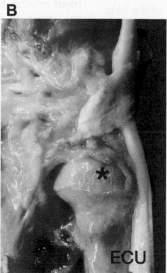

Fig. 2. (*A*) The neuromuscular stability of the DRUJ is primarily determined by (*A*) the PQ, in particular the deep head, which wraps around the volar forearm just proximal to the DRUJ. (*B*) The ECU with its subsheath (SS) similarly plays a role in the dynamic stability of both the DRUJ and the carpus as a whole. The asterisk indicates the ulnar head. (*From* Hagert E, Chim H, Moran SL. Anatomy of the distal radioulnar joint. In: JA G, editor. Ulnar sided wrist pain: A master skills publication. Rosemont: American Society for Surgery of the Hand; 2013. p. 11-22; with permission.)

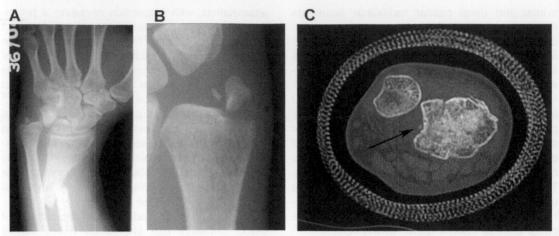

Fig. 3. (A–C) There are several radiographic indicators of potential DRUJ instability. (A) A fracture within 7.5 cm of the radius articular surface can be an indication of a Galeazzi fracture. (B) A proximal ulnar styloid fracture, which may indicate a disruption of the foveal insertion of the deep fibers of the dorsal and volar radioulnar ligaments. (C) Axial CT of a close reduced distal radius fracture with concomitant dorsal dislocation of the ulnar. Arrow points to an avulsion fracture fragment attached to volar radioulnar ligament.

described and have some utility for assessing static and dynamic instability.[40–42] However, MRI has largely supplanted CT because of its ability to detect the specific soft tissue lesions causing DRUJ instability.[43] CT is the study of choice for intra-articular DRFs to assess the congruency of the sigmoid facet and to facilitate operative planning (Fig. 3).[42,44] CT should also be used if malunion or osseous anatomy is thought to contribute to DRUJ instability.

Intraoperative assessment of the DRUJ has primarily relied on arthroscopic evaluation. Radiographic dynamic parameters of instability have been described. Specifically, the DRUJ ballottement test has been described to evaluate DRUJ instability intraoperatively. To perform the test, force is applied to the palmar surface of the ulna and dorsal displacement is assessed on a lateral

radiograph. Significant instability is suggested with displacement of more than 9 mm. However, this test requires comparison with the normal side and has not been validated in a clinical series.[45] Until dynamic intraoperative radiographic evaluation improves, wrist arthroscopy will remain the gold standard for assessment of TFCC injury. With the use of DRUJ portals, surgeons may also evaluate the foveal insertion, signs of impaction, and associated ligamentous injury.[46–48]

Acute Distal Radioulnar Joint Dislocation

Isolated acute dislocation of the DRUJ is uncommon.[37,44] DRUJ dislocation is, by convention, described in terms of the position of the ulnar head relative to the sigmoid notch, even though the ulna is the fixed unit of the forearm. Therefore, in a dorsal dislocation of the DRUJ, the ulnar head

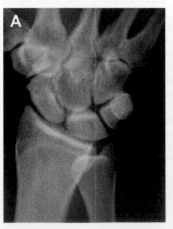
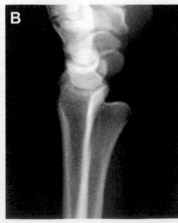

Fig. 4. Isolated palmar dislocation of the ulna in relation to the radius. AP radiograph (A) shows overlap of the ulna and radius at the sigmoid notch, whereas lateral radiograph (B) show anterior displacement of ulna in relation to the radius. Such an injury involves an injury to the dorsal radioulnar ligaments, in addition to the palmar radioulnar ligament and IOM.

is prominent dorsally (see **Fig. 3**C). Although the TFCC can be completely disrupted in DRUJ dislocation, case reports have noted restoration of stability with simple reduction of the dislocation.[49,50] In volar dislocation, the dorsal radioulnar ligaments and volar capsule are often disrupted, whereas in dorsal dislocations the palmar radioulnar ligaments and dorsal capsule are often disrupted (see **Fig. 4**).[51–53] Closed reduction of the DRUJ is performed under local anesthesia with or without sedation. Gentle traction and pressure on the ulnar head are often enough to reduce the joint. Reduction of volar dislocations can be more difficult because of the pull of the deep head of the PQ. In these cases, distraction of the radius from the ulna coupled with pronation and volar pressure assists reduction.

DRUJ dislocations have been classified as simple or complex. In complex dislocations the DRUJ cannot be reduced following reduction and stabilization of the radius. In simple dislocations, the DRUJ can be reduced.[49,54–57] Clinicians should be cognizant of complex dislocation that cannot be closed reduced because of interposition of tendons, most commonly the ECU tendon.[44,49,58] When closed reduction is difficult or incomplete, it is best to proceed with an open, or arthroscopic-assisted, reduction to allow extraction of interposed structures.

If DRUJ stability is restored following closed reduction, management in a Munster-style splint or cast with the forearm in the position of stability (supination for dorsal dislocations; pronation for volar dislocations) is recommended. However, if open reduction is required, direct repair of the TFCC to its foveal insertion is recommended using a suture anchor or bone tunnels. When the ulnar

head is dislocated and protrudes through the skin, the diagnosis of associated TFCC injury/avulsion is easy. The authors recommend placing a suture anchor in the fovea before reduction to facilitate TFCC repair. Following repair, the arm is still immobilized in a Munster-style splint or cast for 4 to 6 weeks. The authors prefer immobilization in neutral rotation as opposed to full supination or full pronation. Stiffness in full supination or pronation can cause more morbidity than stiffness in a neutral position. In addition, studies have failed to show superiority of splinting in the extremes of pronation or supination compared with neutral forearm positioning.[59]

Triangular Fibrocartilage Complex Injuries

TFCC injuries are the most common cause of ulnar-sided wrist pain and can be a cause of acute or chronic DRUJ instability. Traumatic tears of the TFCC occur with axial load on an extended and ulnar-deviated wrist or with an axial load and extremes of pronation or supination.[60] Palmer[61] classified TFCC tears as traumatic or degenerative, central or peripheral (**Fig. 5**, **Table 1**). A complete review of sources of ulnar-sided wrist pain is beyond the scope of this article; however, DRUJ instability with TFCC tears or degeneration are a common cause of ulnar-sided wrist pain. Instability of the DRUJ requires either disruption or laxity of the radioulnar ligaments, often with disruption or disorder of the secondary stabilizers (DOB, ECU subsheath, ulnotriquetral ligament, DRUJ capsule).

Treatment of DRUJ instability caused by TFCC injury focuses on diagnosis, tightening, and repair or reconstruction of the radioulnar ligaments and/

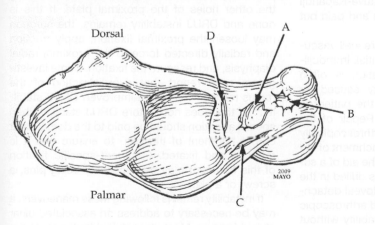

Dorsal

Palmar

Common TFC Tears

Fig. 5. TFCC injuries following trauma can occur within the articular disc (*A*), ulnar periphery (*B*), palmar periphery (*C*), and along the radial attachment (*D*). TFCC tears which result in instability occur in areas B and C. TFCC detachment from the radius (a type D Palmar lesion) could also theoretically result in DRUJ instability if the tear proceeds palmarly or dorsally through the palmar or dorsal radioulnar ligaments respectively. Arthroscopic evaluation needs to be combined with physical exam to verify the diagnosis of a destabilizing TFCC injury.

Table 1
Palmer classification of triangular fibrocartilage complex injuries

Traumatic Lesions:	
Class 1A	Central rupture
Class 1B	Disruption of insertion of radioulnar ligaments at ulnar fovea and/or styloid (with or without ulnar styloid fracture)
Class 1C	Avulsion/tear of the ulnocarpal ligaments
Class 1D	Disruption of radial origins of radioulnar ligaments (with or without sigmoid notch fracture)
Degenerative Lesions:	
Class 2A	TFCC wear
Class 2B	TFCC wear with lunate and/or ulnar chondromalacia
Class 2C	TFCC perforation with lunate and/or ulnar chondromalacia
Class 2D	Class 2C plus lunotriquetral ligament perforation
Class 2E	Class 2D plus ulnocarpal arthritis

or secondary stabilizers. Before repairing, reconstructing, or tightening these structures, surgeons should ensure that bony alignment is correct and there is no arthritis of the DRUJ to avoid causing pain in the process of improving stability. If arthritis does already exist, it must be addressed with denervation, interposition arthroplasty, hemiarthroplasty, or whole-joint arthroplasty.[62–66] Resection arthroplasty (Darrach or Sauve-Kapandji procedure) may resolve the arthritis and pain but does not address instability.[67]

The fovea and peripheral TFCC are well vascularized and have good healing potential. Immobilization in neutral pronation-supination is often adequate to treat DRUJ instability caused by TFCC injury and can be trialed if the patient is reluctant to undergo surgery.[59,68] Repair of the radioulnar ligaments can be done arthroscopically or as an open procedure.[69–71] Reattachment of the TFCC to the fovea is achieved with the aid of a suture anchor, or through bone tunnels drilled in the ulna using arthroscopic imaging of foveal detachment, hook test, trampoline test, and arthroscopic repair. In the setting of chronic instability without DRUJ arthritis, the radioulnar ligaments can be reconstructed with tendon graft with good success[72–74] (**Fig. 6**).

Distal Radius Fractures and Distal Radioulnar Joint Instability

Patients presenting with a DRF also have a TFCC or DRUJ injury in 43% to 84% of cases.[75,76] Therefore, it is essential to examine for DRUJ instability in all patients with DRF. However, because the volar and dorsal radioulnar ligaments originate from the distal radius, this will necessarily be unstable until the fracture has been fixated. DRFs affect the DRUJ anatomy and stability in 3 major ways: (1) dorsal tilt of the distal radius alters the orientation of the sigmoid notch, causing incongruity with the ulnar head; (2) shortening of the distal radius slackens the radioulnar ligaments and the DOB; and (3) failure to secure the volar or dorsal ulnar fragments of an intra-articular fragment results in uncoupling of the radius and ulna at the DRUJ through the radioulnar ligaments.[34,77] For this reason, proper identification, restoration of alignment, and fixation of both the volar and dorsal ulnar-sided fragments of a DRF is imperative, especially if early motion or short arm immobilization is planned.[78]

However, following fixation of a DRF, if instability of the DRUJ remains, there is no accepted algorithm for management.[79] Lindau and colleagues[80,81] showed worse outcomes 12 months or more after DRF fixation in patients with DRUJ instability or partial or complete TFCC tears diagnosed arthroscopically but treated with immobilization rather than fixation. Therefore, our practice is to address DRUJ instability at the time of DRF fixation. We do this by first checking our reduction to ensure that we have adequately restored radial length and corrected radial translation of the distal fragment. To do so, it is essential to check for DRUJ stability after securing a volar locking plate proximally with the oblong hole but before drilling the other holes of the proximal plate. If this is done and DRUJ instability remains, the surgeon may loosen the proximal fixation, apply traction and radially directed force to the proximal radial diaphysis, and resecure the fixation. Some investigators even report that overdistracting of the radius relative to the ulna improved DRUJ stability.[82] If this does not restore DRUJ stability, then special attention should be paid to the dorsal ulnar corner fragment of the DRF to ensure that it is reduced and fixated. Fragment-specific fixation of this fragment may be necessary using pins, a screw, or a plate.[77]

If instability remains following these maneuvers, it may be necessary to address an associated ulnar styloid fracture. Most ulnar styloid fractures do not require fixation, and association of ulnar styloid fractures and TFCC injury has not been

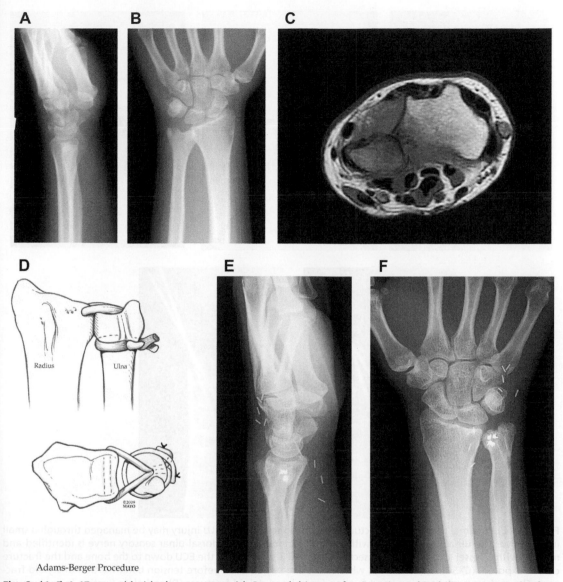

Fig. 6. (A–F) A 17-year-old girl who presents with 3-month history of wrist pain and inability to rotate the forearm. (A) AP radiograph shows overlapping of the radius and ulna. (B) The original lateral radiograph is of poor quality and may have resulted in delay in diagnosis by primary physician; however, (C) MRI showed palmar dislocation of the ulna in relation to the radius. (D) The Adams-Berger procedure was used for reconstruction of the DRUJ in the setting of chronic dislocation (Used with permission of Mayo Foundation for Medical Education and Research, all rights reserved). (E, F) ten-year results with preservation of reduction and excellent motion and pain relief.

established.[80,83] However, nonunion and malunion of the ulnar styloid have been associated with poor outcomes.[84,85] Several investigators have shown that large fragments, especially those displaced 2 mm or more, are associated with disruption of the foveal insertion of the radioulnar ligaments.[37–39] Therefore, the authors acutely repair all large ulnar styloid fragments, especially those associated with DRUJ instability. This repair

is most easily achieved through a 2-cm to 3-cm incision made directly over the ulnar styloid. The TFCC is secured to the fovea using a suture anchor through this incision and the styloid fragment can be repaired with a Kirschner wire (K-wire) and tension band[9,86] (Fig. 7). If there is not an ulnar styloid fragment requiring fixation, the authors prefer to perform an arthroscopy of the radiocarpal joint, assess for TFCC injury, and repair that as indicated.

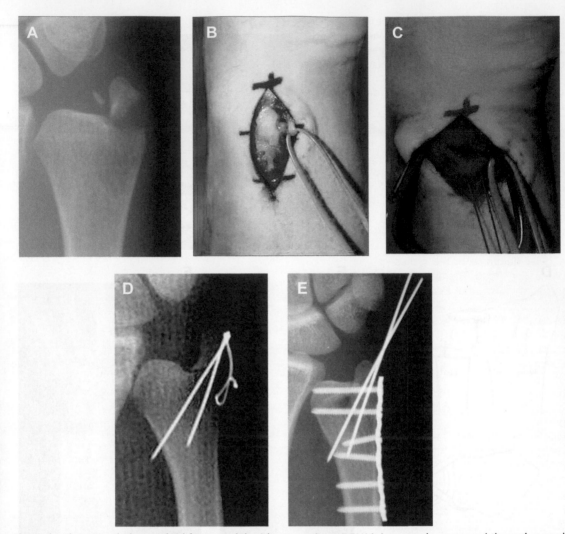

Fig. 7. (*A–E*) Proximal ulnar styloid fractures (*A*) with concomitant DRUJ injury may be managed through a small incision over the ulnar styloid in line with the ECU tendon. (*B*) The dorsal ulnar sensory nerve is identified and marked with a vessel loop and then dissection is carried just palmar to the ECU down to the bone and the fracture can be exposed. (*C*) Suture placement, which is used to secure TFCC before tension band fixation of styloid fracture. The authors prefer tension band fixation for isolated styloid fractures (*D*) and plate fixation in conjunction with tension band (*E*) for ulnar head or metaphyseal fractures with concomitant ulnar styloid fractures.

Distal Ulnar Fractures and Distal Radioulnar Joint Instability

Isolated fractures of the distal ulna are rare but can be a cause of DRUJ instability.[87–89] Fractures of the ulnar head and neck associated with DRFs have been shown to have increased complications relative to fractures isolated to the radius and ulnar styloid.[90–92] Following stable locked fixation of DRFs, many ulnar head and neck fractures are stable and can be managed with immobilization in a Munster-type splint or cast.[88,93] However, stability should be checked with fluoroscopy following DRF fixation. Unstable, comminuted, or displaced

fractures likely benefit from surgical treatment. Operative fixation can be achieved with percutaneous K-wire fixation in young, nonosteoporotic patients without comminution. Open reduction and internal fixation (ORIF) provides more secure fixation and the option for earlier motion but is often challenging because fragments of the distal ulna are often small and osteoporotic (see **Fig. 7**). Plates need to be low profile and carefully positioned to avoid irritating the dorsal cutaneous branch of the ulnar nerve and mechanically interfering with DRUJ rotation, respectively. ORIF is achieved with a condylar plate or locking 2.0-mm plate, and good results have been reported with both.[93,94] Associated styloid fractures or foveal avulsions should be repaired at the same time. The most important step for obtaining a reduced ulna is properly reducing an associated DRF.

Galeazzi Fractures and Distal Radioulnar Joint Instability

A Galeazzi fracture is a diaphyseal fracture of the radius, occurring at least 4 to 5 cm proximal to the radiocarpal joint with an associated DRUJ dislocation[95] (see Fig. 3A). These fractures are described in detail Rohit Garg and Chaitanya Mudgal's article, "Galeazzi Injuries," elsewhere in this issue. Briefly, this is a high-energy trauma that is thought to occur with hyperextension and pronation.[36,96] Galeazzi fractures typically present with angular deformity of the radius and prominence of the ulnar head. The ulnar head sometimes protrudes through the skin as an open fracture-dislocation. Radial fractures within 7.5 cm of the midarticular surface are more likely to involve injury to the DRUJ.[96] Clues to DRUJ instability mirror those of DRF: ulnar styloid base fracture, DRUJ widening on true AP radiographs, dislocation of the ulna on true lateral radiographs, and greater than 5 mm of radial shortening.

This fracture requires ORIF because it is unstable and immobilization alone has been associated with poor outcomes.[97–100] Galeazzi fractures, like DRFs, are often fixed with a volar plate through a modified Henry incision in the forearm. As with DRFs, reduction of the DRUJ and its stability should be checked following reduction and stable fixation of the radius. If the DRUJ is unstable, the surgeon should repair an ulnar styloid fragment, the TFCC, or both.

Like acute DRUJ dislocation, Galeazzi fractures have been classified as simple or complex[49,54–57] because of interposition of soft tissues, most commonly the ECU tendon.[101–103] If unable to reduce the DRUJ following radial fracture fixation and a mushy feeling is encountered, proceed to an open, or arthroscopically assisted, reduction of the DRUJ.[104]

Essex-Lopresti Fractures and Distal Radioulnar Joint Instability

As mentioned earlier, but frequently forgotten, pronation and supination of the forearm occur through 2 joints that function as 1, the DRUJ and PRUJ.[105] Essex-Lopresti[106] described 2 cases of radial head fracture in combination with DRUJ dislocation in 1951. This injury pattern is the reason why the elbow should always be examined along with the wrist when assessing wrist injuries. Clinicians should specifically assess for elbow stability and associated coronoid fracture or a medial collateral ligament injury.

The Essex-Lopresti injury is described in detail elsewhere in this issue, and includes disruption of the DRUJ, the IOM, and the PRUJ because of axial compression that causes longitudinal radioulnar disruption. Radial head excision in the case of Essex-Lopresti injury results in proximal migration of the radius, ulnar impingement of the carpus, and radial impingement of the capitellum.[107–109] The radius pull test is a useful maneuver to assess for Essex-Lopresti injury, in which the radius is pulled proximally while imaging the DRUJ with fluoroscopy. Proximal migration of the radius suggests Essex-Lopresti injury.[110] Timely diagnosis of this injury is important because delayed management is associated with worse outcomes.[111,112] Following stabilization of the forearm, the DRUJ should be assessed for stability. If the DRUJ remains unstable, the surgeon should then repair the TFCC arthroscopically, or open, in addition to addressing the other sites of instability.[113–120]

SUMMARY

Pronation and supination (axial rotation) occur through both the PRUJ and DRUJ, which function as 1 unit. Instability of the DRUJ acutely may occur in the setting of injury to the TFCC and may be associated with fractures of the distal radius and ulna. Furthermore, clinicians should be cognizant of the possibility of concomitant injury to the forearm axis, including the elbow. Thus it is important to examine not only the wrist but also the forearm and elbow when presented with patients with acute distal radioulnar instability.

DISCLOSURE

The authors have nothing to disclose.

REFERENCES

1. Ray RD, Johnson RJ, Jameson RM. Rotation of the forearm; an experimental study of pronation and supination. J Bone Joint Surg Am 1951;33-A(4): 993–6.
2. Linscheid RL. Biomechanics of the distal radioulnar joint. Clin Orthop Relat Res 1992;(275):46–55.
3. Houdek MT, Wagner ER, Moran SL, et al. Disorders of the distal radioulnar joint. Plast Reconstr Surg 2015;135(1):161–72.
4. Epner RA, Bowers WH, Guilford WB. Ulnar variance–the effect of wrist positioning and roentgen filming technique. J Hand Surg 1982;7(3):298–305.
5. Palmer AK, Werner FW. Biomechanics of the distal radioulnar joint. Clin Orthop Relat Res 1984;187: 26–35.

6. Drobner WS, Hausman MR. The distal radioulnar joint. Hand Clin 1992;8(4):631–44.

7. Stuart PR, Berger RA, Linscheid RL, et al. The dorsopalmar stability of the distal radioulnar joint. J Hand Surg Am 2000;25(4):689–99.

8. Tolat AR, Stanley JK, Trail IA. A cadaveric study of the anatomy and stability of the distal radioulnar joint in the coronal and transverse planes. J Hand Surg Br 1996;21(5):587–94.

9. Tham SK, Bain GI. Sigmoid notch osseous reconstruction. Tech Hand Up Extrem Surg 2007;11(1):93–7.

10. Palmer AK, Werner FW. The triangular fibrocartilage complex of the wrist–anatomy and function. J Hand Surg Am 1981;6(2):153–62.

11. Hagert E, Chim H, Moran SL. Anatomy of the distal radioulnar joint. In: JA G, editor. Ulnar sided wrist pain: a master skills publication. Rosemont (IL): American Society for Surgery of the Hand; 2013. p. 11–22.

12. Hagert CG. Distal radius fracture and the distal radioulnar joint–anatomical considerations. Handchir Mikrochir Plast Chir 1994;26(1):22–6.

13. Kleinman WB. Stability of the distal radioulna joint: biomechanics, pathophysiology, physical diagnosis, and restoration of function what we have learned in 25 years. J Hand Surg Am 2007;32(7):1086–106.

14. Xu J, Tang JB. In vivo changes in lengths of the ligaments stabilizing the distal radioulnar joint. J Hand Surg Am 2009;34(1):40–5.

15. af Ekenstam F. Anatomy of the distal radioulnar joint. Clin Orthop Relat Res 1992;(275):14–8.

16. Schuind F, An KN, Berglund L, et al. The distal radioulnar ligaments: a biomechanical study. J Hand Surg Am 1991;16(6):1106–14.

17. Kihara H, Short WH, Werner FW, et al. The stabilizing mechanism of the distal radioulnar joint during pronation and supination. J Hand Surg Am 1995;20(6):930–6.

18. Rose-Innes AP. Anterior dislocation of the ulna at the inferior radio-ulnar joint. Case report, with a discussion of the anatomy of rotation of the forearm. J Bone Joint Surg Br 1960;42-B:515–21.

19. Hui FC, Linscheid RL. Ulnotriquetral augmentation tenodesis: a reconstructive procedure for dorsal subluxation of the distal radioulnar joint. J Hand Surg 1982;7(3):230–6.

20. Buterbaugh GA, Palmer AK. Fractures and dislocations of the distal radioulnar joint. Hand Clin 1988;4(3):361–75.

21. Johnson RK, Shrewsbury MM. The pronator quadratus in motions and in stabilization of the radius and ulna at the distal radioulnar joint. J Hand Surg 1976;1(3):205–9.

22. Stuart PR. Pronator quadratus revisited. J Hand Surg Br 1996;21(6):714–22.

23. Moritomo H, Noda K, Goto A, et al. Interosseous membrane of the forearm: length change of ligaments during forearm rotation. J Hand Surg 2009;34(4):685–91.

24. Noda K, Goto A, Murase T, et al. Interosseous membrane of the forearm: an anatomical study of ligament attachment locations. J Hand Surg 2009;34(3):415–22.

25. Watanabe H, Berger RA, Berglund LJ, et al. Contribution of the interosseous membrane to distal radioulnar joint constraint. J Hand Surg Am 2005;30(6):1164–71.

26. Hohenberger GM, Schwarz AM, Weiglein AH, et al. Prevalence of the distal oblique bundle of the interosseous membrane of the forearm: an anatomical study. J Hand Surg Eur Vol 2018;43(4):426–30.

27. Trehan SK, Gould HP, Meyers KN, et al. The effect of distal radius fracture location on distal radioulnar joint stability: a cadaveric study. J Hand Surg 2019;44(6):473–9.

28. Kim YH, Gong HS, Park JW, et al. Magnetic resonance imaging evaluation of the distal oblique bundle in the distal interosseous membrane of the forearm. BMC Musculoskelet Disord 2017;18(1):47.

29. Dy CJ, Jang E, Taylor SA, et al. The impact of coronal alignment on distal radioulnar joint stability following distal radius fracture. J Hand Surg 2014;39(7):1264–72.

30. Arimitsu S, Moritomo H, Kitamura T, et al. The stabilizing effect of the distal interosseous membrane on the distal radioulnar joint in an ulnar shortening procedure: a biomechanical study. J Bone Joint Surg Am 2011;93(21):2022–30.

31. Rampazzo A, Gharb BB, Brock G, et al. Functional outcomes of the aptis-scheker distal radioulnar joint replacement in patients under 40 years old. J Hand Surg 2015;40(7):1397–403.e3.

32. Bellevue KD, Thayer MK, Pouliot M, et al. Complications of semiconstrained distal radioulnar joint arthroplasty. J Hand Surg 2018;43(6):566.e1-e9.

33. Ruch DS, Weiland AJ, Wolfe SW, et al. Current concepts in the treatment of distal radial fractures. Instr Course Lect 2004;53:389–401.

34. Adams BD. Effects of radial deformity on distal radioulnar joint mechanics. J Hand Surg Am 1993;18:492–8.

35. Moore TM, Klein JP, Patzakis MJ, et al. Results of compression-plating of closed Galeazzi fractures. J Bone Joint Surg Am 1985;67(7):1015–21.

36. Giannoulis FS, Sotereanos DG. Galeazzi fractures and dislocations. Hand Clin 2007;23(2):153–63, v.

37. Mikic ZD. Treatment of acute injuries of the triangular fibrocartilage complex associated with distal radioulnar joint instability. J Hand Surg Am 1995;20(2):319–23.

38. Nakamura R, Horii E, Imaeda T, et al. Ulnar styloid malunion with dislocation of the distal radioulnar joint. J Hand Surg Br 1998;23(2):173–5.

39. May MM, Lawton JN, Blazar PE. Ulnar styloid fractures associated with distal radius fractures: incidence and implications for distal radioulnar joint instability. J Hand Surg Am 2002;27(6): 965–71.

40. Park MJ, Kim JP. Reliability and normal values of various computed tomography methods for quantifying distal radioulnar joint translation. J Bone Joint Surg Am 2008;90(1):145–53.

41. Mino DE, Palmer AK, Levinsohn EM. The role of radiography and computerized tomography in the diagnosis of subluxation and dislocation of the distal radioulnar joint. J Hand Surg 1983;8(1): 23–31.

42. Amrami KK, Moran SL, Berger RA, et al. Imaging the distal radioulnar joint. Hand Clin 2010;26(4): 467–75.

43. Coggins CA. Imaging of ulnar-sided wrist pain. Clin Sports Med 2006;25(3):505–26.

44. Carlsen BT, Dennison DG, Moran SL. Acute dislocations of the distal radioulnar joint and distal ulna fractures. Hand Clin 2010;26(4):503–16.

45. Gil JA, Kosinski LR, Shah KN, et al. Distal radioulnar joint instability: assessment of three intraoperative radiographic stress tests. Hand (N Y) 2019. https://doi.org/10.1177/1558944719875487. 1558944719875487.

46. Park A, Lutsky K, Matzon J, et al. An evaluation of the reliability of wrist arthroscopy in the assessment of tears of the triangular fibrocartilage complex. J Hand Surg 2018;43(6):545–9.

47. Brogan DM, Berger RA, Kakar S. Ulnar-sided wrist pain: a critical analysis review. JBJS Rev 2019;7(5):e1.

48. Ochman S, Wieskotter B, Langer M, et al. High-resolution MRI (3T-MRI) in diagnosis of wrist pain: is diagnostic arthroscopy still necessary? Arch Orthop Trauma Surg 2017;137(10):1443–50.

49. Bruckner JD, Lichtman DM, Alexander AH. Complex dislocations of the distal radioulnar joint. Recognition and management. Clin Orthop Relat Res 1992;(275):90–103.

50. Heiple KG, Freehafer AA, Van'T Hof A. Isolated traumatic dislocation of the distal end of the ulna or distal radio-ulnar joint. J Bone Joint Surg Am 1962;44-A:1387–94.

51. Hagert CG. The distal radioulnar joint. Hand Clin 1987;3(1):41–50.

52. Hagert CG. The distal radioulnar joint in relation to the whole forearm. Clin Orthop Relat Res 1992;(275):56–64.

53. Bruckner JD, Alexander AH, Lichtman DM. Acute dislocations of the distal radioulnar joint. Instr Course Lect 1996;45:27–36.

54. Cetti NE. An unusual cause of blocked reduction of the Galeazzi injury. Injury 1977;9(1):59–61.

55. Alexander A, Lichtman DM. Treatment of acute injuries of the distal radioulnar joint. In: Lichtman D, Alexander AH, editors. The wrist and its disorders. Philadelphia: WB Saunders; 1997.

56. Jenkins NH, Mintowt-Czyz WJ, Fairclough JA. Irreducible dislocation of the distal radioulnar joint. Injury 1987;18(1):40–3.

57. Hanel DP, Scheid DK. Irreducible fracture-dislocation of the distal radioulnar joint secondary to entrapment of the extensor carpi ulnaris tendon. Clin Orthop Relat Res 1988;(234):56–60.

58. Garrigues GE, Aldridge JM 3rd. Acute irreducible distal radioulnar joint dislocation. A case report. J Bone Joint Surg Am 2007;89(7):1594–7.

59. Park MJ, Pappas N, Steinberg DR, et al. Immobilization in supination versus neutral following surgical treatment of Galeazzi fracture-dislocations in adults: case series. J Hand Surg 2012;37(3): 528–31.

60. Henry MH. Management of acute triangular fibrocartilage complex injury of the wrist. J Am Acad Orthop Surg 2008;16(6):320–9.

61. Palmer AK. Triangular fibrocartilage complex lesions: A classification. J Hand Surg Am 1989; 14A:594–606.

62. Hohenberger GM, Maier MJ, Dolcet C, et al. Sensory nerve supply of the distal radio-ulnar joint with regard to wrist denervation. J Hand Surg Eur volume 2017;42(6):586–91.

63. Kakar S, Noureldin M, Elhassan B. Ulnar head replacement and sigmoid notch resurfacing arthroplasty with a lateral meniscal allograft: 'calamari procedure. J Hand Surg Eur volume 2017;42(6): 567–72.

64. Clark NJ, Munaretto N, Elhassan BT, et al. Ulnar head replacement and sigmoid notch resurfacing arthroplasty with minimum 12-month follow-up. J Hand Surg Eur volume 2019;44(9):957–62.

65. Savvidou C, Murphy E, Mailhot E, et al. Semiconstrained distal radioulnar joint prosthesis. J Wrist Surg 2013;2(1):41–8.

66. Kachooei AR, Chase SM, Jupiter JB. Outcome assessment after aptis distal radioulnar joint (DRUJ) implant arthroplasty. Arch Bone Jt Surg 2014;2(3):180–4.

67. Jochen-Frederick H, Pouyan Y, Khosrow BA, et al. Long-term functional outcome and patient satisfaction after ulnar head resection. J Plast Reconstr Aesthet Surg 2016;69(10):1417–23.

68. Faucher GK, Zimmerman RM, Zimmerman NB. Instability and arthritis of the distal radioulnar joint: a critical analysis review. JBJS Rev 2016;4(12). 01874474.

69. Argintar E, Mantovani G, Pavan A. TFCC reattachment after traumatic DRUJ instability: a simple

alternative to arthroscopic management. Tech Hand Up Extrem Surg 2010;14(4):226–9.

70. Atzei A, Luchetti R, Braidotti F. Arthroscopic foveal repair of the triangular fibrocartilage complex. J Wrist Surg 2015;4(1):22–30.

71. Anderson ML, Larson AN, Moran SL, et al. Clinical comparison of arthroscopic versus open repair of triangular fibrocartilage complex tears. J Hand Surg Am 2008;33(5):675–82.

72. Kakar S, Carlsen BT, Moran SL, et al. The management of chronic distal radioulnar instability. Hand Clin 2010;26(4):517–28.

73. Gillis JA, Soreide E, Khouri JS, et al. Outcomes of the Adams-Berger ligament reconstruction for the distal radioulnar joint instability in 95 consecutive cases. J Wrist Surg 2019;8(4):268–75.

74. Adams BD, Berger RA. An anatomic reconstruction of the distal radioulnar ligaments for posttraumatic distal radioulnar joint instability. J Hand Surg 2002; 27(2):243–51.

75. Geissler WB, Fernandez DL, Lamey DM. Distal radioulnar joint injuries associated with fractures of the distal radius. Clin Orthop Relat Res 1996;(327):135–46.

76. Lindau T, Arner M, Hagberg L. Intraarticular lesions in distal fractures of the radius in young adults. A descriptive arthroscopic study in 50 patients. J Hand Surg Br 1997;22(5):638–43.

77. Rhee PC, Medoff RJ, Shin AY. Complex distal radius fractures: an anatomic algorithm for surgical management. J Am Acad Orthop Surg 2017;25(2):77–88.

78. Medoff RJ. Essential radiographic evaluation for distal radius fractures. Hand Clin 2005;21(3): 279–88.

79. Carlsen B, Rizzo M, Moran S. Soft-tissue injuries associated with distal radius fractures. Oper Tech Orthop 2009;19(2):107–18.

80. Lindau T, Adlercreutz C, Aspenberg P. Peripheral tears of the triangular fibrocartilage complex cause distal radioulnar joint instability after distal radial fractures. J Hand Surg Am 2000;25(3):464–8.

81. Lindau T, Hagberg L, Adlercreutz C, et al. Distal radioulnar instability is an independent worsening factor in distal radial fractures. Clin Orthop Relat Res 2000;376:229–35.

82. Wang JP, Huang HK, Fufa D. Radial distraction to stabilize distal radioulnar joint in distal radius fixation. J Hand Surg 2018;43(5):493.e1-4.

83. Richards RS, Bennett JD, Roth JH, et al. Arthroscopic diagnosis of intra-articular soft tissue injuries associated with distal radial fractures. J Hand Surg Am 1997;22(5):772–6.

84. Knirk JL, Jupiter JB. Intra-articular fractures of the distal end of the radius in young adults. J Bone Joint Surg Am 1986;68(5):647–59.

85. af Ekenstam F, Jakobsson OP, Wadin K. Repair of the triangular ligament in Colles' fracture. No effect in a prospective randomized study. Acta Orthop Scand 1989;60(4):393–6.

86. Chen AC, Chiu CH, Weng CJ, et al. Early and late fixation of ulnar styloid base fractures yields different outcomes. J Orthop Surg Res 2018;13(1):193.

87. Richards TA, Deal DN. Distal ulna fractures. J Hand Surg 2014;39(2):385–91.

88. Moloney M, Farnebo S, Adolfsson L. Incidence of distal ulna fractures in a Swedish county: 74/ 100,000 person-years, most of them treated non-operatively. Acta Orthop 2020;91(1):104–8.

89. Ciminero M, Yohe N, Garofolo-Gonzalez G, et al. Isolated distal ulna fracture with distal radioulnar joint dislocation: a novel fracture pattern. Hand (N Y) 2019. https://doi.org/10.1177/1558944719856116. 1558944719856116.

90. Lafontaine M, Hardy D, Delince P. Stability assessment of distal radius fractures. Injury 1989;20(4):208–10.

91. Biyani A, Simison AJ, Klenerman L. Fractures of the distal radius and ulna. J Hand Surg Br 1995;20(3): 357–64.

92. McKee MD, Waddell JP, Yoo D, et al. Nonunion of distal radial fractures associated with distal ulnar shaft fractures: a report of four cases. J Orthop Trauma 1997;11(1):49–53.

93. Dennison DG. Open reduction and internal locked fixation of unstable distal ulna fractures with concomitant distal radius fracture. J Hand Surg 2007;32(6):801–5.

94. Ring D, McCarty LP, Campbell D, et al. Condylar blade plate fixation of unstable fractures of the distal ulna associated with fracture of the distal radius. J Hand Surg 2004;29(1):103–9.

95. Faierman E, Jupiter JB. The management of acute fractures involving the distal radio-ulnar joint and distal ulna. Hand Clin 1998;(14):213–29.

96. Rettig ME, Raskin KB. Galeazzi fracture-dislocation: a new treatment-oriented classification. J Hand Surg Am 2001;26(2):228–35.

97. Anderson LD, Meyer FN. Fractures of the shafts of the radius and ulna. In: Rockwood CA, Green DP, editors. Fractures in adults. 3rd edition. Philadelphia: JB Lippincott Co; 1991. p. 728.

98. Hughston JC. Fracture of the distal radial shaft. Mistakes in management. J Bone Joint Surg Am 1957;39:249–64.

99. Mikic ZDJ. Galeazzi fracture-dislocations. J Bone Joint Surg 1975;57A:1071–80.

100. Reckling FW. Unstable fracture-dislocations of the forearm (Montaggia and Galeazzi lesions). J Bone Joint Surg Am 1982;64:857–63.

101. Paley D, Rubenstein J, McMurtry RY. Irreducible dislocation of distal radial ulnar joint. Orthop Rev 1986;15(4):228–31.

102. Itoh Y, Horiuchi Y, Takahashi M, et al. Extensor tendon involvement in Smith's and Galeazzi's fractures. J Hand Surg 1987;12(4):535–40.

103. Yohe NJ, De Tolla J, Kaye MB, et al. Irreducible Galeazzi Fracture-Dislocations. Hand (N Y) 2019; 14(2):249–52.

104. Iwamae M, Yano K, Kaneshiro Y, et al. Arthroscopic reduction of an irreducible distal radioulnar joint in Galeazzi fracture-dislocation due to a fragment of the ulnar styloid: a case report. BMC Musculoskelet Disord 2019;20(1):354.

105. Elzinga K, Chung K. Evolution of the ring concept for the forearm and its implication on treatment: from galeazzi, monteggia, essex-lopresti, and darrach to the current era. J Hand Surg Asian Pac Vol 2019;24(3):251–7.

106. Essex-Lopresti P. Fractures of the radial head with distal radio-ulnar dislocation; report of two cases. J Bone Joint Surg Br 1951;33B(2):244–7.

107. Shepard MF, Markolf KL, Dunbar AM. Effects of radial head excision and distal radial shortening on load-sharing in cadaver forearms. J Bone Joint Surg Am 2001;83(1):92–100.

108. Shepard MF, Markolf KL, Dunbar AM. The effects of partial and total interosseous membrane transection on load sharing in the cadaver forearm. J Orthop Res 2001;19(4):587–92.

109. Taylor TK, O'Connor BT. The Effect Upon the Inferior Radio-Ulnar Joint of Excision of the Head of the Radius in Adults. J Bone Joint Surg Br 1964; 46:83–8.

110. Smith AM, Urbanosky LR, Castle JA, et al. Radius pull test: predictor of longitudinal forearm instability. J Bone Joint Surg Am 2002;84-A(11):1970–6.

111. Trousdale RT, Amadio PC, Cooney WP, et al. Radioulnar dissociation. A review of twenty cases. J Bone Joint Surg Am 1992;74(10):1486–97.

112. Schnetzke M, Porschke F, Hoppe K, et al. Outcome of early and late diagnosed essex-lopresti injury. J Bone Joint Surg Am 2017;99(12):1043–50.

113. Moro JK, Werier J, MacDermid JC, et al. Arthroplasty with a metal radial head for unreconstructible fractures of the radial head. J Bone Joint Surg Am 2001;83-A(8):1201–11.

114. Edwards GS Jr, Jupiter JB. Radial head fractures with acute distal radioulnar dislocation. Essex-Lopresti revisited. Clin Orthop Relat Res 1988; 234:61–9.

115. Gaspar MP, Adams JE, Zohn RC, et al. Late reconstruction of the interosseous membrane with bone-patellar tendon-bone graft for chronic essex-lopresti injuries: outcomes with a mean follow-up of over 10 years. J Bone Joint Surg Am 2018; 100(5):416–27.

116. Masouros PT, Apergis EP, Babis GC, et al. Essex-Lopresti injuries: an update. EFORT Open Rev 2019;4(4):143–50.

117. Kam CC, Jones CM, Fennema JL, et al. Suture-button construct for interosseous ligament reconstruction in longitudinal radioulnar dissociations: a biomechanical study. J Hand Surg 2010;35(10): 1626–32.

118. Gaspar MP, Kearns KA, Culp RW, et al. Single-versus double-bundle suture button reconstruction of the forearm interosseous membrane for the chronic Essex-Lopresti lesion. Eur J Orthop Surg Traumatol 2018;28(3):409–13.

119. Hackl M, Andermahr J, Staat M, et al. Suture button reconstruction of the central band of the interosseous membrane in Essex-Lopresti lesions: a comparative biomechanical investigation. J Hand Surg Eur volume 2017;42(4):370–6.

120. de Vries EN, Walenkamp MM, Mulders MA, et al. Minimally invasive stabilization of the distal radioulnar joint: a cadaveric study. J Hand Surg Eur volume 2017;42(4):363–9.

Chronic Distal Radioulnar Joint Instability

Logan W. Carr, MD*, Brian Adams, MD

KEYWORDS

- Distal radioulnar joint • Chronic DRUJ instability • DRUJ ligament reconstruction

KEY POINTS

- The ligaments and surrounding muscles and tendons are the principal stabilizers of the distal radio-ulnar joint (DRUJ), with the radioulnar ligaments being the most important.
- DRUJ instability often results from osseous injuries that alter forearm and wrist alignment and that also compromise the actions of the ligaments.
- Imaging modalities are helpful in assessing DRUJ instability; however, a thorough history and physical examination is the foundation for the diagnosis.
- DRUJ ligament reconstruction is indicated when the native ligaments are not reparable, but it is contraindicated in the presence of radius or ulna bony deformity or arthritis of the DRUJ.
- Many DRUJ ligament reconstructive techniques have been described; however, a technique that closely mimics normal anatomy is usually preferred.

INTRODUCTION

Distal radioulnar joint (DRUJ) instability can be described as acute or chronic, and as dorsal, volar, or multidirectional. Instability can occur in isolation or concomitantly with osseous trauma, resulting from dislocations, fractures, ligament injuries, or malunions. Triangular fibrocartilage complex (TFCC) tears, extensor carpi ulnaris (ECU) tendonitis, lunotriquetral ligament tears, or ulnocarpal abutment can occur simultaneously. Untreated instability alters wrist and forearm kinematics, leading to pain, weakness, and possibly degenerative arthritis.

DRUJ instability is typically defined by increased translation of the ulna relative to the radius compared with the contralateral wrist. Although dorsal subluxation of the ulna is more commonly unstable, volar or bidirectional subluxation can cause greater symptoms, especially during lifting and heavy loading. Understanding, accurately diagnosing, and properly treating DRUJ instability requires a comprehensive understanding of the bony and soft tissue anatomy.

ANATOMY

There are key anatomic features of the DRUJ that are important in effectively treating chronic instability. The sigmoid notch is shallow and has a much greater radius of curvature than the ulnar head, resulting in both rotational and translational motion and natural laxity.[1,2] In full supination, there is only a few millimeters (10%) of articular surface contact.[1] There is substantial individual variation in the shape of the sigmoid notch. Tolat and colleagues[3] defined 4 morphologic notch types: flat (42%), C type (30%), ski slope (14%), and S type (14%) (**Fig. 1**). A fibrocartilaginous labrum, which augments the bony rims, was also described.[3] A cadaveric study found the joint geometry provided about 20% of the DRUJ stability, leaving the surrounding soft tissues responsible for the remainder.[4] Thus, a flat or damaged sigmoid notch

Department of Orthopedic Surgery, Baylor College of Medicine, 7200 Cambridge, Suite 10A, Houston, TX 77044, USA
* Corresponding author.
E-mail address: Lcarr61350@gmail.com

Hand Clin 36 (2020) 443–453
https://doi.org/10.1016/j.hcl.2020.07.004
0749-0712/20/© 2020 Elsevier Inc. All rights reserved.

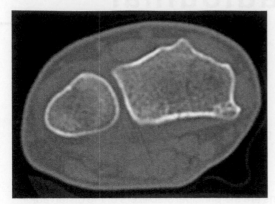

Fig. 1. Flat sigmoid notch.

causes added mechanical disadvantage to joint stability and greater reliance on the ligaments, which may indicate the need for augmentation with a concurrent osseous procedure.

The TFCC comprises the radioulnar ligaments, articular disc, meniscus homolog, ulnocarpal ligaments, and the ECU subsheath (**Fig. 2**). In addition to its ligamentous function, it also transmits load between the carpus and the forearm. In neutral forearm and wrist position, the avascular, central articular disc carries 16% of axial wrist loads.[1] Ulnar deviation causes additional load through the articular disk and ulnar head. When the radius further shortens in pronation, even greater load is transmitted through the ulnocarpal joint.[5] Although the central disk is avascular, the periphery and fovea are well vascularized.[6] Because of these mechanical features, an acquired or developmental positive ulnar variance places additional load across the ulnocarpal joint that may substantially compromise any ligament reconstructive procedure.

DRUJ stabilizers can be described as extrinsic or intrinsic in relation to its capsule. Extrinsic stability is provided dynamically by the ECU tendon and pronator quadratus, whereas the distal interosseous membrane (DIOM) and ECU subsheath provide static constraint.[7] The DIOM has a thickened band, known as the distal oblique band (DOB), which travels obliquely from the ulnar shaft to the distal radius.[8] The presence of a distal DOB results in a significantly more stable DRUJ if the TFCC is torn.[8,9] The importance of each structure to DRUJ stability was demonstrated in a study showing continued near-normal kinematics after dividing the radioulnar ligaments and preserving the remaining soft tissue constraints.[10] Thus, reconstructive procedures should aim to preserve all uninjured structures to maximize the outcome.

Although multiple structures contribute to DRUJ stability, the stout radioulnar ligaments, which comprise the volar and dorsal margins of the TFCC, are the most important.[11] Each radioulnar ligament includes a superficial and deep component (**Fig. 3**). The deep fibers (ligamentum subcruentum) attach to the fovea, through which the axis of forearm motion passes. The deep fibers have an obtuse approach to the fovea, whereas the superficial fibers take a more direct course to the ulnar styloid base. In maximum supination, the dorsal deep fibers and volar superficial fibers become taught and resist dorsal subluxation of the ulna, whereas the opposite tensions occur in these fibers in full pronation. At the extremes of

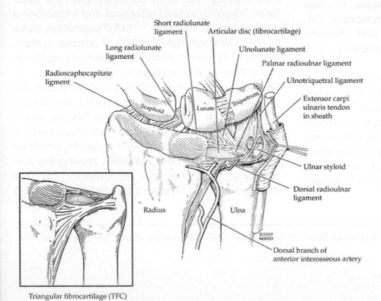

Fig. 2. Anatomy of the TFCC and soft tissue–stabilizing structure. (*From* Carlsen BT, Rizzo M, Moran SL. Soft-Tissue Injuries Associated With Distal Radius Fractures. Operative Techniques in Orthopaedics. 2009 Apr;19(2):107-118; with permission.)

Short radiolunate ligament
Long radiolunate ligament
Radioscaphocapitate ligment
Articular disc (fibrocartilage)
Ulnolunate ligament
Palmar radioulnar ligament
Ulnotriquetral ligament
Extensor carpi ulnaris tendon in sheath
Scaphoid
Lunate
Triquetrum
Ulnar styloid
Dorsal radioulnar ligament
Radius
Ulna
Dorsal branch of anterior interosseous artery
Triangular fibrocartilage (TFC)

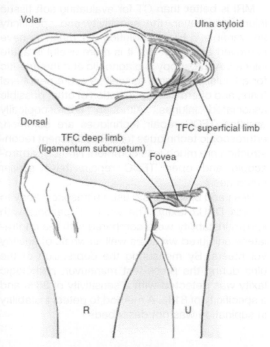

Fig. 3. Radioulnar ligaments of the TFCC. R, radius; U, ulna. (*From* Adams B: Distal radioulnar joint. In Trumble TE, ed: Hand surgery update 3: Hand, elbow, and shoulder, Rosemont, IL, 2003, American Society for Surgery of the Hand, p.147–157; with permission.)

pronation and supination, the superficial radioulnar fibers are less effective than the deep fibers.[12] The anatomic and mechanical importance of the fovea should be recognized in the design and surgical precision of a ligament reconstruction.

CAUSES OF INSTABILITY

Instability can result from seemingly minor injuries in individuals with generalized ligament laxity caused by connective tissue aberrancy or inflammatory arthritis. Inherent laxity caused by hypermobility or sigmoid notch anatomy requires special consideration because reconstructive outcomes are less predictable.[13] The most common causes of acquired instability are missed diagnosis or failed treatment of an injury. An isolated TFCC tear caused by a rotatory force or a fall on the outstretched hand is often initially diagnosed as a simple wrist sprain, but, if inadequately treated, can result in instability if the secondary restraints are also sprained.

A variety of extra-articular and intra-articular fractures of the distal radius can result in DRUJ instability. Both dorsal and volar fractures of the lunate facet can cause incongruency of the sigmoid notch.[14,15] Distal radius malunions with metaphyseal deformity can substantially alter sigmoid notch alignment, resulting in subluxation and instability. A malunion with a combination of radius shortening, radial translation, and dorsal angulation is particularly at risk for instability.[16–18] Radial translation has received increased emphasis because it reduces the stabilizing effect of the interosseous membrane and inhibits the radioulnar ligaments from healing to the ulnar fovea.[11,19,20]

Distal third radial shaft fractures with DRUJ injury (Galeazzi) can cause chronic instability, particularly if radius alignment is not anatomically restored. Extensive interosseous membrane tearing, which is commonly the result of an Essex-Lopresti injury, can produce both longitudinal and translational instability.

EVALUATION
Clinical

Diagnosis of DRUJ instability is challenging because the signs and symptoms are often unclear. When instability is suspected, a history of prior trauma should be sought, particularly a fall or twisting event. Although pain at rest and swelling resolve, ulnar-sided wrist pain associated with forearm rotation persists. In severe instability, clunking can occur when the ulna dislocates and reduces. Weakness and avoidance of stressful hand use is common.

On examination, clunking may be visualized during active motion or felt during passive manipulation when the ulna is compressed against the radius during pronation-supination. Resisted pronation and supination is often painful. The piano key sign describes a dorsal resting position of the ulna that translates volar with applied stress.[21,22] Wijffels and colleagues[22] reported a sensitivity of 66% and specificity of 68% for the sign. Volar subluxation produces slight fullness on the volar aspect of the wrist with a corresponding depression dorsally.

Subluxation is more subtle and difficult to detect than frank dislocation, and thus it is imperative to compare findings with the contralateral, normal side, especially because normal laxity differs considerably among individuals. Point tenderness is common over the fovea, known as the fovea sign, which is located between the styloid process and flexor carpi ulnaris tendon.[23] Because this site can be naturally sensitive, tenderness should be compared with the other wrist.

The DRUJ stress test or ballottement test was originally described with the forearm in neutral rotation.[24] Shucking the ulna relative to the radius is painful and/or grossly unstable in symptomatic patients. The test has high specificity (96%), but only moderate sensitivity (59%).[25] Because more laxity is naturally present with the forearm in neutral rotation, accuracy can be improved by also testing in pronation and supination. In addition, the radiocarpal joint should be held stable during the test to eliminate it as a source of translation and pain. This test can be performed with injection of local anesthetic to eliminate guarding.[26]

The press test is performed by having the patient push up with the affected wrist from a seated position using the arm rest, which causes exacerbation of ulnar-sided wrist pain.[27] The test was reported to have a sensitivity of 100% for the diagnosis of TFCC injuries.[22,27] A modification described by Adams[28,29] has the patient remain seated and apply downward force to the examination table located in front of the patient. Comparatively increased depression of the ulnar head on the affected side shows instability. The maneuver may also invoke pain.

Imaging

Importantly, the diagnosis of DRUJ instability is made clinically and corroborated by imaging studies. Standard wrist radiographs may show specific findings, such as joint widening on the posteroanterior (PA) view or displacement of the ulnar head relative to the radius on the lateral view. A radioulnar distance of greater than 6 mm on the PA view suggests instability.[22,30] Although slight degrees of rotation can alter the interpretation of standard radiographs, the dorsal tangential view showed high intraobserver and interobserver reliability in a cadaver study.[31] Furthermore, interpretation was independent of forearm position in identifying dislocation as well as subluxation. Radiographs are also used to identify distal radius malunion, ulnar styloid nonunion, ulnocarpal impaction, and arthrosis.

Computed topography (CT) scanning provides important useful information, including a direct comparison with the other side in multiple joint positions. The forearm is typically scanned in neutral, full supination, and full pronation.[32] There are several described methods to quantify instability: the Mino method, congruency method, epicenter method, and radioulnar ratio method.[33] The Mino and congruency methods have resulted in high false-positive rates, especially in the presence of malunions.[34,35] The epicenter method takes into consideration physiologic translation, making it the most specific and most used.[34,35] Combining this method of measurement with contralateral comparison reduces radiographic overestimation of stability.[36]

MRI is better than CT for evaluating soft tissue injuries; however, the sensitivity and specificity are variable.[12] High-resolution 3-T magnets have improved accuracy, but it is more useful in acute injuries. Arthroscopy is diagnostic and therapeutic for articular disc tears as well as acute peripheral tears, and offers direct evaluation of other possible associated injuries. Although arthroscopically assisted TFCC repair techniques are common, arthroscopic techniques for DRUJ ligament reconstruction are much less common. Notably, arthroscopic and open TFCC repairs have similar outcomes.[37]

Hess and colleagues[38] used ultrasonography to assess DRUJ laxity. The wrists in patients with known instability were compared with the contralateral uninjured wrists as well as wrists of healthy volunteers. By measuring the depression of the ulna during the press-test maneuver, pathologic laxity was detected with a sensitivity of 88% and a specificity of 81%. A method to detect instability in supination was not described.

MANAGEMENT

Although nonsurgical management is less successful in chronic DRUJ instability, it may be appropriate for mild instability in lower-demand patients. An exercise program to strengthen the forearm and wrist is often included in nonoperative management and rehabilitation following surgery. Functional bracing, using one of a variety of flexible braces designed for the DRUJ, helps to limit translation but may also limit motion.[39]

The goal of surgical management is to restore stability while preserving forearm and wrist motion. A successful long-term outcome from ligament repair or reconstruction requires proper bony alignment. A corrective osteotomy of a distal radius malunion will often restore stability and negates the need for a ligament reconstruction. However, reconstruction may still be required if intraoperative testing following bony correction reveals persistent instability. The condition of the TFCC dictates whether a delayed TFCC repair versus a ligament reconstruction using a graft is required. Patients with negative ulnar variance are more likely to have robust TFCCs that are repairable even in chronic tears. MRI can show the thickness of the TFCC and the severity of its retraction from the fovea. A variety of techniques, both arthroscopic and open, can be used to repair the TFCC directly to the fovea. Use of transosseous sutures exiting the ulnar neck is common repair method that provides reliable tension and fixation.

The outcome of a repair or ligament reconstruction is less predictable when the sigmoid notch is flat. Osteoplasty can be performed concomitantly to increase stability (**Fig. 4**). Delayed sigmoid notch osteoplasty may also be considered if the DRUJ remains unstable after a ligament reconstruction.[40] Coexisting ulnar impaction syndrome likely increases the risk of failure of a soft tissue procedure because of the heightened forces the tissues must resist. Thus, prior or concurrent ulnar shortening osteotomy is considered to improve the outcome of the procedure.[41,42]

Arthrosis of the DRUJ is a relative contraindication to radioulnar ligament reconstruction because the procedure is designed to increase the joint contact force, which may exacerbate the arthrosis. Nevertheless, reconstruction may still be attempted in active individuals with arthrosis who are not likely to have a good result from a salvage procedure, particularly because a salvage could be performed later if the reconstruction fails.

SURGICAL PROCEDURES

Ligament reconstructive procedures can be categorized as extra-articular or intra-articular. Extra-articular procedures do not attempt to reconstruct the normal anatomy but create a direct tether between the radius and ulna or indirectly tether the joint using a nearby tenodesis. Intra-articular

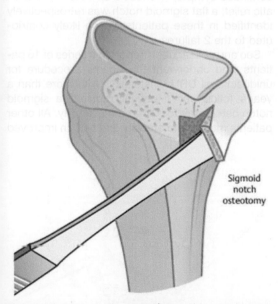

Sigmoid notch osteotomy

Fig. 4. Sigmoid notch osteoplasty: this can be performed through the osseous tunnel, but before the tendon graft is passed. The graft then helps secure the bone graft supporting the osteoplasty. (*From* Neumeister M., Sauerbier M. Problems in Hand Surgery. Thieme NY. 2020; with permission.)

procedures attempt to closely mimic the normal radioulnar ligaments. Although anatomic reconstruction is widely practiced, the procedure is usually more complex and requires intact articular surfaces and bony alignment, whereas nonanatomic procedures can often accommodate bony deformities.

Extra-Articular Reconstruction

Fulkerson and Watson[43] first described a technique to stabilize the ulna against the radius by means of an extra-articular radioulnar tether using a long tendon graft passed through a hole drilled in the radius at the level of the ulnar neck just proximal to the TFCC. The technique is less technically demanding than intra-articular techniques, but its functional outcome and long-term success have not been well established. In a small series of 5 patients with an average of 15 months' follow-up, stability was achieved but produced limitation of pronosupination.[44] The graft also caused circumferential bone resorption of the ulnar neck. The brachioradialis has been used similarly and takes advantage of its normal insertion as a tether point.[45]

In a series of 21 patients, a reconstruction was performed by passing the pronator quadratus around the ulna. Patient function was improved without a significant loss of motion.[46] Although the technique was less technically demanding, postoperative instability in pronation was not corrected.

Techniques have been described to create or reinforce the DOB using a tendon autograft or allograft passed through bone tunnels in the radius and ulna.[47] Securing the graft to the radius and ulna can be difficult.[48] Two of 14 patients had recurrent instability requiring reoperation, and another sustained an ulnar fracture at the bone tunnel.

Hui and Linscheid[49] used a cadaver model to study dorsal DRUJ instability. Sectioning the dorsal radioulnar ligaments produced dorsal instability in pronation, and instability in supination was evident when the ulnocarpal ligaments were sectioned. These findings led to the design of an ulnocarpal sling using a distally based strip of the flexor carpi ulnaris passed dorsally through the pisotriquetral ligament and then dorsally through a bone tunnel at the fovea. The tendon strip is then passed under the ECU tendon and secured back to itself. The technique causes reduced pronation, and biomechanical studies showed it to be less effective than other techniques.[21]

Using a similar concept to Hui and Linscheid,[49] a capsulorrhaphy technique using part of the extensor retinaculum was described. The technique was originally used to improve the stability of an ulnar head implant.[50,51] An ulnar-based extensor retinaculum flap is attached to the ulnar border of the radius. Stanley and Herbert[51] reported good to excellent results in most of their patients, with few complications related to the retinacular flap. Ouellette and Makowski[50] modified the technique by altering the direction of the flap, with the intention to address both the DRUJ and the ulnocarpal joint.

Intra-articular Reconstruction

Scheker and colleagues[26] and others described techniques to reconstruct 1 or both radioulnar ligaments. These techniques required extensive dissection and multiple passes of the tendon graft through bone tunnels. Stability was usually restored but many patients had limited forearm rotation.

Adams[28,29] described a reconstructive technique that closely mimics the natural origins and insertions of both radioulnar ligaments using less invasive dissection (**Fig. 5**). The DRUJ is exposed using an L-shaped capsulotomy through the floor of the fifth extensor compartment (see **Fig. 5**). The integrity of the TFCC is inspected to determine whether a repair or ligament reconstruction is indicated. The floor of the fourth extensor compartment is elevated to expose an area that will allow a 3.5-mm tunnel to be drilled in the radius from dorsal to volar parallel to the sigmoid notch and several millimeters proximal to the lunate fossa.

Another 3.5-mm to 4.5-mm tunnel is drilled in the distal ulna to create an oblique tunnel from the fovea to the ulnar neck (**Fig. 6**). The tendon graft is passed from dorsal to volar through the radius tunnel and retrieved through a separate volar incision (**Fig. 7**). The graft end is pulled

back through the volar DRUJ capsule using a straight hemostat punctured from dorsally near to the ulnar styloid and proximal to any TFCC remnant. By partially encircling a substantial segment of the volar capsule with the graft, the procedure not only reconstructs the volar radioulnar ligament but it also increases tension in the volar DRUJ capsule and ulnocarpal ligaments, resulting in additional DRUJ and ulnocarpal stability (**Fig. 8**). Both graft ends are passed through the ulnar tunnel and secured under tension with the forearm in neutral rotation. A variety of techniques have been used to fix the graft to the ulnar neck. If graft length is sufficient, 1 end can be passed around the neck and tied directly to the other end. Some surgeons prefer to make divergent bony tunnels from the fovea to the ulnar neck and tie the graft ends over the bony bridge between the tunnel openings. Another method is to loop 1 graft end around the ECU sheath after extracting the tendon at the ulnar neck, but leaving the tendon within the ulnar groove more distally (**Fig. 9**). The extensor digiti quinti is left subcutaneous and the extensor retinaculum and dorsal capsule are closed in a single layer. Of the 14 patients described in the original series with an average 2-year follow-up, instability was resolved in 12 patients, who returned to previous activities.[28] One patient required another soft tissue stabilization procedure and another with continued symptoms chose a splint for symptomatic relief; a flat sigmoid notch was retrospectively identified in these patients, which likely contributed to the 2 failures.

Seo and colleagues[52] reported a series of 16 patients who underwent the Adams procedure for unidirectional DRUJ instability. With more than a year's follow-up, 1 patient required a sigmoid notch osteotomy for recurrent instability. All other patients maintained stability and had an improved

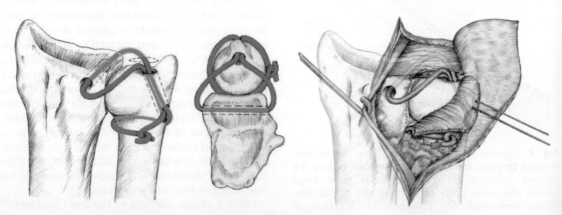

Fig. 5. Adams anatomic radioulnar reconstruction with tendon graft.

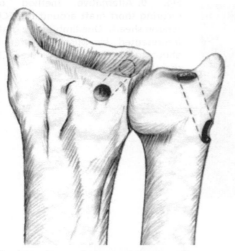

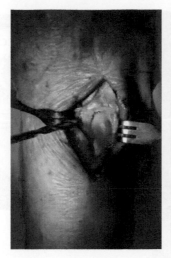

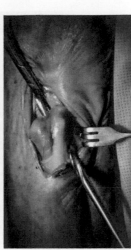

Fig. 6. Radius and ulna osseous tunnels.

Modified Mayo Wrist Score (MMWS). Kootstra and colleagues[53] identified 74 patients who underwent the Adams procedure, 22 of whom were examined after an average of 5 years. Compared with the opposite side, patients recovered approximately 90% of pronosupination and grip strength. DASH (disabilities of the arm, shoulder and hand) and PRWHE (patient-rated wrist/hand evaluation) scores were comparable with healthy working individuals. Interestingly, failures occurred in 3 patients, caused by detachment of the tendon grafts.

Meyer and colleagues[54] retrospectively reviewed 48 patients who underwent anatomic reconstruction. They used 2 diverging bone tunnels from the fovea and tied the graft over the osseous bridge. Some patients had concomitant ulnar shortening. At an average of 16 months' follow-up, stability was restored in 44 patients. Patients had approximately 10° greater loss of both pronation and supination compared with the series of Adams and Berger.[28]

Gillis and colleagues[55] have the largest series, including 95 wrists in 93 patients with an average follow-up of 5.5 years. The Adams reconstruction was used as originally described, except the tendon graft was secured using 3 different methods (sutures alone, suture anchors, or an

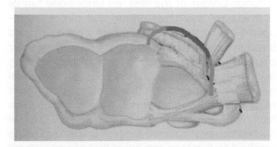

Fig. 8. Path of tendon graft encompassing volar capsule and ulnocarpal ligaments. Dark green represents segment of graft encircling ulnocarpal ligaments.

Fig. 7. Volar incision.

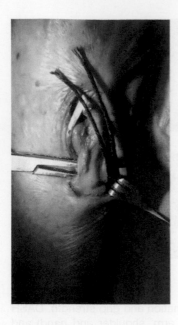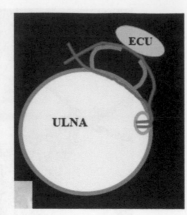

Fig. 9. Alternative method of securing short graft around the ECU tendon sheath. One limb of the graft (represented by purple suture) is about to be pulled under the ECU sheath by a hemostat.

interference screw) and allograft was used in approximately half. A 14% failure rate was reported. Failure was independent of age, chronicity of injury, sigmoid notch shape, and number of prior surgeries. No complications were judged to be caused by the allograft. Revision was more likely if an interference screw was used and in female patients. The study highlights the importance of graft tensioning and secure fixation. Furthermore, female patients are more likely to have hyperlaxity, which may have contributed to the increased failure rate in women.

Tse and colleagues[56] described a technique for arthroscopic-assisted anatomic reconstruction. Using the standard wrist arthroscopy portals, the TFCC was evaluated and debrided without violating the DRUJ capsule. If reconstruction was necessary, the 4-5 portal is extended to create the radial tunnel dorsally and a volar incision is made as described for the open procedure (**Fig. 10**). Using a 3-cm incision over the subcutaneous border of the ulna, an ulnar bone tunnel is made by antegrade drilling and direct arthroscopic visualization. Graspers were placed through the tunnels, as well as the dorsal and volar capsules, to pass the tendon graft. After retrieving both graft ends at the ulnar incision, an additional bone tunnel was made transversely to pass 1 graft limb and tie the graft over the bony bridge. The limb was immobilization in a long arm cast in neutral forearm rotation for first 3 weeks. During weeks 4 to 6, a long arm splint that allowed elbow motion was used, and both active and passive forearm rotation were performed under a therapist's supervision. After 7 weeks, strengthening

and mobilizing exercises were started. Fifteen patients with an average follow-up of 7 years were reviewed. Two ruptures, thought to be caused by trauma, occurred at 14 and 18 months after surgery. Pronosupination improved following surgery but remained limited compared with the opposite side. Almost all patients returned to work or previous activities. The MMWS, visual analogue scale (VAS), and grip strength significantly improved from preoperative to postoperative. Arthroscopy was performed on 2 patients at 9 and 21 months after reconstruction, which showed intact reconstructions and synovial-like tissue covering the grafts; mild graft fraying was seen in 1.

Luchetti and Atzei[57] treated 11 patients by arthroscopic-assisted anatomic reconstruction using a tendon graft. An interference screw was used to secure the tendon graft, which caused an ulnar styloid fracture in 1 patient. Follow-up averaged more than 5 years, with 1 patient having recurrent instability that required a second reconstructive procedure. All other patients resumed previous activities and had improved DASH, MMWS, VAS, and PRWHE scores. Wrist and forearm motion were maintained, whereas grip strength increased from 54% to 96% of the opposite side. The rehabilitation program was very similar to that used for open techniques. The wrist and elbow were immobilized for 3 to 4 weeks.[53,55,57] Kirschner wires were placed across the DRUJ in select patients. Full elbow motion and limited forearm rotation were started between 3 and 6 weeks. Strengthening was started after 8 weeks; however, heavy loading was delayed for 4 to 6 months.

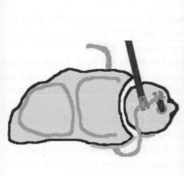

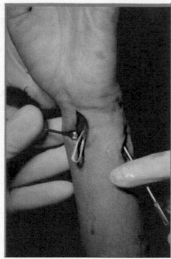

Fig. 10. Arthroscopic-assisted Adams procedure: trocars and graspers are used to pass the tendons through the dorsal and volar capsule to be delivered into the ulnar wound, tensioned, and secured. (*From* Tse WL, Lau SW, Wong WY, et al. Arthroscopic reconstruction of triangular fibrocartilage complex (TFCC) with tendon graft for chronic DRUJ instability. Injury. 2013 Mar;44(3):386-90; with permission.)

SUMMARY

Proper bony alignment is a prerequisite to restore DRUJ stability. Peripheral TFCC tears that cause DRUJ instability can often be repaired primarily if the injury is identified acutely and the radioulnar ligaments are robust. Ligament reconstruction may be required for injuries with more extensive damage or in chronic injuries with advanced attenuation of the stabilizing soft tissues. The addition of a sigmoid notchplasty may be required if the notch is flat. Patients can expect reduced pain and improved grip strength following surgical treatment but may develop DRUJ stiffness following a ligament reconstruction. The outcome of anatomic reconstructive procedures is less predictable in patients with generalized ligamentous laxity or gross posttraumatic laxity. A salvage procedure should be considered in patients with substantial arthrosis or uncorrected bony deformity.

DISCLOSURE

The authors have nothing to disclose.

REFERENCES

1. af Ekenstam F, Hagert CG. Anatomical studies on the geometry and stability of the distal radio ulnar joint. Scand J Plast Reconstr Surg 1985;19(1): 17–25.

2. af Ekenstam FW, Palmer AK, Glisson RR. The load on the radius and ulna in different positions of the wrist and forearm. A cadaver study. Acta Orthop Scand 1984;55(3):363–5.

3. Tolat AR, Stanley JK, Trail IA. A cadaveric study of the anatomy and stability of the distal radioulnar joint

in the coronal and transverse planes. J Hand Surg Br 1996;21(5):587–94.

4. Stuart PR, Berger RA, Linscheid RL, et al. The dorsopalmar stability of the distal radioulnar joint. J Hand Surg Am 2000;25(4):689–99.

5. Faucher GK, Zimmerman RM, Zimmerman NB. Instability and Arthritis of the Distal Radioulnar Joint: A Critical Analysis Review. JBJS Rev 2016;4(12). 01874474-201612000-00001.

6. Bednar MS, Arnoczky SP, Weiland AJ. The microvasculature of the triangular fibrocartilage complex: its clinical significance. J Hand Surg Am 1991;16(6): 1101–5.

7. Hotchkiss RN, An KN, Sowa DT, et al. An anatomic and mechanical study of the interosseous membrane of the forearm: pathomechanics of proximal migration of the radius. J Hand Surg Am 1989;14(2 Pt 1):256–61.

8. Moritomo H. The Function of the Distal Interosseous Membrane and its Relevance to the Stability of the Distal Radioulnar Joint: An Anatomical and Biomechanical Review. Handchir Mikrochir Plast Chir 2015;47(5):277–80.

9. Arimitsu S, Moritomo H, Kitamura T, et al. The stabilizing effect of the distal interosseous membrane on the distal radioulnar joint in an ulnar shortening procedure: a biomechanical study. J Bone Joint Surg Am 2011;93(21):2022–30.

10. Gofton WT, Gordon KD, Dunning CE, et al. Soft-tissue stabilizers of the distal radioulnar joint: an in vitro kinematic study. J Hand Surg Am 2004; 29(3):423–31.

11. Kleinman WB. Stability of the distal radioulna joint: biomechanics, pathophysiology, physical diagnosis, and restoration of function what we have learned in 25 years. J Hand Surg Am 2007;32(7): 1086–106.

12. Omokawa S, Iida A, Kawamura K, et al. A Biomechanical Perspective on Distal Radioulnar Joint Instability. J Wrist Surg 2017;6(2):88–96.

13. Kakar S, Carlsen BT, Moran SL, et al. The management of chronic distal radioulnar instability. Hand Clin 2010;26(4):517–28.

14. Cole DW, Elsaidi GA, Kuzma KR, et al. Distal radioulnar joint instability in distal radius fractures: the role of sigmoid notch and triangular fibrocartilage complex revisited. Injury 2006;37(3):252–8.

15. Kleinman WB. Distal radius instability and stiffness: common complications of distal radius fractures. Hand Clin 2010;26(2):245–64.

16. Adams BD. Effects of radial deformity on distal radioulnar joint mechanics. J Hand Surg Am 1993;18(3):492–8.

17. Kihara H, Palmer AK, Werner FW, et al. The effect of dorsally angulated distal radius fractures on distal radioulnar joint congruency and forearm rotation. J Hand Surg Am 1996;21(1):40–7.

18. Nishiwaki M, Welsh MF, Gammon B, et al. Effect of Volarly Angulated Distal Radius Fractures on Forearm Rotation and Distal Radioulnar Joint Kinematics. J Hand Surg Am 2015;40(11):2236–42.

19. Dy CJ, Jang E, Taylor SA, et al. The impact of coronal alignment on distal radioulnar joint stability following distal radius fracture. J Hand Surg Am 2014;39(7):1264–72.

20. Fujitani R, Omokawa S, Akahane M, et al. Predictors of distal radioulnar joint instability in distal radius fractures. J Hand Surg Am 2011;36(12):1919–25.

21. Glowacki KA, Shin LA. Stabilization of the unstable distal ulna: the Linscheid-Hui procedure. Tech Hand Up Extrem Surg 1999;3(4):229–36.

22. Wijffels M, Brink P, Schipper I. Clinical and nonclinical aspects of distal radioulnar joint instability. Open Orthop J 2012;6:204–10.

23. Tay SC, Tomita K, Berger RA. The "ulnar fovea sign" for defining ulnar wrist pain: an analysis of sensitivity and specificity. J Hand Surg Am 2007;32(4):438–44.

24. King GJ, McMurtry RY. Physical examination of the wrist and hand. Philadelphia: WB Saunders; 1996. p. 5–18.

25. Lindau T, Adlercreutz C, Aspenberg P. Peripheral tears of the triangular fibrocartilage complex cause distal radioulnar joint instability after distal radial fractures. J Hand Surg Am 2000;25(3):464–8.

26. Scheker LR, Belliappa PP, Acosta R, et al. Reconstruction of the dorsal ligament of the triangular fibrocartilage complex. J Hand Surg Br 1994;19(3):310–8.

27. Lester B, Halbrecht J, Levy IM, et al. Press test" for office diagnosis of triangular fibrocartilage complex tears of the wrist. Ann Plast Surg 1995;35(1):41–5.

28. Adams BD, Berger RA. An anatomic reconstruction of the distal radioulnar ligaments for posttraumatic distal radioulnar joint instability. J Hand Surg Am 2002;27(2):243–51.

29. Adams BD. Anatomic reconstruction of the distal radioulnar ligaments for DRUJ instability. Tech Hand Up Extrem Surg 2000;4(3):154–60.

30. Nakamura R, Horii E, Imaeda T, et al. Distal radioulnar joint subluxation and dislocation diagnosed by standard roentgenography. Skeletal Radiol 1995;24(2):91–4.

31. El Naga AN, Jordan ME, Netscher DT, et al. Reliability of the dorsal tangential view in assessment of distal radioulnar joint reduction in the neutral, pronated, and supinated positions in a cadaver model. J Hand Surg Am 2020;45(4):359.e1-8.

32. Mino DE, Palmer AK, Levinsohn EM. The role of radiography and computerized tomography in the diagnosis of subluxation and dislocation of the distal radioulnar joint. J Hand Surg Am 1983;8(1):23–31.

33. Squires JH, England E, Mehta K, et al. The role of imaging in diagnosing diseases of the distal radioulnar joint, triangular fibrocartilage complex, and distal ulna. AJR Am J Roentgenol 2014;203(1):146–53.

34. Chiang CC, Chang MC, Lin CF, et al. Computerized tomography in the diagnosis of subluxation of the distal radioulnar joint. Zhonghua Yi Xue Za Zhi (Taipei) 1998;61(12):708–15.

35. Nakamura R, Horii E, Imaeda T, et al. Criteria for diagnosing distal radioulnar joint subluxation by computed tomography. Skeletal Radiol 1996;25(7):649–53.

36. Wijffels M, Stomp W, Krijnen P, et al. Computed tomography for the detection of distal radioulnar joint instability: normal variation and reliability of four CT scoring systems in 46 patients. Skeletal Radiol 2016;45(11):1487–93.

37. Anderson ML, Larson AN, Moran SL, et al. Clinical comparison of arthroscopic versus open repair of triangular fibrocartilage complex tears. J Hand Surg Am 2008;33(5):675–82.

38. Hess F, Farshad M, Sutter R, et al. A novel technique for detecting instability of the distal radioulnar joint in complete triangular fibrocartilage complex lesions. J Wrist Surg 2012;1(2):153–8.

39. Millard GM, Budoff JE, Paravic V, et al. Functional bracing for distal radioulnar joint instability. J Hand Surg Am 2002;27(6):972–7.

40. Kim BS, Song HS, Jung KH, et al. Distal radioulnar joint volar instability after ligament reconstruction failure treated with sigmoid notch osteotomy. Orthopedics 2012;35(6):e984–7.

41. Moritomo H. The distal interosseous membrane: current concepts in wrist anatomy and biomechanics. J Hand Surg Am 2012;37(7):1501–7.

42. Nishiwaki M, Nakamura T, Nakao Y, et al. Ulnar shortening effect on distal radioulnar joint stability: a biomechanical study. J Hand Surg Am 2005;30(4):719–26.

43. Fulkerson JP, Watson HK. Congenital anterior subluxation of the distal ulna. A case report. Clin Orthop Relat Res 1978;(131):179–82.

44. Pürisa H, Sezer İ, Kabakaş F, et al. Ligament reconstruction using the Fulkerson-Watson method to treat chronic isolated distal radioulnar joint instability: short-term results. Acta Orthop Traumatol Turc 2011;45(3):168–74.

45. Burke CS, Zoeller KA, Waddell SW, et al. Assessment of distal radioulnar joint stability after reconstruction with the brachioradialis wrap. Hand (N Y) 2018;13(4):455–60.

46. Lee SK, Lee JW, Choy WS. Volar stabilization of the distal radioulnar joint for chronic instability using the pronator quadratus. Ann Plast Surg 2016;76(4): 394–8.

47. Riggenbach MD, Wright TW, Dell PC. Reconstruction of the distal oblique bundle of the interosseous membrane: a technique to restore distal radioulnar joint stability. J Hand Surg Am 2015;40(11):2279–82.

48. Brink PR, Hannemann PF. Distal oblique bundle reinforcement for treatment of DRUJ instability. J Wrist Surg 2015;4(3):221–8.

49. Hui FC, Linscheid RL. Ulnotriquetral augmentation tenodesis: a reconstructive procedure for dorsal subluxation of the distal radioulnar joint. J Hand Surg Am 1982;7(3):230–6.

50. Dy CJ, Ouellette EA, Makowski AL. Extensor retinaculum capsulorrhaphy for ulnocarpal and distal radioulnar instability: the Herbert sling. Tech Hand Up Extrem Surg 2009;13(1):19–22.

51. Stanley D, Herbert TJ. The Swanson ulnar head prosthesis for post-traumatic disorders of the distal radio-ulnar joint. J Hand Surg Br 1992;17(6):682–8.

52. Seo KN, Park MJ, Kang HJ. Anatomic reconstruction of the distal radioulnar ligament for posttraumatic distal radioulnar joint instability. Clin Orthop Surg 2009;1(3):138–45.

53. Kootstra TJM, van Doesburg MH, Schuurman AH. Functional effects of the adams procedure: a retrospective intervention study. J Wrist Surg 2018;7(4): 331–5.

54. Meyer D, Schweizer A, Nagy L. Anatomic reconstruction of distal radioulnar ligaments with tendon graft for treating distal radioulnar joint instability: surgical technique and outcome. Tech Hand Up Extrem Surg 2017;21(3):107–13.

55. Gillis JA, Soreide E, Khouri JS, et al. Outcomes of the Adams-Berger ligament reconstruction for the distal radioulnar joint instability in 95 consecutive cases. J Wrist Surg 2019;8(4):268–75.

56. Tse WL, Lau SW, Wong WY, et al. Arthroscopic reconstruction of triangular fibrocartilage complex (TFCC) with tendon graft for chronic DRUJ instability. Injury 2013;44(3):386–90.

57. Luchetti R, Atzei A. Arthroscopic assisted tendon reconstruction for triangular fibrocartilage complex irreparable tears. J Hand Surg Eur Vol 2017;42(4): 346–51.

Galeazzi Injuries

Rohit Garg, MD*, Chaitanya Mudgal, MD

KEYWORDS

- Galeazzi • Forearm fracture • DRUJ

KEY POINTS

- Galeazzi injuries are unstable fracture dislocations involving fracture of radial shaft and distal radio-ulnar joint (DRUJ) disruption.
- Surgical management is needed to achieve optimal outcomes.
- DRUJ stability needs to be carefully assessed.

GALEAZZI INJURIES

Fracture of the radius shaft associated with a dislocation of the distal radioulnar joint (DRUJ) is termed the Galeazzi fracture[1] (**Fig. 1**). This fracture was first described by Sir Astley Cooper in 1822 but the eponym Galeazzi fracture is based on a series of 18 patients described in 1934 by an Italian surgeon, Riccardo Galeazzi.[2,3] This injury pattern has also been described as fracture of necessity, signifying the need for surgical management to obtain optimal results.[1,4] Hughston[4] in 1957 described poor results from nonoperative management of these fractures in the Piedmont Orthopedic Society, which gave this injury pattern another eponym of Piedmont fractures. Other eponyms used are reverse Monteggia fracture, and Darrach-Hughston-Milch fracture.[3]

Certain injury patterns are Galeazzi equivalent lesions. In children, a fracture of the radial shaft may be associated with separation of the distal ulnar epiphysis without disruption of the DRUJ. In adults, a fracture of the radial shaft may be associated with an additional fracture of the distal ulna. These injuries are considered Galeazzi equivalents and are treated the same way as a Galeazzi injury. Closed reduction and management can often be successful in the pediatric population; however, in adults, closed treatment is associated with poor outcomes.[1,4,5] Treatment in adults consists of fixation of the radius shaft and stabilization of the DRUJ.

ANATOMY AND CLASSIFICATION

The forearm is a complex joint formed between the radius and ulna. It consists of the proximal radioulnar joint (PRUJ), interosseous membrane (IOM), and DRUJ (**Fig. 2**). The forearm axis may be drawn proximally from the radial head and distally to the DRUJ. The radius functions similarly to a bucket/crank handle because it has a proximal valgus, distal varus, and a distal flare. This anatomy creates the radial bow, which is on an average 15.3 ± 0.3 mm and present at around 60% of the length of radius measured from bicipital tuberosity proximally to DRUJ distally.[6] Restoration of the radial bow is critical in restoring normal forearm anatomy and motion.[6,7] The ulna has a reversed orientation in the forearm compared with the radius (see **Fig. 2**). Mechanically, the radius rotates around a relatively fixed ulna, although language to describe the relationship between the forearm bones seems to suggest otherwise, by convention. Proximally, these 2 bones form the PRUJ with its surrounding annular ligament. Pure rotation occurs at the PRUJ. Distally, they form the DRUJ, which includes the volar and dorsal radioulnar ligaments and triangular fibrocartilaginous complex (TFCC). Both rotation

Hand and Upper Extremity Surgery, Department of Orthopaedics, Massachusetts General Hospital, 55 Fruit Street, Boston, MA 02114, USA
* Corresponding author.
E-mail address: Rgarg2@mgh.harvard.edu

Hand Clin 36 (2020) 455–462
https://doi.org/10.1016/j.hcl.2020.07.006

hand.theclinics.com

A   **B**

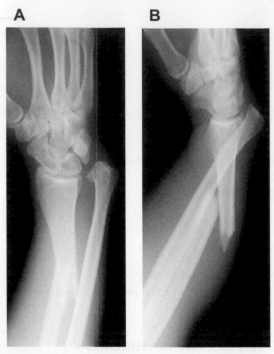

Fig. 1. Anteroposterior (AP) (*A*) and lateral (*B*) radiographs of the wrist. There is a fracture of distal radius shaft with displacement, shortening, widening of DRUJ on AP view, positive ulnar variance, and dislocation of DRUJ on lateral view. These findings are consistent with a Galeazzi fracture dislocation.

and translation occur at the DRUJ. In between, the 2 bones are connected by the IOM (see **Fig. 2**). The IOM maintains the interosseous space, helps in loading both radius and ulna, and contributes to the longitudinal stability of the forearm. The IOM consists of distal, central, and proximal portions (see **Fig. 2**). The distal oblique band (DOB) arises from the dorsal ulna, approximately at the level of pronator quadratus, and is attached to the inferior rim of sigmoid notch and DRUJ capsule.

In terms of stability, the radial head is the primary contributor to longitudinal forearm stability, with secondary contributions from the IOM and the TFCC.[7–9] The DOB of the IOM is involved in stability of the DRUJ. The central portion, with its most functionally important component, the central band, confers longitudinal forearm stability (see **Fig. 2**).

Galeazzi fractures involve fracture of the radial shaft and disruption of the DRUJ. Cadaveric studies[10,11] have determined which critical stabilizers of the DRUJ are disrupted when the radius shortens in Galeazzi injuries. Moore and colleagues[10] produced Galeazzi fractures in cadavers

by cutting the radius distal to insertion of the pronator teres. There was no disruption of DRUJ for shortening up to 5 mm. Shortening more than 10 mm required injury to both TFCC and IOM. Intermediate shortening occurred with disruption of either TFCC or IOM. Maculé Beneyto and colleagues[12] classified these injuries into 3 types. Type I has a radius fracture within 10 cm of the styloid process. Type II has a radius fracture between 10 and 15 cm, and type III greater than 15 cm from the styloid process. They used both nonsurgical treatments and a variety of surgical methods to fix these fractures; however, the worst results were obtained for patients with a type I injury. Rettig and Raskin[13] classified these fractures into 2 types based on location of fracture from the midarticular surface of the distal radius. Type I fractures occurred within 7.5 cm from the midarticular surface of distal radius and had a higher incidence of DRUJ instability requiring operative fixation (55%, 12 patients). The investigators postulated that these fractures occur through a high-impact hyperextension mechanism that results in a direct continuum of injury through TFCC and IOM, which predisposes the DRUJ to residual dorsal subluxation despite anatomic and rigid radial shaft fixation. Type II fractures were greater than 7.5 cm from the midarticular surface of the distal radius and rarely required fixation of the DRUJ (6%, 1 patient). The investigators suggested that an indirect pronation force is incurred with incomplete soft tissue disruption for fractures through the middle third of the radial shaft. Presence of a substantially intact central portion of the IOM might also have a role to play and hence there is a higher likelihood of DRUJ stabilization after fracture fixation in type II injuries.

Ring and colleagues[14] showed in their retrospective series that isolated radius shaft fractures without disruption of the DRUJ might be more common than true Galeazzi injuries. The results of this study were similar to those of the study by Rettig and Raskin,[13] because most of the fractures in this investigation were middle third or proximal radius shaft fractures, and, in fractures involving the distal third of the radius shaft, there was a higher incidence of DRUJ instability. Similar to classifications discussed earlier, Korompilias and colleagues[15] proposed a classification system for Galeazzi injuries to predict DRUJ instability. According to this classification, type I fractures are located at the distal third of radius (from the point at which the diaphysis begins to straighten to the metaphyseal flare), type II fractures are of the middle third of the radius (from the beginning to the end of radial bow), and type III fractures occurred at the proximal third of the radius (from radial

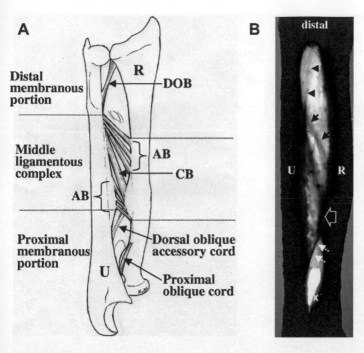

Fig. 2. (*A*) Structure of the IOM. Right forearm viewed from the anterior aspect. The IOM consists of distal, middle, and proximal portions. The middle portion is a ligamentous complex (middle ligamentous complex) that is further divisible into the central band (CB) and the accessory band (AB). Distal and proximal portions on either side of the middle portion comprise transparent membranous tissue (distal and proximal membranous portions) with holes for perforation of the interosseous artery. The DOB is present within the distal membranous portion. The proximal oblique cord is present on the anterior side of the forearm and the dorsal oblique accessory cord on the posterior side in the proximal membranous portion. (*B*) Backlit view of IOM ligaments. Asterisks indicate the CB as part of the middle ligamentous complex, which originates from the interosseous crest of the radius (*white arrow*), runs distally and ulnarly, and inserts into the interosseous border of the ulna. Black arrows indicate the AB, which runs in a similar way to the CB. Black arrowheads indicate the DOB within the distal membranous portion, which originates from around the distal one-sixth of the ulnar shaft and inserts into the inferior rim of the sigmoid notch of the radius. Broken white arrows indicate the dorsal oblique accessory cord on the posterior aspect of the forearm, which originates from around the distal two-thirds of the ulnar shaft and inserts into the interosseous crest of the radius. The proximal oblique cord cannot be distinguished here because this cord is in contact with the surface of the radial tuberosity (*X*). R, radius; U, ulna. (*From Noda K, Goto A, Murase T, et al. Interosseous membrane of the forearm: an anatomical study of ligament attachment locations. J Hand Surg Am. 2009;34(3):415e422; with permission.*)

tuberosity to the beginning of radial bow). Stabilization of DRUJ was required in 54% of patients with type I injury, and only 12% (2 patients) and 11% (1 patient) with type II and III injuries respectively. All these studies show that incidence of instability of DRUJ after fracture fixation is higher as the fracture line moves from proximal to distal. However, fracture location should not be seen in isolation, and the stability of the DRUJ is likely determined by a combination of fracture location, mechanism of injury, and degree of shortening/displacement. Although these associations are helpful, careful intraoperative assessment of the DRUJ is critical to determine stability after fracture fixation.[16]

CLINICAL EVALUATION

Galeazzi injuries usually occur as a result of high-energy trauma, such as motor vehicle accidents, athletic injuries, and falls from a height.[13] Other mechanisms include a fall on an outstretched and pronated hand.[1] The patients usually present with swelling and deformity of the forearm. Neurovascular damage is rare. It is essential to get good anteroposterior (AP) and lateral radiographs of the forearm. Orthogonal views of the wrist and elbow should be obtained as well. The radiographic signs that suggest disruption of the DRUJ are fracture at the base of ulnar styloid, widening of the DRUJ space (on a true AP view), dislocation of the radius relative to the ulna (on a true lateral view), and more than 5 mm of shortening of radius relative to the ulna,[17] although radiographic predictors of instability remain imperfect[16](see **Fig. 1**). Although injury to the distal radioulnar ligaments can be accompanied by a bony fracture of the styloid, injury to the DRUJ can also be purely ligamentous. A computed tomography scan or a radiograph of the contralateral wrist can also be useful tools for assessment of the DRUJ.

TREATMENT

Treatment in adults is uniformly surgical and involves anatomic and rigid fixation of the radius

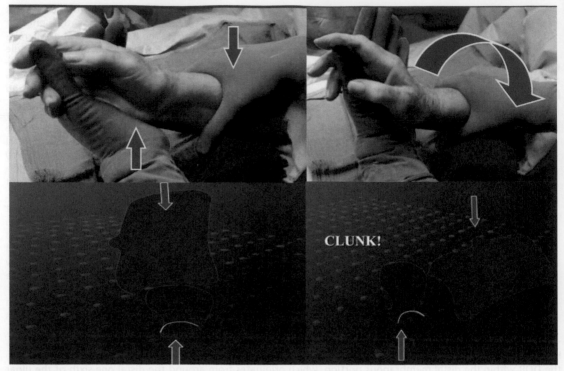

Fig. 3. Assessment of DRUJ stability. DRUJ is stabilized and gently compressed between the 2 hands of the examiner and the forearm is passively rotated to evaluate for any audible or palpable clunk at DRUJ. (*Courtesy of* Jesse Jupiter MD.)

and stabilization of DRUJ. Conservative management results in a high percentage of failure.[1,4,5] Hughston[4] noted various deforming forces that lead to failure of conservative management. These forces include the brachioradialis, which tends to shorten the radius, and pronator quadratus, which rotates the distal fragment toward the ulna. The weight of the hand also acts as a strong volar force causing subluxation of the DRUJ. Thumb abductors and extensors tend to shorten the radial side of the wrist by relaxing the radial collateral ligaments.[4] These deforming forces make it difficult to control these fractures in a cast and hence operative treatment is recommended for optimal results. Further, the forearm is a joint and articular fractures require anatomic reduction and rigid fixation. It has been shown in some series that surgery within 10 days of injury gives improved outcomes compared with delayed surgery.[15,17] The goal of treatment is restoration of radial bow, anatomic reduction with rigid fixation of radius, and stability of the DRUJ. Plate and screw fixation is the preferred method of treatment. Alternative fixation options, including Kirschner wires (K-wires) and intramedullary pins, are not rigid enough to resist the deforming forces outlined

earlier. They also allow shortening of the radius and are unable to control rotation.

SURGICAL TECHNIQUE

The volar Henry approach is used to expose the fracture site. Periosteal elevation should be minimized and soft tissue attachments need to be preserved to intermediate fragments. A 3.5-mm limited-contact dynamic compression (LCDC) plate is used to obtain a minimum of 6 cortices of fixation on either side of the fracture. Initially, the plate is fixed with 2 screws, and radiographs are obtained to confirm the accuracy of fracture reduction and precision of DRUJ reduction. DRUJ stability is assessed after anatomic reduction of radius shaft fracture has been obtained. The DRUJ is stabilized and gently compressed between the 2 hands of the examiner as the forearm is passively rotated to evaluate for any audible or palpable clunk at the DRUJ (**Fig. 3**).

If the DRUJ is immediately stable, then postoperative immobilization for 4 weeks is not mandatory and rehabilitation can be started soon after surgery. For an unstable but reducible DRUJ, multiple treatment options exist. One option is a long arm cast with forearm in semisupination for 4 weeks without the need for transfixing K-wires. This option has been shown to be sufficient for DRUJ healing in some series.[17,18] Transfixing K-wires are also a reasonable option for unstable and reducible DRUJs. K-wire size must be at least 1.57 mm (0.062 inch) to ensure adequate fixation and avoid bending or breakage. They are placed proximal to the sigmoid notch and should be passed from ulnar to radial, and should extend out of both radius and ulna. In case the wires break, it makes retrieval of the broken wires much easier (**Fig. 4**). If a small ulnar styloid fracture is present in cases of unstable and reducible DRUJ, then fixation of that fragment with K-wires and/or tension band wires or a small screw can be performed (**Fig. 5**). Long arm cast in semisupination is also a reasonable option for ulnar styloid fractures if the DRUJ is reducible.

If the DRUJ is not reducible, then careful assessment of the radius shaft reduction should be performed. In most circumstances, anatomic reduction of the radius shaft fracture obtains reduction of the DRUJ. Rarely, the DRUJ can be irreducible because of interposition of soft tissue. There are multiple case reports where tendons of the extensor carpi ulnaris, extensor digitorum communis, or extensor digit minimi are interposed and prevent reduction.[19–22] Other causes can be a metaphyseal fragment that is dislocated through a

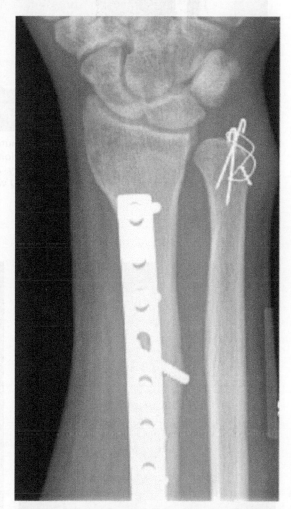

Fig. 4. Two 1.57-mm (0.062-inch) K-wires transfixing radius and ulna with reduced DRUJ position. They are placed proximal to sigmoid notch and should be passed out of both radius and ulna in case the wire breaks. (*Courtesy of* Marco Rizzo MD.)

Fig. 5. A Galeazzi fracture dislocation that has been treated by open reduction with internal fixation (ORIF) of the ulnar styloid, using K-wires with a tension band and ORIF of the radius. (*Courtesy of* Jesse Jupiter MD.)

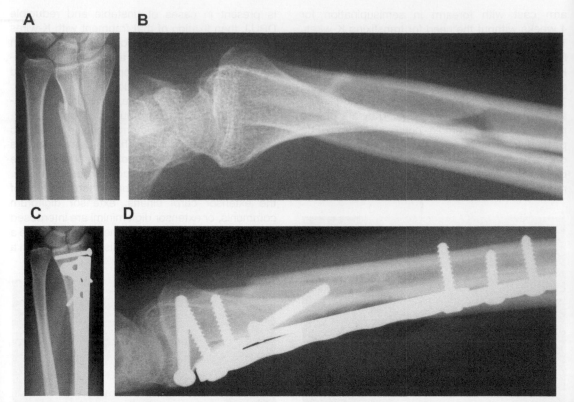

Fig. 6. AP (*A*) and lateral (*B*) views showing a comminuted distal radius fracture extending into the distal radius shaft with disruption of DRUJ. This fracture is a transitional lesion with a combination of both a distal radius fracture and Galeazzi injury. (*C, D*) Fixation of this injury. Articular portion was reduced and fixed first and then stacked plating was used to fix the radius shaft. DRUJ was reduced and stable after fixation of radius.

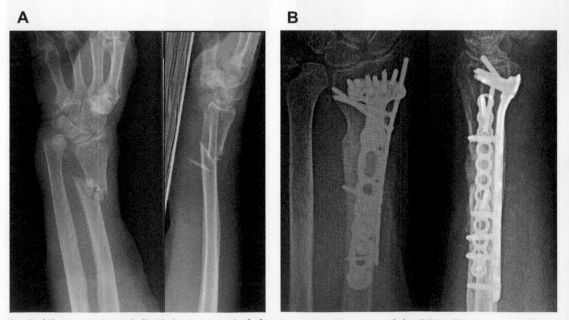

Fig. 7. (*A*) A comminuted distal third radius shaft fracture with dislocation of the DRUJ. Fixation was achieved using orthogonal plates (*B*).

capsular buttonhole, periosteal tissue, or a bony fragment from an avulsion fracture of the fovea,[23] which necessitates a dorsal approach to the DRUJ, removal of interposed structures, and open reduction of the DRUJ. The TFCC is repaired with either sutures placed through bone tunnels or a suture anchor, and transfixing K-wires with the forearm in neutral position are used to protect the TFCC repair.

THE TRANSITIONAL LESION

There are certain high-energy metadiaphyseal injuries that are essentially a combination of distal radius fracture and Galeazzi injuries (**Fig. 6**A, B). Distal radius articular restoration is performed first and then these are treated as standard Galeazzi fracture dislocations. Stacked plating for these fractures has also been described[24] (**Fig. 6**C, D).

ADDRESSING COMMINUTION

In the presence of comminution, longer than usual plates are selected, typically placed in an orthogonal arrangement. Smaller plates (2.4 or 2.7 mm) can be used as reduction tools (**Fig. 7**), applied out of the plane of the major plate (ie, orthogonal to the major plate) to act as a reduction tool. In most circumstances, the smaller plate as a reduction tool is applied along the radial border. After confirming reduction of the DRUJ, the 3.5-mm LCDC plate is then applied to the volar surface of the radius as described earlier.

GALEAZZI EQUIVALENTS

In adults, fractures of the radial shaft can be associated with fractures of the distal ulna. **Fig. 8** shows an example of a transitional and Galeazzi equivalent lesion with a distal radius fracture extending into a fracture of the radius shaft, distal ulna fracture, and disruption of the DRUJ. The metaphyseal component of the radius was fixed using orthogonal plates with a metadiaphyseal plate (Synthes, Paoli, PA) spanning the metaphyseal area with the shaft of the distal radius. An additional cannulated screw was placed to obtain fixation of the distal radius fracture. A separate approach was made along the subcutaneous border of the ulna to perform fixation of the distal ulnar fracture using a 2.0-mm locking plate.

OUTCOMES

Excellent restoration of wrist motion, forearm rotation, strength, and functional scores can be obtained with anatomic reduction and rigid fixation of the fracture and reduction of the DRUJ.[25] Complications of these injuries are similar to those of other forearm fractures and include nonunion, delayed union, malunion, nerve injuries, and infection. Plate removal is not routinely done, and, if needed, should not be done before 18 months because of the risk of refracture. Risk of refracture after plate removal is higher with the use of 4.5-mm plates, removal before 12 months, comminuted and displaced fracture

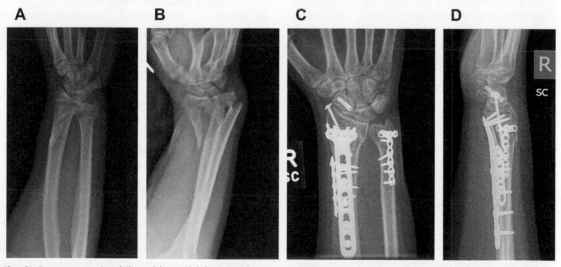

Fig. 8. Posteroanterior (*A*) and lateral (*B*) views show a transitional and Galeazzi equivalent lesion with both a distal radius fracture extending into a fracture of the radius shaft, distal ulna fracture, and disruption of DRUJ. The metaphyseal component of the radius was fixed using orthogonal plates with a metadiaphyseal plate spanning the metaphyseal area with the shaft of distal radius. An additional cannulated screw was placed to obtain fixation of the distal radius fracture. A separate approach was made along subcutaneous border of ulna to perform fixation of distal ulna fracture using a 2.0-mm locking plate (*C, D*).

pattern, and unrestricted activity immediately after plate removal.[26–28]

SUMMARY

Fractures of the radial shaft associated with disruption of the DRUJ are termed Galeazzi injuries. These fractures are unstable injuries requiring open reduction and internal fixation to achieve optimal outcomes. DRUJ stability should be carefully assessed intraoperatively and addressed accordingly.

DISCLOSURE

The authors have nothing to disclose.

REFERENCES

1. Mikić ZD. Galeazzi fracture-dislocations. J Bone Joint Surg Am 1975;57(8):1071–80.
2. Galeazzi R. Di una particolare syndrome traumatica dello scheletro dell 'avambraccio. Atti e memorie della Societa' lombarda di chirurgia 1934;2:663–6.
3. Sebastin SJ, Chung KC. A historical report on Riccardo Galeazzi and the management of Galeazzi fractures. J Hand Surg Am 2010;35(11):1870–7.
4. Hughston JC. Fracture of the distal radial shaft; mistakes in management. J Bone Joint Surg Am 1957; 39-A(2):249–64.
5. Reckling FW. Unstable fracture-dislocations of the forearm (Monteggia and Galeazzi lesions). J Bone Joint Surg Am 1982;64(6):857–63.
6. Schemitsch EH, Richards RR. The effect of malunion on functional outcome after plate fixation of fractures of both bones of the forearm in adults. J Bone Joint Surg Am 1992;74(7):1068–78.
7. Adams JE. Forearm Instability: Anatomy, Biomechanics, and Treatment Options. J Hand Surg Am 2017;42(1):47–52.
8. Sowa DT, Hotchkiss RN, Weiland AJ. Symptomatic proximal translation of the radius following radial head resection. Clin Orthop Relat Res 1995;317: 106–13.
9. Noda K, Goto A, Murase T, et al. Interosseous membrane of the forearm: an anatomical study of ligament attachment locations. J Hand Surg Am 2009; 34(3):415–22.
10. Moore TM, Lester DK, Sarmiento A. The stabilizing effect of soft-tissue constraints in artificial Galeazzi fractures. Clin Orthop Relat Res 1985;194:189–94.
11. Schneiderman G, Meldrum RD, Bloebaum RD, et al. The interosseous membrane of the forearm: structure and its role in Galeazzi fractures. J Trauma 1993;35(6):879–85.
12. Maculé Beneyto F, Arandes Renú JM, Ferreres Claramunt A, et al. Treatment of Galeazzi fracture-dislocations. J Trauma 1994;36(3):352–5.
13. Rettig ME, Raskin KB. Galeazzi fracture-dislocation: a new treatment-oriented classification. J Hand Surg Am 2001;26(2):228–35.
14. Ring D, Rhim R, Carpenter C, et al. Isolated radial shaft fractures are more common than Galeazzi fractures. J Hand Surg Am 2006;31(1):17–21.
15. Korompilias AV, Lykissas MG, Kostas-Agnantis IP, et al. Distal radioulnar joint instability (Galeazzi type injury) after internal fixation in relation to the radius fracture pattern. J Hand Surg Am 2011; 36(5):847–52.
16. Tsismenakis T, Tornetta P. Galeazzi fractures: Is DRUJ instability predicted by current guidelines? Injury 2016;47(7):1472–7.
17. Moore TM, Klein JP, Patzakis MJ, et al. Results of compression-plating of closed Galeazzi fractures. J Bone Joint Surg Am 1985;67(7):1015–21.
18. Strehle J, Gerber C. Distal radioulnar joint function after Galeazzi fracture-dislocations treated by open reduction and internal plate fixation. Clin Orthop Relat Res 1993;(293):240–5.
19. Alexander AH, Lichtman DM. Irreducible distal radioulnar joint occurring in a Galeazzi fracture - case report. J Hand Surg Am 1981;6(3):258–61.
20. Jenkins NH, Mintowt-Czyz WJ, Fairclough JA. Irreducible dislocation of the distal radioulnar joint. Injury 1987;18(1):40–3.
21. Biyani A, Bhan S. Dual extensor tendon entrapment in Galeazzi fracture-dislocation: a case report. J Trauma 1989;29(9):1295–7.
22. Hanel DP, Scheid DK. Irreducible fracture-dislocation of the distal radioulnar joint secondary to entrapment of the extensor carpi ulnaris tendon. Clin Orthop Relat Res 1988;234:56–60.
23. Kikuchi Y, Nakamura T. Irreducible Galeazzi fracture-dislocation due to an avulsion fracture of the fovea of the ulna. J Hand Surg Br 1999;24(3): 379–81.
24. Mudgal CS, Ring D. Stacked plating for metadiaphyseal fractures of the distal radius: a technique report. J Orthop Trauma 2007;21(1):63–6.
25. van Duijvenbode DC, Guitton TG, Raaymakers EL, et al. Long-term outcome of isolated diaphyseal radius fractures with and without dislocation of the distal radioulnar joint. J Hand Surg Am 2012;37(3): 523–7.
26. Hidaka S, Gustilo RB. Refracture of bones of the forearm after plate removal. J Bone Joint Surg Am 1984;66(8):1241–3.
27. Yao C-K, Lin K-C, Tarng Y-W, et al. Removal of forearm plate leads to a high risk of refracture: decision regarding implant removal after fixation of the forearm and analysis of risk factors of refracture. Arch Orthop Trauma Surg 2014;134(12):1691–7.
28. Beaupre GS, Csongradi JJ. Refracture risk after plate removal in the forearm. J Orthop Trauma 1996;10(2):87–92.

The Essex-Lopresti Injury:
Evaluation and Treatment Considerations

Julie E. Adams, MD[a],*, A. Lee Osterman, MD[b]

KEYWORDS

- Essex-Lopresti • Longitudinal instability of the forearm • Axial instability of the forearm

KEY POINTS

- Essex-Lopresti injuries occur with injury to structures at the wrist, elbow, and forearm.
- Instability of the forearm may present immediately or be apparent over time because the interosseous membrane may attenuate.
- Early recognition and treatment is associated with improved outcomes.

INTRODUCTION

The Essex-Lopresti injury results from an axial loading injury to the forearm, with injuries to structures at the wrist, forearm, and elbow.

The injury at the lateral aspect of the elbow is typically a radial head fracture, although a fracture dislocation or dislocation may also occur. The forearm injury involves disruption of the interosseous membrane (IOM) and what is thought to be the most important portion, the central band of the IOM. At the wrist, there is typically a triangular fibrocartilage complex (TFCC) tear with distal radioulnar joint (DRUJ) instability.[1,2]

Clinical evaluation hinges on awareness and recognition of the injury. It is a truth universally acknowledged that, in patients in whom an injury occurs to the elbow, an examination should also be performed at the wrist and forearm; nevertheless, these injuries often go unrecognized, either from lack of recognition by the examining physician or because of distracting injury sustained by the patient. In addition, patients may have forearm instability at the time of injury or alternatively may develop instability over time. It is for this reason that an estimated nearly two-thirds of patients may fail to have the diagnosis made.[3,4]

ACUTE PRESENTATION

In the acute setting, patients often present with a radial head fracture, and the examiner and patient may be distracted by the obvious radiographic findings and elbow findings, without appreciating more subtle complaints at the wrist or forearm.

Typically, if instability is present right away, this radial head fracture will be one in which there is evidence of axial loading and the radial head may be excavated out because of the neck impinging on the metaphyseal bone from the axial load or parts of the radial head widely displaced and extruded because of the pressure of the axial load from the forearm. However, in more subtle patterns, occasionally the radial head injury appears relatively innocuous.

At the wrist, patients often have evidence of a DRUJ dislocation or ulnar positivity.

At the forearm, patients may have vague discomfort or swelling along the forearm axis.

Imaging of the elbow and wrist is typically routine, and includes usually only anteroposterior, lateral, and oblique dedicated views each of the elbow and wrist. Occasionally comparison views of the contralateral normal wrist or elbow can be helpful, and occasionally axial imaging such as

a University of Tennessee College of Medicine - Chattanooga, Erlanger Orthopedic Institute, 975 East 3rd Street, Suite C 225, Chattanooga, TN 37403, USA; b Thomas Jefferson University, Philadelphia Hand to Shoulder Center, 834 Chestnut St G114, Philadelphia, PA 19107, USA
* Corresponding author.
E-mail address: Adams.julie.e@gmail.com

Hand Clin 36 (2020) 463–468
https://doi.org/10.1016/j.hcl.2020.07.012
0749-0712/20/© 2020 Elsevier Inc. All rights reserved.

computed tomography scan or MRI scanning can be helpful at the elbow or wrist. Imaging of the forearm is more difficult. Although some investigators have described protocols to evaluate for IOM injury at the forearm with ultrasonography or MRI, imaging findings are often subtle (edema, fluid changes, herniation of the muscles through the IOM) or can be nonspecific.[5–8]

In the acute setting, in patients in whom a radial head fracture is treated surgically with excision, with or without plans for replacement, the stability of the forearm may be assessed with the radial pull test. In this situation, the surgeon pulls in-line traction on the radial neck after radial head excision, with fluoroscopic assessment at the wrist for a change in ulnar variance. A change of 3 mm of ulnar variance indicates an injury to the IOM, whereas a change of 6 mm or more suggests injury to IOM and DRUJ/TFCC.[9]

In the chronic setting, patients may have had previous surgery or multiple previous failed procedures.[3,4] Here, radiographs often show impingement of the proximal radius (or a radial head arthroplasty) on the capitellum with subsequent arthritis, ulnar positive variance, and ulnar impaction, and clinical complaints of elbow pain, wrist pain, and forearm discomfort or weakness. In the evaluation of patients with chronic forearm instability, contralateral comparison views of the asymptomatic wrist, forearm, and elbow are often helpful.

TREATMENT

Treatment strategies are focused on the wrist, forearm, and elbow and differ based on the acuity or chronicity of the problem.

In the chronic setting as opposed to the acute setting, there may be arthritic changes at the radiocapitellar joint that alter the treatment options available. In the acute setting, treatment at the elbow may include radial head fixation versus replacement. In the chronic setting, patients with continued axial loading of the forearm may not tolerate a metallic radial head, especially without treatment of the forearm and stabilization of same.[4,10,11] Previously, radiocapitellar replacement arthroplasty had been used at the elbow to resurface both the proximal radius as well as the capitellar joint surface; however, these are no longer available in the United States.[12–14]

In some cases, radial head excision or excision of the radial head implant in the chronic setting is desirable, provided the forearm can be stabilized with reconstruction, to limit the contribution of pain from radiocapitellar impingement at the arthritic joint.

In general, in the acute setting, radial head preservation or replacement is preferred to help restore the normal constraints on axial load of the arm and limit proximal migration of the radius (and thus radiocapitellar impingement and ulnar impaction).[1,4,15–17]

In the acute setting at the wrist, reduction of any DRUJ dislocation and stabilization is performed. This reduction may take the form of an open TFCC repair.

In the chronic setting, wrist pain is from ulnar impaction, and patients may benefit from wrist arthroscopy and debridement and a joint leveling procedure, most commonly ulnar shortening

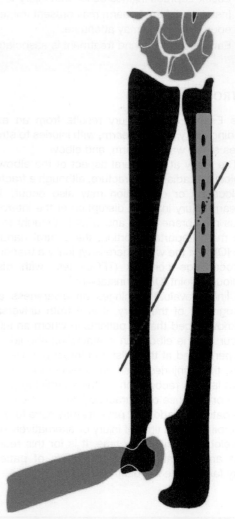

Fig. 1. A forearm after ulnar shortening osteotomy, with the red line representing the orientation of the IOM and the IOM reconstruction. (*From* Gaspar et al. Interosseous membrane reconstruction with a suture-button construct for treatment of chronic forearm instability. J Shoulder Elbow Surg 2016;25:1491-500; with permission.)

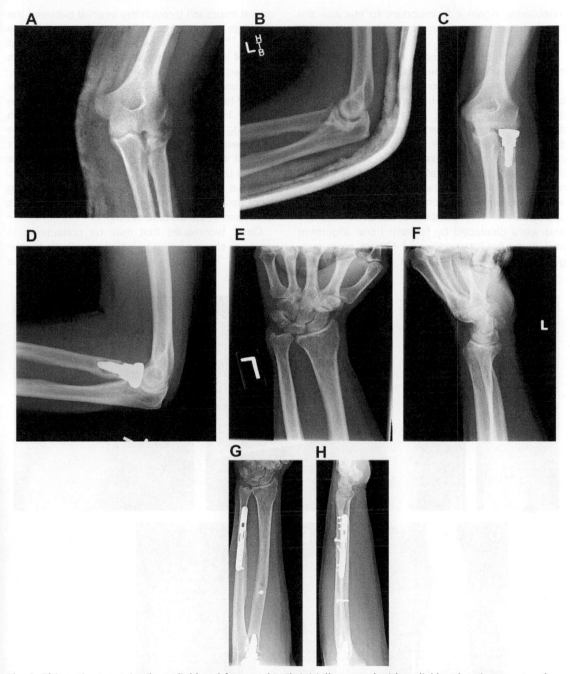

Fig. 2. This patient sustained a radial head fracture (*A, B*), initially treated with radial head replacement arthroplasty (*C, D*). He returned with worsening wrist pain and forearm discomfort and weakness. Radiographs revealed ulnar impaction (*E, F*) caused by axial instability. The patient underwent ulnar shortening osteotomy and reconstruction of the IOM with bone–patellar tendon–bone reconstruction (*G, H*). (*From* Gaspar MP, Adams JE, Zohn RC, Jacoby SM, Culp RW, Osterman AL, Kane PM. Late Reconstruction of the Interosseous Membrane with Bone-Patellar Tendon-Bone Graft for Chronic Essex-Lopresti Injuries: Outcomes with a Mean Follow-up of Over 10 Years. J Bone Joint Surg Am 2018;100:416-27; with permission.)

osteotomy. Again it is important to stabilize the forearm to prevent recurrent axial loading and ulnar impaction.

Treatment of the forearm instability and IOM injury is the most controversial subject.

In the acute setting, some surgeons have advocated simply stabilizing the forearm in an effort to allow the IOM to heal. This treatment may be done with supination splinting, transfixion pinning, or screw fixation of the ulna to radius.[15,18] This procedure can be problematic for several reasons. In series in which exploration of acute IOM injuries have been performed, there is a high rate of midsubstance tears in which the ends did not lie in apposition in any position of forearm rotation, and were displaced by forearm bone alignment and muscular interposition.[3,4] Others have suggested repair of the IOM and have described a dorsal approach through the interval between the extensor digitorum communis and extensor digiti minimi,[19] although 1 series suggests only about 20% of IOM injuries represent bony avulsions as opposed to midsubstance tears.

Interosseous ligament reconstruction with a variety of techniques and substances has been proposed. In the acute setting, reconstruction with rerouting or tendon transfer of autologous tendon has been proposed of a strip of the pronator teres as well as the brachioradialis, as well as other tendon tissue.[18,20,21]

These techniques have the advantage of using local tissue that is rerouted, and are sometimes also used in the chronic setting.

Other techniques that may be considered in acute or chronic settings include synthetic manufactured materials, allogeneic or autologous

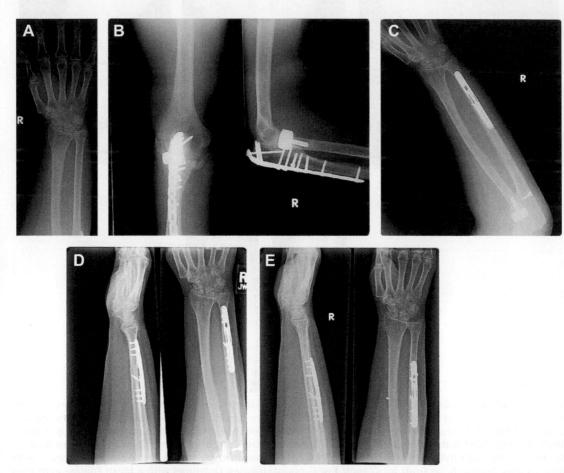

Fig. 3. This patient sustained a forearm injury with initial treatment of radial head replacement and open reduction with internal fixation of the ulna fracture. She presented subsequently with ulnar impaction (*A*) and (*B*) hardware irritation. She underwent hardware removal and ulnar shortening osteotomy (*C*); subsequently, from continued axial instability, she developed recurrent wrist and elbow discomfort and recurrent ulnar positive variance (*D*). She underwent revision ulnar shortening osteotomy and reconstruction of the IOM with a suture button construct (*E*). (*From* Gaspar et al. Interosseous membrane reconstruction with a suture-button construct for treatment of chronic forearm instability. J Shoulder Elbow Surg 2016;25:1491-500; with permission.)

bone–patellar tendon–bone graft, Achilles allograft, and flexor carpi radialis tendon.[4,17,18,21–27]

Whatever the technique or tissue used, the procedures to reconstruct the IOM attempt to replicate the restraining and tethering forces on the forearm, and in general replicate the anatomic pathway of the IOM. The central band of the IOM is a proximal radial to distal ulnarly directed band of tissue, oriented about 21° to the axis of the forearm. The radial origin is located about 40% of the radial length as measured from the radial head distally, and the ulnar insertion is located about two-thirds of the ulnar bone length as measured from the proximal ulna distally[4,28] (**Fig. 1**).

The pronator teres augmentation involves harvesting a distally based strip of the pronator tendon, leaving it attached to the distal radial insertion. The tendon tissue is then rerouted distally, and tunneled dorsally under the extensor tendons and muscles, to attachment at a site on the distal one-third of the ulna.[21]

The bone–patellar tendon–bone reconstructive technique involves placing the graft under the extensor muscles and tendons, tensioning the graft and creating a trough at the radius and ulna to accept the bony ends of the graft, which is usually secured with a screw at either end. It closely replicates the path and size of the native IOM, and more closely approximates the mechanics of the IOM than other allograft or autograft materials[10,22,26,29] (**Fig. 2**).

Recent interest in the use of manufactured materials for stabilization of the forearm has prompted use of a suture button construct for this purpose. The path of the suture button replicates that of the native IOM (**Fig. 3**). One potential advantage is the ability to place the reconstructive device with a limited incision on the radial and ulnar sides in the axis of the bones of the radius and ulna rather than resting on the dorsal side of the forearm. This method also eliminates the passage of a graft under the extensor tendons and muscles, which can be a source of irritation or tethering. The suture button technique is quite strong, and care is taken to ensure there is not overtightening of the construct.[27]

SUMMARY

There is no universal agreement on the optimal treatment of Essex-Lopresti injuries; however, a few observations seem to be readily agreed on. Patients with this constellation of injuries often initially go unrecognized or under-recognized. However, there is commonly a delay in diagnosis. Further, patients in whom the diagnosis is not recognized and or there is a delay in treatment

have poorer ultimate outcomes than those in whom the injury is recognized and treated promptly.[29,30]

Although the literature consists mostly of case series with different techniques or approaches; in the review of these cases, it seems that most successful techniques for treatment of chronic Essex-Lopresti injuries involve assessment and treatment of all 3 sites of disorder (the wrist, forearm and elbow), and that, in most series, satisfactory outcomes involve addressing the forearm instability by some sort of reconstruction of the IOM to prevent recurrent instability. In addition, even reconstruction of the IOM fails to restore forces and biomechanics to normal.[10,22]

REFERENCES

1. Essex-Lopresti P. Fractures of the radial head with distal radio-ulnar dislocation; report of two cases. J Bone Joint Surg Br 1951;33B:244–7.
2. Dodds SD, Yeh PC, Slade JF 3rd. Essex-lopresti injuries. Hand Clin 2008;24:125–37.
3. Osterman AL, Warhold L, Culp RW, et al. Reconstruction of the interosseous membrane using a bone-ligament-bone graft. American Society for Surgery of the Hand 52nd Annual Meeting. Denver, CO, September 11–13, 1997.
4. Marcotte AL, Osterman AL. Longitudinal radioulnar dissociation: identification and treatment of acute and chronic injuries. Hand Clin 2007;23:195–208.
5. Awan H, Goitz R. MRI correlation of radial head fractures and forearm injuries. Hand 2017;12:145–9.
6. Zhao YM, Li W, Tao ZG, et al. Value of MRI in the diagnosis of radial head fracture with forearm interosseous membrane injury. Zhongguo Gu Shang 2014;27:74–7 [in Chinese].
7. Okada K, Moritomo H, Miyake J, et al. Morphological evaluation of the distal interosseous membrane using ultrasound. Eur J Orthop Surg Traumatol 2014; 24:1095–100.
8. Rodriguez-Martin J, Pretell-Mazzini J. The role of ultrasound and magnetic resonance imaging in the evaluation of the forearm interosseous membrane. A review. Skeletal Radiol 2011;40:1515–22.
9. Smith AM, Urbanosky LR, Castle JA, et al. Radius pull test: predictor of longitudinal forearm instability. J Bone Joint Surg Am 2002;84:1970–6.
10. Tejwani SG, Markolf KL, Benhaim P. Graft reconstruction of the interosseous membrane in conjunction with metallic radial head replacement: a cadaveric study. J Hand Surg Am 2005;30:335–42.
11. Heijink A, Morrey BF, Cooney WP 3rd. Radiocapitellar hemiarthroplasty for radiocapitellar arthritis: A report of three cases. J Shoulder Elbow Surg 2008; 17:e12–5.

12. Kachooei AR, Heesakkers NAM, Heijink A, et al. Radiocapitellar prosthetic arthroplasty: short-term to midterm results of 19 elbows. J Shoulder Elbow Surg 2018;27:726–32.

13. Heijink A, Morrey BF, van Riet RP, et al. Delayed treatment of elbow pain and dysfunction following Essex-Lopresti injury with metallic radial head replacement: a case series. J Shoulder Elbow Surg 2010;19:929–36.

14. Watkins CEL, Elson DW, Harrison JWK, et al. Long-term results of the lateral resurfacing elbow arthroplasty. Bone Joint J 2018;100:338–45.

15. Hotchkiss RN, An KN, Sowa DT, et al. An anatomic and mechanical study of the interosseous membrane of the forearm: pathomechanics of proximal migration of the radius. J Hand Surg Am 1989;14(2 Pt 1):256–61.

16. Sowa DT, Hotchkiss RN, Weiland AJ. Symptomatic proximal translation of the radius following radial head resection. Clin Orthop Relat Res 1995;317: 106–13.

17. Skahen JR 3rd, Palmer AK, Werner FW, et al. Reconstruction of the interosseous membrane of the forearm in cadavers. J Hand Surg Am 1997;22:986–94.

18. Ruch DS, Chang DS, Koman LA. Reconstruction of longitudinal stability of the forearm after disruption of interosseous ligament and radial head excision (Essex-Lopresti lesion). J South Orthop Assoc 1999;8:47–52.

19. Failla JM, Jacobson J, van Holsbeeck M. Ultrasound diagnosis and surgical pathology of the torn interosseous membrane in forearm fractures/dislocations. J Hand Surg Am 1999;24:257–66.

20. Apergis EP, Masouros PT, Nikolaou VS, et al. Central band reconstruction for the treatment of Essex-Lopresti injury : A novel technique using the brachioradialis tendon. Acta Orthop Belg 2019;85: 63–71.

21. Chloros GD, Wiesler ER, Stabile KJ, et al. Reconstruction of essex-lopresti injury of the forearm: technical note. J Hand Surg Am 2008;33:124–30.

22. Sellman DC, Seitz WH Jr, Postak PD, et al. Reconstructive strategies for radioulnar dissociation: a biomechanical study. J Orthop Trauma 1995;9: 516–22.

23. Pfaeffle HJ, Stabile KJ, Li ZM, et al. Reconstruction of the interosseous ligament unloads metallic radial head arthroplasty and the distal ulna in cadavers. J Hand Surg Am 2006;31:269–78.

24. Pfaeffle HJ, Stabile KJ, Li ZM, et al. Reconstruction of the interosseous ligament restores normal forearm compressive load transfer in cadavers. J Hand Surg Am 2005;30:319–25.

25. Tomaino MM, Pfaeffle J, Stabile K, et al. Reconstruction of the interosseous ligament of the forearm reduces load on the radial head in cadavers. J Hand Surg Br 2003;28:267–70.

26. Gaspar MP, Adams JE, Zohn RC, et al. Late reconstruction of the interosseous membrane with bone-patellar tendon-bone graft for chronic essex-lopresti injuries: outcomes with a mean follow-up of over 10 years. J Bone Joint Surg Am 2018;100: 416–27.

27. Gaspar MP, Kane PM, Pflug EM, et al. Interosseous membrane reconstruction with a suture-button construct for treatment of chronic forearm instability. J Shoulder Elbow Surg 2016;25:1491–500.

28. Skahen JR 3rd, Palmer AK, Werner FW, et al. The interosseous membrane of the forearm: Anatomy and function. J Hand Surg Am 1997;22:981–5.

29. Adams JE, Culp RW, Osterman AL. Interosseous membrane reconstruction for the Essex-Lopresti injury. J Hand Surg Am 2010;35:129–36.

30. Troudale RT, Amadio PC, Cooney WP, et al. Radio-ulnar dissociation. A review of twenty cases. J Bone Joint Surg Am 1992;74:1486–97.

Management of Monteggia Injuries in the Pediatric Patient

Tyler C. Miller, MD, Felicity G. Fishman, MD*

KEYWORDS

- Pediatric Monteggia • Radial head dislocation • Ulnar osteotomy • Annular ligament

KEY POINTS

- Monteggia fracture-dislocations in the pediatric population have unique patterns of injury that require distinct considerations in diagnosis and management.
- Successful treatment of acute pediatric Monteggia fracture-dislocations depends on early diagnosis with appropriate radiographic assessment followed by prompt and stable reduction of the ulna fracture and radiocapitellar joint.
- Corrective ulnar osteotomy is a key component in the reconstruction of chronic Monteggia lesions, whereas additional procedures such as annular ligament repair or reconstruction may provide secondary stabilization.

INTRODUCTION

In 1814, Giovanni Battista Monteggia first described a fracture of the ulna with associated dislocation of the radiocapitellar joint and disruption of the proximal radioulnar joint.[1,2] Although our understanding of the now eponymous Monteggia injury has improved since its first description, evaluation and management of this condition remains a challenge. Despite often being grouped together with the adult counterpart, Monteggia fracture-dislocations in the pediatric population can have unique injury patterns that require particular attention and consideration in diagnosis and management. The primary focus of any treatment is stable reduction of the radiocapitellar joint, typically guided by anatomic reduction of the ulna. In adults, this injury pattern typically warrants surgical stabilization due to the associated complete and often comminuted ulna fracture. However, the nature of fractures in the immature bone of children results in a variety of injury patterns that may influence treatment. Incomplete or plastically deformed fractures are often more stable and may allow maintenance of anatomic reduction in a cast. Therefore, in children, operative intervention is reserved for comminuted or length unstable fractures. When diagnosis and appropriate treatment are accomplished in the acute setting, outcomes are generally favorable, with recovery of forearm and elbow motion and fracture union. If radial head dislocation or subluxation is not recognized or adequately treated, it can lead to progressive instability, deformity, loss of motion, as well as tardy ulnar and/or radial nerve palsies.[3–9] Although chronic Monteggia lesions may necessitate more complex surgical reconstructions and are associated with less predictable outcomes, the principles of restoring ulnar length and radiocapitellar stability remain.[10,11]

CLASSIFICATION

Bado's original classification based on the direction of the radial head dislocation and the direction of the apex of the associated ulna fracture

Department of Orthopaedic Surgery & Rehabilitation, Loyola University Medical Center, 2160 South First Avenue, Maguire Center, Suite 1700, Maywood, IL 60153, USA
* Corresponding author.
E-mail address: Felicity.fishman@lumc.edu

Hand Clin 36 (2020) 469–478
https://doi.org/10.1016/j.hcl.2020.07.001

remains the most commonly used method of categorizing Monteggia fracture-dislocations. This system, which describes 4 true Monteggia types, has been expanded on with the subsequent publication of numerous case reports describing various Monteggia-equivalent lesions based on similar mechanism of injury. These equivalent lesions are especially notable in children due to the pliability of skeletally immature bone and the possibility of associated physeal fractures. An alternative classification was proposed by Letts and colleagues[12] that accommodates the unique nature of these pediatric injuries (**Fig. 1**). Their classification highlighted the possibility of radial head dislocation in the presence of plastic deformation or incomplete fracture of the ulna in children.

DIAGNOSIS

The standard evaluation of a Monteggia fracture-dislocation should include anteroposterior (AP) and lateral radiographs of the forearm and elbow. The importance of being able to evaluate the alignment of the radiocapitellar joint is paramount. Although oblique views can often augment the examiner's understanding of the injury, the relationship between the radial head and the capitellum is best interpreted on a true lateral of the elbow. Forearm radiographs are carefully evaluated for any disruption in the ulna, including altered bowing of the dorsal border that may signal disruption of the proximal radioulnar joint. Obtaining similar radiographs of the uninjured, contralateral extremity can provide a helpful comparison that may facilitate identifying subtle side-to-side differences. Occasionally fluoroscopic imaging, ultrasound or MRI can provide additional information to make or exclude the diagnosis.

Evaluating the pediatric elbow and appropriate joint alignment on conventional radiographs can be especially challenging in younger children due to the initially absent and subsequent dynamic ossification of cartilage during development.[13] First described by Storen,[14] the radiocapitellar line has long served as a method of recognizing deviations from the normal anatomic alignment of the pediatric elbow. The radiocapitellar line, drawn through the center of the radial neck and head, is expected to intersect the capitellum on a lateral radiograph regardless of the degree of flexion or extension of the elbow[14,15] (**Fig. 2**). Patient age, forearm positioning, and obliquity of the radiograph may affect the accuracy of the radiocapitellar line. Much discussion exists concerning the method in which the line should be drawn on the radius as well as how it should intersect the capitellum and whether the relationship holds true on additional elbow radiographic views.[13,16–18] Despite these limitations, the radiocapitellar line remains a useful tool in the initial evaluation of pediatric elbow injuries that may potentially identify radiocapitellar joint dislocation.

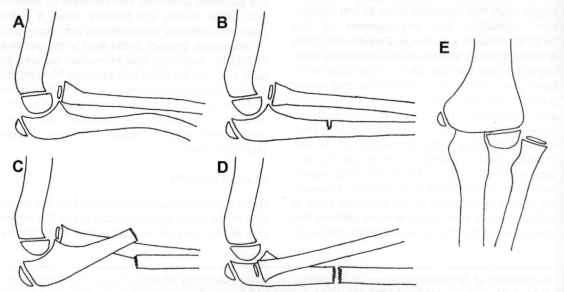

Fig. 1. Letts classification of pediatric Monteggia fracture-dislocation. (*A*) Anterior dislocation of radial head with plastic deformation of ulna. (*B*) Anterior dislocation of radial head with greenstick fracture of ulna. (*C*) Anterior dislocation of radial head with complete fracture of the ulna. (*D*) Posterior dislocation of the radial head with complete fracture of the ulna. (*E*) Lateral dislocation of the radial head with greenstick fracture of the ulna.

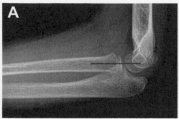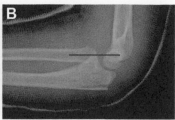

Fig. 2. (*A*) Lateral radiograph of an uninjured elbow demonstrating the radiocapitellar line, drawn through the center of the radial neck and head, intersecting the capitellum. (*B*) Lateral radiograph of a Monteggia injury with anterior radial head subluxation demonstrating the radiocapitellar line passing anterior to the capitellum.

MANAGEMENT

All Monteggia injuries warrant a formal reduction; however, the optimal approach to achieve the reduction as well as indications for nonoperative versus operative treatment are matters of debate. Despite a lack of consensus on a standard treatment protocol, there is general agreement that successful treatment of acute pediatric Monteggia fractures depends on early diagnosis and stable reduction of the ulna fracture and radiocapitellar joint.

Historically, treatment algorithms for both adult and pediatric injuries have been guided by the Bado classification in terms of how the fracture deformation should be approached to achieve stable reduction of the radiocapitellar joint. Closed reduction and casting has been successful in treating pediatric Monteggia fractures of all types.[10,12,19] However, an understanding of the risk for loss of reduction and potential for recurrent instability with cast immobilization alone is required of both the physician and family. A discussion regarding this possibility and the need for close follow-up with weekly radiographs for at least the first 3 weeks will help manage expectations.

Acute Monteggia Fractures

Nonoperative

Nonoperative treatment in the form of closed reduction and long arm casting is best accomplished in the acute setting. Attempts at closed reduction have been met with failure as early as 2 weeks after the injury.[9] In contrast, some cases of closed reduction and casting may still be successful in patients diagnosed up to 4 weeks after their initial injury.[3] No specific time interval separating successful and unsuccessful attempts at closed reduction has been established. However, most investigators agree that injuries greater than 4 weeks old represent chronic Monteggia lesions, and nonoperative treatment is likely to be unsuccessful.[20–22]

Anatomic reduction of the ulna fracture is achieved through a combination of longitudinal traction, forearm rotation, and manual manipulation to correct any angular deformity or plastic deformation. Once ulnar length has been reestablished, the radiocapitellar joint will often reduce spontaneously, or reduction can be aided by appropriately directed pressure on the radial head and positioning of the elbow depending on lesion type (**Fig. 3**). Inability to reduce the radial head or the need for application of significant force should raise suspicion for interposed soft tissue blocking the reduction and the potential need for an open reduction of the radiocapitellar joint. Furthermore, excessive hyperflexion of the elbow to maintain reduction should be used with caution, as this may lead to nerve injury, vascular insult, and subsequent compartment syndrome. Injuries necessitating extreme positioning to maintain reduction may be better treated with surgery.

Reduction Maneuvers Based on Bado Type

- Bado type 1 fractures are immobilized in 90° to 110° elbow flexion and near full forearm

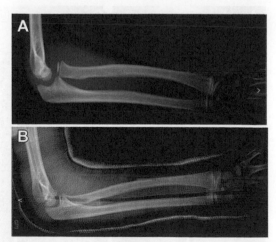

Fig. 3. (*A*) An 8-year-old boy with acute Monteggia injury with plastic deformation of the ulna and anterior dislocation of the radial head. (*B*) Following closed reduction and casting with correction of the ulnar deformity and reestablishment of radiocapitellar alignment. (Images Courtesy of Sarah Sibbel, MD.)

supination to tighten the interosseous membrane and relax the biceps tendon.[23]

- Bado type 2 fractures are treated in elbow extension to relax the triceps and maintain reduction of the ulna.
- Bado type 3 injuries may also be treated in elbow extension with the addition of a valgus mold; however, relative flexion may be required depending on the direction of radial head displacement.[10]
- Bado type 4 injuries are treated in a similar manner as other Bado types with aims of conversion to a type 1 lesion but can be complicated by a free-floating proximal radial fragment.[15]

In all cases, appropriate reduction should be confirmed under fluoroscopy and a long arm cast applied. The child should be seen in follow-up weekly to evaluate alignment and confirm maintenance of reduction with serial radiographs. Immobilization is continued for 4 to 6 weeks to allow for bony healing before cast removal, initiation of elbow range-of-motion exercises, and progressive return to activity.

Operative

The primary operative indications for any Monteggia fracture include inability to obtain or maintain reduction of either the ulnar fracture or the radiocapitellar joint. Debate continues regarding which injuries require initial operative management versus a trial of closed reduction and casting.[2,10,24] However, with appreciation for the importance of stable anatomic reduction of the ulna to optimize outcome,[25,26] some investigators have advocated a treatment strategy based on the type of ulna fracture.[2,15,23,24]

Using this treatment algorithm, first proposed by Ring and Waters,[2] incomplete or length stable fractures, including plastic deformation or greenstick fractures, are treated with closed reduction and casting as previously described.

Patients with complete, yet length-stable fractures such as transverse or short oblique ulna fractures may remain unstable after closed reduction (**Fig. 4**A, B). In this clinical scenario, intramedullary (IM) fixation of the ulna is recommended to facilitate stable reduction and help maintain ulnar length and alignment as well as radiocapitellar reduction.[11] Depending on the child's age and weight, an appropriately sized K-wire or flexible nail is selected. The lateral view of the forearm can be used to measure the isthmus and select a nail approximately two-thirds of this diameter. A small incision is made over the tip of the olecranon just radial to the center to accommodate for the radial bow of the proximal ulna. A drill sleeve protector is inserted through the triceps, and the cortex of the proximal ulna is opened with a drill bit slightly larger than the chosen flexible nail or K-wire (**Fig. 5**). The wire or nail is then inserted with a T-handled chuck through the opening in the cortex and advanced across the fracture site after a reduction is obtained. Serendipitous reduction of the radiocapitellar joint often occurs or may

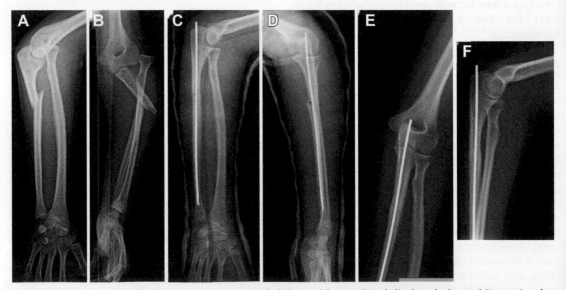

Fig. 4. (*A, B*) A 12-year-old girl with acute Monteggia injury with associated displaced, short-oblique ulna fracture. (*C, D*) Following closed reduction and IM nail fixation of the ulna. (*E, F*) Three-month follow-up demonstrating cortical healing of the ulna fracture and maintenance of radiocapitellar alignment.

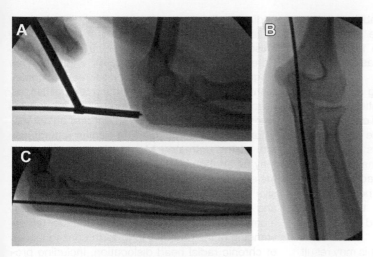

Fig. 5. Operative technique for IM stabilization of ulna fracture. (*A*) Cortex of the proximal ulna is opened using a drill bit protected by a drill sleeve inserted through a small incision made over the tip of olecranon. (*B, C*) Following fracture reduction, a flexible nail or K-wire is passed into the canal, and positioning is confirmed on AP and lateral radiographs.

be performed simultaneously. The nail can be bent and cut outside the skin to facilitate easy removal in the office in 6 weeks or cut beneath the skin for future removal in the operating room. A long arm cast is applied with the elbow in 90° of flexion and the forearm in supination (**Fig. 4**C, D). Immobilization is continued for 4 to 6 weeks and may be discontinued (and the IM nail removed if left outside the skin) on confirmation of bony healing on radiographs. In children, although the fracture line may still be visible at 6 weeks, adequate healing is represented by visible callous on at least 3 cortices on orthogonal radiographs (**Fig. 4**E, F).

In contrast to short oblique or transverse ulna fractures, long oblique and comminuted fractures are considered "length unstable" and therefore are treated with plate and screw fixation to avoid shortening and malalignment, which are more likely to occur with alternative treatment methods, including IM fixation (**Fig. 6**A, B). Reduction is performed through a longitudinal incision along the subcutaneous border of the ulna. An appropriate plate is chosen based on the size of the child and applied using standard techniques. In these cases in which the goal is to maintain length of the ulna, 4 to 6 cortices of fixation on either side

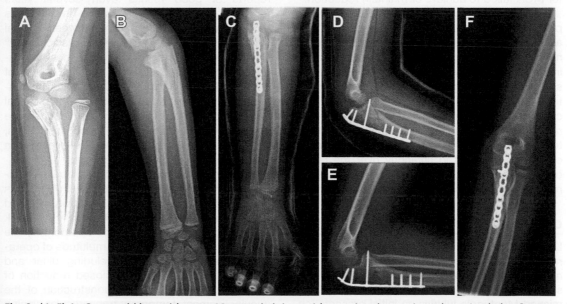

Fig. 6. (*A, B*) An 8-year-old boy with acute Monteggia injury with associated comminuted proximal ulna fracture. (*C, D*) Following open reduction internal fixation of the ulna. (*E, F*) Six-month follow-up demonstrating complete healing of the ulna fracture and maintenance of radiocapitellar alignment.

of the fracture provide adequate stability, as this will be augmented by postoperative immobilization. Radiocapitellar joint reduction is achieved and confirmed in a similar manner as previously described (**Fig. 6**C–F).

With this treatment algorithm, Ring and Waters reported excellent results in all 28 patients treated within 24 hours of injury.[2] Ramski and colleagues[24] retrospectively evaluated 112 acute Monteggia fractures and found no subluxations or dislocations of the radial head or loss of ulnar fixation in 57 patients treated with this ulnar fracture-based treatment strategy, whereas 6 of these failures occurred in a group of 32 patients treated less rigorously with closed reduction and casting for complete fractures.

However, some surgeons believe this may result in overtreatment of these injuries and contend that most acute pediatric Monteggia fractures can be treated nonoperatively with favorable outcomes. Foran and colleagues[10] evaluated a more conservative approach for 94 acute Monteggia fractures and found an 83% success rate with initial closed reduction and casting. Bado type (II and III) and increased ulnar angulation were identified as risk factors for loss of reduction and the potential need for secondary surgical stabilization. In another study, Leonidou and colleagues[19] reported excellent outcomes at an average follow-up of 4.6 years in 32 of 40 acute Monteggia fractures treated with manipulation under anesthesia (MUA) and casting. The remaining 8 patients underwent open reduction internal fixation only after MUA failed to achieve or maintain reduction.

In some cases closed reduction of the radiocapitellar joint is unable to be achieved even after appropriately reestablishing ulnar length and alignment. The treating surgeon must not accept imperfect reductions and should consider the possibility of annular ligament or periosteal interposition that prevents reduction. In these circumstances, open reduction with careful exploration of the joint and removal of interposed structures is warranted. A displaced annular ligament can often be reduced anteriorly over the radius or if necessary, partially incised, and subsequently repaired following appropriate reduction.

Chronic Monteggia Lesions

Late presentation of a Monteggia injury or missed radial head dislocation following injury in a child is not an uncommon occurrence.[3,6,27] Multiple reasons have been proposed for the high rate of missed Monteggia injuries on initial presentation, including inadequate initial radiographs, difficulty interpreting the various ossification centers of the pediatric elbow, as well as simply overlooking radial injury while focusing on ulnar displacement (misdiagnosed isolated ulnar fracture).[6,9,25,28] Careful scrutiny of high-quality AP and lateral radiographs of both the elbow and forearm, supplemented with alternative imaging modalities as needed, will minimize the number of missed injuries and lead to better treatment and outcomes.

Earlier reports suggested a benign natural history of the untreated Monteggia lesion,[15] which may be attributable to the remodeling capacity of the skeletally immature child as well as a progressive nature in symptoms with continued growth and increasing functional demands.[6,7] However, a paradigm shift has occurred with a better understanding of the potential long-term consequences of chronic radial head dislocation, including progressive dysplasia of both the radial head and the distal humerus, instability, deformity, loss of motion, arthritis, as well as tardy ulnar and radial nerve palsies.[3–9] Presently, nonoperative management has a limited role in the treatment of chronic Monteggia lesions.[7,29,30]

A consensus for successful treatment of chronic Monteggia lesions has not been achieved and a review of the current literature will demonstrate a wide variety of treatment indications and approaches. Specific operative indications include pain, decreased range of motion, progressive deformity, and functional disability.[8,9,15,31] Reports also vary regarding the time interval between injury and treatment as well as patient age at the time of surgical intervention.[7,8,22,25,32] Although there are reports of good results even several years following the initial injury, some investigators have demonstrated a correlation between surgical success and duration of radial head dislocation.[7,8] Despite the lack of specific criteria, most investigators agree that surgical reconstruction of chronic Monteggia lesions is best suited for patients with minimal dysplastic changes of the radial head or capitellum.[7,22,33,34] In the younger age group before complete radial head ossification, an MRI may be necessary to evaluate for dysplasia when considering operative treatment.

Controversy exists regarding appropriate treatment of chronic Monteggia lesions with high rates of complications and recurrent instability reported following operative reconstruction.[9,35,36] The lack of a standard protocol is made apparent by the proposal and modification of a multitude of operative procedures,[8,28,32,33,37] including ulnar and radial osteotomies, open or closed reduction of the radial head, repair or reconstruction of the annular ligament, temporary transarticular pinning of the radiocapitellar joint, or a combination of these. The complexity and frequently unpredictable results of surgical reconstruction for chronic Monteggia lesions highlight the importance of appropriate initial recognition and treatment.[8,10]

Despite the variability in proposed approaches for management of the chronic pediatric Monteggia, the unifying principle is restoration of the radiocapitellar articulation and correction of the persistent ulnar deformity. Ulnar osteotomy is used to restore both ulnar length and axis in order to reestablish the normal anatomic relationship between the radius and the ulna, particularly at the proximal radioulnar joint. Early reports have demonstrated success but also highlighted the complexity and potential complications associated with these procedures.[9,38] Numerous case series have subsequently been published on the successful use of ulnar osteotomies in the treatment of chronic Monteggia lesions.

Surgical treatment is typically performed through a single posterolateral incision (Boyd[3,21,22,35,38] or Kocher approach[8,9,39]) that allows exposure of both the proximal ulna and the radiocapitellar joint.

In order to ensure a concentric radiocapitellar joint, most investigators advocate open reduction to release capsular contractures, excise interposed tissue, and identify any remnant annular ligament.[8,21,22,36,37] Using an alternative technique, some argue that open reduction of the radial head may not be necessary, reporting successful closed reduction with the use of external fixation and gradual lengthening through an ulnar osteotomy.[31,40] Use of this method may be less

invasive and may allow for guided adjustments in the postoperative period to achieve and maintain reduction of the radial head; however, the prolonged periods of external fixation necessary may limit its utility.

Osteotomy is most commonly performed in the metaphysis of the proximal ulna where blood supply is robust but can also be performed at the site of the previous fracture if an obvious deformity persists (**Fig. 7**). A posterior opening wedge osteotomy addresses the most common ulnar malunion associated with an anteriorly dislocated radial head, although anterior- or lateral-based osteotomies may better address some lesions depending on the direction of dislocation. Hubbard and colleagues[6] advocated for a crescentic osteotomy to minimize risk of nonunion. Although some have described an osteotomy at the center of rotation of angulation,[7,36,41,42] remodeling of the ulna over time can make the exact location difficult to determine, and in cases where this may result in diaphyseal cuts, there may be an increased risk for nonunion.[41]

Through the osteotomy, the ulna is lengthened and/or angulated in a manner to facilitate reduction of the radial head. Previous studies described simple correction of the ulna to its anatomic position[20,43] versus overcorrection resulting in a more angulated position.[21,22,40,41] Review of the recent literature offers the recommendation that the degree of angular correction is best determined by the position that allows for stable reduction of the radial head throughout elbow and forearm range of motion.[8,21,37,41,44] The osteotomy site is

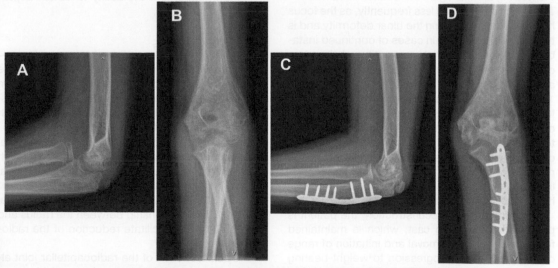

Fig. 7. (A, B) A 8-year-old boy with chronic Monteggia Lesion showing persistent radial head dislocation without significant dysplastic changes. (C, D) Following corrective ulnar osteotomy and reestablishment of radiocapitellar alignment. (Images Courtesy of Sarah Sibbel, MD.)

typically rigidly fixed with a plate-and-screw construct[8,9,21,22,36,38,41,44] although other methods have been used including Kirschner wire[3,9,20,43] and external fixation.[31,37,39,40]

Following ulnar osteotomy and successful reduction of the radiocapitellar joint, debate continues regarding the necessity and method of maintaining stability of the radial head in the treatment of pediatric chronic Monteggia lesions. Many investigators advocate for annular ligament repair or reconstruction as part of the treatment strategy to increase stability of the joint.[8,12,21,22,25,45] Although the remnant annular ligament may be used or augmented if present, multiple methods of ligament reconstruction have been described, including the use of a strip of triceps tendon,[7,22,35,36,45] a fascial loop,[12,20,25,42] and a free palmaris tendon graft.[8]

In contrast, some investigators argue that correction of the ulnar deformity facilitates stability of the radial head through tensioning of the interosseous membrane, and annular ligament reconstruction may not be necessary in every case.[21,37,38] In a direct comparison of ulnar osteotomy and open reduction of the radiocapitellar joint with and without annular ligament reconstruction, Delpont and colleagues[44] found no significant difference in clinical functional outcomes and concluded that annular ligament reconstruction does not guarantee radial head stability and is not beneficial in conjunction with ulnar osteotomy in the treatment of chronic Monteggia lesions.

In the past, some investigators have used temporary pinning of the radiocapitellar joint as a means of maintaining reduction and protecting the healing annular ligament reconstruction.[22,25,36] This technique is used less frequently, as the focus has shifted to correcting the ulnar deformity and is typically only be used in cases of continued instability despite appropriate correction of the ulnar deformity and repair or reconstruction of the annular ligament.[37,44]

In the operative reconstruction of a chronic Monteggia lesion, a safe approach may involve continually reassessing stability of the radiocapitellar joint following open reduction and ulnar osteotomy, making necessary adjustments to the position of the osteotomy or considering annular ligament repair or reconstruction to ensure radial head stability postoperatively.

Following surgical reconstruction, the patient is placed in a long arm cast, which is maintained for 6 weeks before removal and initiation of range of motion. Further progression to weight-bearing and activity should be dictated by clinical and radiographic evaluation of osteotomy healing and regaining motion. Additional procedures may be required to address hardware irritation as well as the possibility of recurrent radial head instability.

SUMMARY

The understanding and treatment of Monteggia lesions has continued to evolve over the last several decades. The unique patterns of this injury seen in children make them distinct from the adult counterpart and require special consideration in almost every aspect of diagnosis and treatment. Additional clarification of best management practices for acute and chronic pediatric Monteggia lesions will require prospective, comparative research studies. Despite ongoing debate and lack of consensus on many elements of management, there are several principles that may guide a surgeon treating a Monteggia fracture-dislocation in a skeletally immature individual.

Acute Monteggia

- Pediatric forearm and elbow injuries require radiographic assessment of a true AP and lateral view of both the elbow and forearm with careful evaluation of radiocapitellar alignment.
- The presence of an ulna fracture or plastic deformation should prompt suspicion for radial head dislocation and visa versa.
- Successful treatment depends on early diagnosis and stable reduction of the ulna fracture and radiocapitellar joint.
- Nonoperative and operative treatment should be dictated by the injury pattern, stability of the fracture, and the ability to obtain appropriate reduction.

Chronic Monteggia

- Chronic Monteggia lesions necessitate more complex surgical reconstructions and are associated with less predictable outcomes, yet the principles of restoring ulnar length and radiocapitellar stability remain.
- Although no specific criteria exist, surgical reconstruction is best suited for patients with minimal dysplastic changes of the radial head or capitellum.
- Ulnar osteotomy is used to restore the normal anatomic relationship between the radius and the ulna and facilitate reduction of the radiocapitellar joint.
- Open reduction of the radiocapitellar joint allows excision of interposed tissue, release of capsular contractures, and identification of remnant annular ligament into which the radial

head may be reduced for secondary stabilization.

- Additional procedures to maintain stability of the radial head including annular ligament incision and repair or reconstruction should be dictated by persistent radiocapitellar instability following reassessment of the adequacy of the corrective ulnar osteotomy.

Future management of chronic pediatric Monteggia lesions may use patient-specific templating of complex ulnar deformities. Computed tomography (CT)-based 3-dimensional modeling allows for precise preoperative planning and is subsequently combined with 3-dimensional printing of patient-specific drill and osteotomy guides. This technology is increasingly being explored in orthopedics and in one study has demonstrated to be a safe and effective method for precise corrections of complex forearm deformities in children.[46] Disadvantages include the need for standardized CT images of both the affected and unaffected extremities for templating purposes, time constraints between modeling and operative intervention associated with continued development in a skeletally immature patient, and overall cost. Further research and development will help streamline this process and may prove this technology to be a valuable tool in treatment of complex chronic pediatric Monteggia lesions in the future.

DISCLOSURE

The authors have nothing to disclose.

REFERENCES

1. Bado J. The Monteggia lesion. Clin Orthop Relat Res 1967;(50):71–86.
2. Ring D, Waters P. Operative fixation of Montggia fractures in children. J Bone Joint Surg Br 1996; 78-B(5):734–9.
3. David-West KS, Wilson NI, Sherlock DA, et al. Missed Monteggia injuries. Injury 2005;36(10): 1206–9.
4. Dormans J, Rang M. The problem of Monteggia fracture-dislocations in children. Orthop Clin North Am 1990;21(2):251–6.
5. Holst-Nielsen F, Jensen V. Tardy posterior interosseous nerve palsy as a result of an unreduced radial head dislocation in Monteggia fractures: A report of two cases. J Hand Surg 1984;9(4):572–5.
6. Hubbard J, Chauhan A, Fitzgerald R, et al. Missed Pediatric Monteggia Fractures. JBJS Rev 2018; 6(6):e2.
7. Kim HT, Conjares JNV, Suh JT, et al. Chronic radial head dislocation in children, part 1: pathologic changes preventing stable reduction and surgical correction. J Pediatr Orthop 2002;22:583–90.
8. Nakamura K, Hirachi K, Uchiyama S, et al. Long-term clinical and radiographic outcomes after open reduction for missed Monteggia fracture-dislocations in children. J Bone Joint Surg Am 2009;91(6):1394–404.
9. Rodgers WB, Waters PM, Hall JE. Chronic monteggia lesions in children, complications and results of reconstruction. J Bone Joint Surg Am 1996;78-A(9):1322–9.
10. Foran I, Upasani VV, Wallace CD, et al. Acute pediatric monteggia fractures: a conservative approach to stabilization. J Pediatr Orthop 2017;37(6):e335–41.
11. Waters PM, Bae DS. Monteggia fracture dislocations. In: Waters PM, Bae DS, editors. Pediatric hand and upper limb surgery: a practical guide. Philadelphia: Lippincott Williams & Wilkins; 2012. p. 351–65.
12. Letts M, Locht R, Wiens J. Monteggia fracture-dislocations in children. J Bone Joint Surg Br 1985; 67-B(5):724–7.
13. Fader LM, Laor T, Eismann EA, et al. Eccentric Capitellar ossification limits the utility of the radiocapitellar line in young children. J Pediatr Orthop 2016; 36(2):161–6.
14. Storen G. Traumatic dislocation of the radial head as an isolated lesion in children; Report of one case with special regard to roentgen diagnosis. Acta Chir Scand 1959;116:144–7.
15. Shah AS, Waters PM. Monteggia fracture-dislocation in children. In: Flynn JM, Skaggs DL, Waters PM, editors. Rockwood and Wilkins' fractures in children. 8th edition. Philadelphia: Wolters Kluwer Health; 2015. p. 527–63.
16. Kunkel S, Cornwall R, Little K, et al. Limitations of the radiocapitellar line for assessment of pediatric elbow radiographs. J Pediatr Orthop 2011;31(6): 628–32.
17. Miles KA, Finlay DB. Disruption of the radiocapitellar line in the normal elbow. Injury 1989;20:365–7.
18. Wang C, Su Y. An alternative to the traditional radiocapitellar line for pediatric forearm radiograph assessment in Monteggia fracture. J Pediatr Orthop 2020;40(3):e216–21.
19. Leonidou A, Pagkalos J, Lepetsos P, et al. Pediatric Monteggia fractures: a single-center study of the management of 40 patients. J Pediatr Orthop 2012;32(4):352–6.
20. Hui JHP, Sulaiman AR, Lee H, et al. Open reduction and annular ligament reconstruction with fascia of the forearm in chronic Monteggia lesions in children. J Pediatr Orthop 2005;25(4):501–6.
21. Song KS, Ramnani K, Bae KC, et al. Indirect reduction of the radial head in children with chronic Monteggia lesions. J Orthop Trauma 2012;26(10): 597–601.

22. Stoll TM, Willis RB, Paterson DC. Treatment of the missed Monteggia fracture in the child. J Bone Joint Surg Br 1992;74-B(3):436–40.

23. Ring D, Jupiter J, Waters P. Monteggia fractures in children and adults. J Am Acad Orthop Surg 1998; 6(4):215–24.

24. Ramski D, Hennriku W, Bae D, et al. Pediatric Monteggia fractures: a multicenter examination of treatment strategy and early clinical and radiographic results. J Pediatr Orthop 2015;35(2):115–20.

25. Fowles J, Sliman N, Kassab M, et al. The Monteggia lesion in children. Fracture of the ulna and dislocation of the radial head. J Bone Joint Surg Br 1983; 65-A(9):1276–83.

26. OB W, Menelaus MB. Monteggia and equivalent lesions in childhood. J Pediatr Orthop 1989;9:219–23.

27. Gleeson AP, Beattie TF. Monteggia fracture-dislocation in children. J Accid Emerg Med 1994; 11:192–4.

28. Wang Q, Du MM, Pei XJ, et al. External fixator-assisted ulnar osteotomy: a novel technique to treat missed monteggia fracture in children. Orthop Surg 2019;11(1):102–8.

29. Kim HT, Park BG, Suh JT, et al. Chronic radial head dislocation in children, part 2: results of open treatment and factors affecting final outcome. J Pediatr Orthop 2002;22:591–7.

30. Take M, Tomori Y, Sawaizumi T, et al. Ulnar osteotomy and the ilizarov mini-fixator for pediatric chronic monteggia fracture-dislocations. Medicine (Baltimore) 2019;98(1):e13978.

31. Bor N, Rubin G, Rozen N, et al. Chronic anterior monteggia lesions in children: report of 4 cases treated with closed reduction by ulnar osteotomy and external fixation. J Pediatr Orthop 2015;35(1): 7–10.

32. Seel MJ, Peterson HA. Management of chronic post-traumatic radial head dislocation in children. J Pediatr Orthop 1999;19(3):306–12.

33. Goyal T, Arora SS, Banerjee S, et al. Neglected Monteggia fracture dislocations in children: a systematic review. J Pediatr Orthop B 2015;24(3):191–9.

34. Oka K, Murase T, Moritomo H, et al. Morphologic evaluation of chronic radial head dislocation: three-dimensional and quantitative analyses. Clin Orthop Relat Res 2010;468(9):2410–8.

35. Oner FC, Diepstraten AFM. Treatment of chronic post-traumatic dislocation of the radial head in children. J Bone Joint Surg Br 1993;75-B(4):577–81.

36. Best TN. Management of old unreduced monteggia fracture dislocations of the elbow in children. J Pediatr Orthop 1994;14(2):193–9.

37. Lu X, Wang Y, Zhang J, et al. Management of missed monteggia fractures with ulnar osteotomy, open reduction, and dual-socket external fixation. J Pediatr Orthop 2013;33(4):398–402.

38. Hirayama T, Takemitsu T, Yagihara K, et al. Operation for chronic dislocation of the radial head in children, reduction by osteotomy of the ulna. J Bone Joint Surg Br 1987;69-B(4):639–42.

39. Hasler CC, Von Laer L, Hell AK. Open reduction, ulnar osteotomy and external fixation for chronic anterior dislocation of the head of the radius. J Bone Joint Surg Br 2003;87-B(1):88–94.

40. Exner GU. Missed chronic anterior monteggia lesion, closed reduction by gradual lengthening and angulation of the ulna. J Bone Joint Surg Br 2001;83-B(4):547–50.

41. Ladermann A, Ceroni D, Lefevre Y, et al. Surgical treatment of missed Monteggia lesions in children. J Child Orthop 2007;1(4):237–42.

42. Wang MN, Chang W. Chronic posttraumatic anterior dislocation of the radial head in children, thirteen cases treated by open reduction, ulnar osteotomy, and annular ligament reconstruction through a boyd incision. J Orthop Trauma 2006;20(1):1–5.

43. Inoue G, Shionoya K. Corrective ulnar osteotomy for malunited anterior Monteggia lesions in children. 12 patients followed for 1-12 years. Acta Orthop Scand 1998;69(1):73–6.

44. Delpont M, Jouve JL, Sales de Gauzy J, et al. Proximal ulnar osteotomy in the treatment of neglected childhood Monteggia lesion. Orthop Traumatol Surg Res 2014;100(7):803–7.

45. Bell Tawse AJ. The treatment of malunited anterior monteggia fractures in children. J Bone Joint Surg Br 1965;47(4):718–23.

46. Bauer AS, Storelli DAR, Sibbel SE, et al. Preoperative computer simulation and patient-specific guides are safe and effective to correct forearm deformity in children. J Pediatr Orthop 2017;37(7):504–10.

Management of Monteggia Injuries in the Adult

Midhat Patel, MD[a,*], Niloofar Dehghan, MD, FRCS[b]

KEYWORDS

• Monteggia fracture • Ulna fracture • Elbow fracture • Elbow dislocation • Radial head

KEY POINTS

• Monteggia fractures-dislocations in adults require open reduction and internal fixation for optimal outcomes.
• Restoration of the native ulnar anatomy is critical for a good outcome, and attention should be given to the proximal ulnar dorsal angulation and the proximal varus angulation of the ulna.
• The elbow should be evaluated closely for associated fractures or ligamentous injuries, and these should be treated at the time of ulna fixation.

INTRODUCTION

Monteggia injuries were originally described in 1814.[1] A Monteggia injury refers to a fracture of the proximal ulna with associated dislocation of the radial head, with or without an associated fracture of the radial head or proximal radial shaft. The ulna fracture is generally distal to the coronoid, with disruption of the radiocapitellar and proximal radioulnar joints.

ANATOMY

The radius and the ulna are connected proximally by the annular and quadrate ligaments. In a Monteggia fracture, these ligaments are disrupted, leading to dissociation of the proximal radioulnar joint (PRUJ).[2] Distally, the interosseous membrane and triangular fibrocartilage complex remain intact. These soft tissue anchors lead to restoration of the PRUJ with anatomic reduction of the ulna except in the rare case of soft-tissue interposition.[3]

The proximal ulnar-humeral articulation is a hinge joint (ginglymus), consisting of the trochlea and greater sigmoid notch allowing flexion and extension.[4] The anatomy of the proximal ulna is complex, with angulation in the varus-valgus and dorsal-volar planes that must be accounted for during surgical fixation. The varus angulation (VA) and proximal ulna dorsal angulation (PUDA) must be considered when reconstructing the ulna[5] (Fig. 1).

The varus angulation of the ulna can be measured as the angle between a line parallel to the olecranon and a line parallel to the ulnar shaft. It has been shown in cadaveric studies to be a mean of 18° in most specimens.[6,7]

The PUDA is measured as the angle between lines along the subcutaneous border of the olecranon and the ulnar shaft. In a radiographic study of 100 bilateral elbow radiographs, Rouleau and colleagues[8] found that the average PUDA in their population was 5.7°, at an average of 47 mm distal to the olecranon tip. They also identified a strong correlation between the PUDA in contralateral limbs and recommended imaging of the contralateral limb to determine individual patient parameters.

[a] Department of Orthopedic Surgery, University of Arizona College of Medicine – Phoenix, 1320 North 10th Street Suite A, Phoenix, AZ 85006, USA; [b] The CORE Institute, 18444 North 25th Avenue #210, Phoenix, AZ 85023, USA
* Corresponding author.
E-mail address: midhatpatel@email.arizona.edu
Twitter: @midpatelmd (M.P.)

Hand Clin 36 (2020) 479–484
https://doi.org/10.1016/j.hcl.2020.07.002

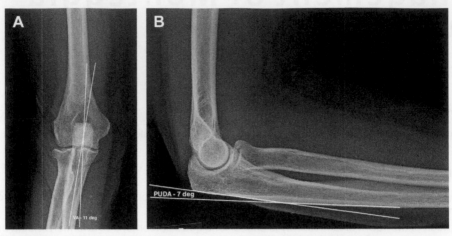

Fig. 1. Measurement of (*A*) VA and (*B*) PUDA on a normal proximal ulna radiograph.

CLASSIFICATION
Bado Classification

Bado originally described 4 main types of Monteggia injuries based on the angulation of the ulna fracture and direction of radial head displacement:[9]

- Type 1: apex anterior proximal ulna fracture with anterior dislocation of the radial head (most common type in pediatric population)
- Type 2: apex posterior proximal ulna fracture with posterior dislocation of the radial head (most common type in adults)

- Type 3: metaphyseal fracture of the proximal ulna with lateral or anterolateral dislocation of the radial head
- Type 4: anterior dislocation of the radial head with ipsilateral proximal radial shaft fracture

The most common type of Monteggia injury is the Type 2 injury, which typically results from an axial load on a partially flexed elbow with a supinated forearm.[10,11]

Jupiter modification
Jupiter noted there were several patterns of posterior Type 2 Monteggia fractures, and further

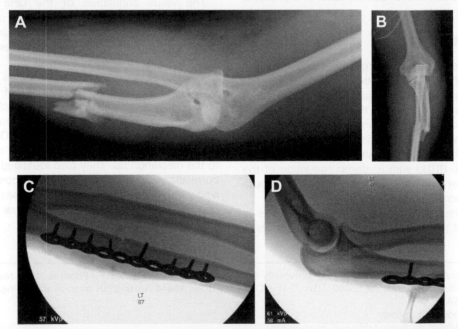

Fig. 2. (*A, B*) Preoperative radiographs demonstrate a Bado Type 2 Monteggia fracture with posterior dislocation of the radial head. (*C, D*) Intraoperative radiographs with reduction of the ulna demonstrate appropriate relocation of the radial head. No additional intervention was necessary in this case.

classified them as types 2A-D based on the ulnar fracture location:[12]

- Type 2A: involves the olecranon and coronoid process
- Type 2B: metaphyseal-diaphyseal junction distal to the coronoid
- Type 2C: diaphyseal fracture
- Type 2D: complex pattern with extension of fracture distally into ulnar shaft

Additionally, he noted that several of these injuries had radial head fractures in addition to radiocapitellar dislocation.

MANAGEMENT

Monteggia injuries in adults are best treated surgically with open reduction and internal fixation of the ulna (followed by fixation or replacement of the radial head, and repair of the lateral ligamentous structures, as needed).[2,5,13–16] Restoration of normal proximal ulnar anatomy is critical to achieving a satisfactory outcome.[5,15]

Technique

A direct posterior incision is made over the olecranon and proximal ulna, and extended distally along the subcutaneous border of the ulna. Full-thickness skin flaps are developed, and the fracture is exposed. Anatomic reduction of the ulna fracture is obtained, and fixation is achieved with standard small-fragment dynamic compression plates or precontoured proximal ulnar plates[1,13] (**Fig. 2**). The plate should be applied dorsally, and contoured to fit over the curve of the olecranon if needed. The use of tubular plates or reconstruction plates should be avoided, as they are not strong enough and can lead to fixation failure or malunion.

In the setting of complex fractures with comminution and fracture of the coronoid process, it is imperative to obtain anatomic reduction and fixation of this anterior coronoid fragment. Lack of reduction and fixation of the coronoid fragment can lead to elbow instability and subsequent dislocation. In such cases fixation of the coronoid fragment can be performed by working through the

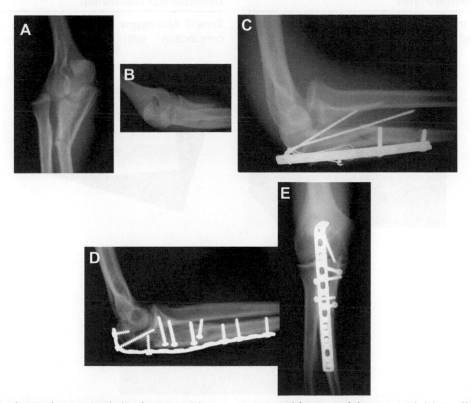

Fig. 3. (*A, B*) Complex proximal ulna fracture with comminution and fracture of the coronoid. (*C*) Insufficient fixation, with lack of fixation of the coronoid fragment, and subsequent failure and radial head dislocation. (*D, E*) Anatomic fixation of the proximal ulna with reduction and fixation of the anterior coronoid fragment with lag screws, and application of a posterior plate.

(posterior) fracture line, which allows direct visualization of the anterior fragments (book the fracture open to visualize the anterior fragments). The anterior fragment can be then reduced and secured with k-wires or lag screws. The posterior fragments can then be reduced and secured with the posteriorly applied plate. The proximal screws in the plate should be long enough to cross the fracture line and obtain bicortical fixation through the anterior cortex[14] (**Fig. 3**).

After fixation of the ulna, anatomic reduction of the radial head should be assessed radiographically, by assessing the radio capitellar joint. If the radial head is not concentrically reduced, the ulna fracture should be reassessed for anatomic reduction. In most cases, persistent radial head subluxation is caused by malreduction of the ulna fracture. After ensuring the ulna is anatomically reduced, persistent radial head dislocation or subluxation may be caused by interposition of the annular ligament, joint capsule, or other soft tissue that should be removed via a separate lateral incision.[1–3,5,13,14]

SPECIAL CONSIDERATIONS
Precontoured Plates

There is increasing interest and utilization of precontoured proximal ulna plates for fixation of proximal ulna fractures. Although these plates can lower the risk of hardware prominence, the risk of hardware irritation and need for hardware removal remain concerns. Studies show that there is significant variability in proximal ulnar angulation, and surgeons must be cautious when utilizing precontoured plates as reduction aides.[17,18]

Proximal Ulna Dorsal Angulation

Restoration of the PUDA is critical for optimal outcomes. The proximal ulna has a dorsal angulation of about 6°, which should be recreated when obtaining reduction and fixation (**Fig. 1**B). Application of a straight plate to the can lead to malalignment of the proximal ulna (and hence persistent dislocation of the radial head) (**Fig. 4**).

A retrospective study of 49 patients who underwent open reduction and internal fixation of proximal ulna fractures compared the PUDA between operative and contralateral limbs. They reported that 29% of patients had a malunion with respect to their PUDA, and had decreased elbow range of motion compared to patients without malunion.[19]

Ulnohumeral Dislocation

Type II Monteggia fracture can rarely occur in conjunction with a posterior ulnohumeral

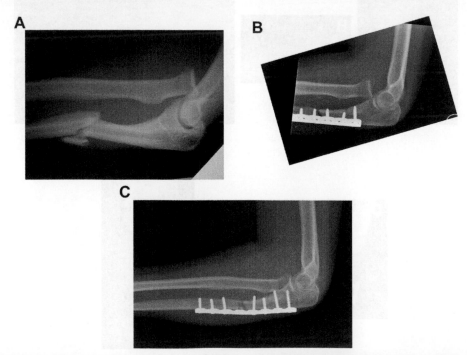

Fig. 4. (*A*) Monteggia injury with proximal ulna fracture and anterior radial head dislocation. (*B*) The proximal ulna fracture was fixed with a straight plate, resulting in malunion of the ulna and subsequent persistent dislocation of the radial head. (*C*) The plate has been contoured to account for the PUDA, resulting in anatomic reduction of the ulna and reduction of the radial head.

dislocation.[20] In these cases, there are often associated fractures of the coronoid, radial head, and disruption of the lateral ligamentous stabilizers of the elbow. It is important to identify and repair these associated lesions; however, limited data suggest that even with appropriate treatment patients with this type of injury have relatively poor functional outcomes when compared to patients with Type II injuries without associated dislocation.[21]

OUTCOMES AND COMPLICATIONS

The key to a successful outcome after Monteggia injuries is early recognition and treatment.[15] The largest series with long-term follow-up contained 47 patients with an average follow-up of 8.4 years. Of these patients, 73% percent had an excellent or good outcome according to the Broberg and Morrey elbow scale, while 8% had a poor outcome. Factors associated with a poor outcome included Bado Type II and Jupiter Type IIa fractures, associated radial head or coronoid fractures, and complications requiring reoperation.[22]

The most common complication that occurs after fixation of Monteggia fractures-dislocations is hardware irritation/prominence.[23] Other complications include elbow stiffness, radial and ulnar neuritis, heterotopic ossification, radioulnar synostosis, and persistent radial head subluxation.[5,24–26]

SUMMARY

Monteggia fractures-dislocations are defined as proximal ulna fractures with associated radial head fracture or dislocation. It is important to have a high index of suspicion for these injuries, as early identification is critical for a good outcome. In adults, these injuries should be managed with open reduction and internal fixation, with an emphasis on anatomic restoration of proximal ulnar anatomy.

DISCLOSURE

M. Patel has nothing to disclose. N. Dehghan has no disclosures relevant to the content of this text. Her disclosures can be found in full on the American Academy of Orthopaedic Surgeons Web site.

REFERENCES

1. Rehim SA, Maynard MA, Sebastin SJ, et al. Monteggia fracture-dislocations: a historical review. J Hand Surg Am 2014;39(7):1384–94.

2. Ring D, Jupiter JB, Waters PM. Monteggia fractures in children and adults. J Am Acad Orthop Surg 1998;6(4):215.

3. Speed JS, Boyd H. Treatment of fractures of ulna with dislocation of head of radius: Monteggia fracture. JAMA 1940;115(20):1699–705.

4. Morrey BF, Llusa-Perez M, Ballesteros-Betancourt J. Anatomy of the elbow joint. In: Morrey B, Sanchez-Sotelo J, Morrey M, editors. Morrey's the elbow and its disorders. 5th edition. Philadelphia: Elsevier; 2018. p. 9–32.

5. Siebenlist S, Buchholz A, Braun KF. Fractures of the proximal ulna: current concepts in surgical management. EFORT Open Rev 2019;4(1):1–9.

6. Grechenig W, Clement H, Pichler W, et al. The influence of lateral and anterior angulation of the proximal ulna on the treatment of a Monteggia fracture: an anatomical cadaver study. J Bone Joint Surg Br 2007;89(6):836–8.

7. Windisch G, Clement H, Grechenig W, et al. The anatomy of the proximal ulna. J Shoulder Elbow Surg 2007;16(5):661–6.

8. Rouleau DM, Faber KJ, Athwal GS. The proximal ulna dorsal angulation: a radiographic study. J Shoulder Elbow Surg 2010;19(1):26–30.

9. Bado JL. The Monteggia lesion. Clin Orthop Relat Res 1967;50:71–86.

10. Bruce HE, Harvey JPJ, Wilson JCJ. Monteggia fractures. J Bone Joint Surg Am 1974;56(8):1563.

11. Suarez R, Barquet A, Fresco R. Epidemiology and treatment of Monteggia lesion in adults: series of 44 cases. Acta Ortop Bras 2016;24(1):48–51.

12. Jupiter JB, Leibovic SJ, Ribbans W, et al. The posterior Monteggia lesion. J Orthop Trauma 1991;5(4): 395–402.

13. Adams JE, Steinmann SP. Olecranon fractures and Monteggia fractures. In: Morrey B, Sanchez-Sotelo J, Morrey M, editors. Morrey's the elbow and its disorders. 5th edition. Philadelphia: Elsevier; 2018. p. 9–32.

14. Ring D. Monteggia Fractures. Orthop Clin 2013; 44(1):59–66.

15. Ring D, Jupiter JB, Simpson NS. Monteggia fractures in adults. J Bone Joint Surg Am 1998;80(12): 1733–44.

16. Ozel O, Demircay E. Review of management of unstable elbow fractures. World J Orthop 2016;7(1): 50–4.

17. Totlis T, Anastasopoulos N, Apostolidis S, et al. Proximal ulna morphometry: which are the "true" anatomical preshaped olecranon plates? Surg Radiol Anat 2014;36(10):1015–22.

18. Puchwein P, Schildhauer TA, Schöffmann S, et al. Three-dimensional morphometry of the proximal ulna: a comparison to currently used anatomically preshaped ulna plates. J Shoulder Elbow Surg 2012;21(8):1018–23.

19. Chapleau J, Balg F, Harvey EJ, et al. Impact of olecranon fracture malunion: study on the importance of PUDA (proximal ulna dorsal angulation). Injury 2016; 47(11):2520–4.

20. Preston CF, Chen AL, Wolinsky PR, et al. Posterior dislocation of the elbow with concomitant fracture of the proximal ulnar diaphysis and radial head: a complex variant of the posterior monteggia lesion. J Orthop Trauma 2003;17(7):530–3.

21. Strauss EJ, Tejwani NC, Preston CF, et al. The posterior Monteggia lesion with associated ulnohumeral instability. J Bone Joint Surg Br 2006;88(1):84–9.

22. Konrad GG, Kundel K, Kreuz PC, et al. Monteggia fractures in adults: long-term results and prognostic factors. J Bone Joint Surg Br 2007;89(3):354–60.

23. Ren Y-M, Qiao H-Y, Wei Z-J, et al. Efficacy and safety of tension band wiring versus plate fixation in olecranon fractures: a systematic review and meta-analysis. J Orthop Surg Res 2016;11(1):137.

24. Foruria AM, Lawrence TM, Augustin S, et al. Heterotopic ossification after surgery for distal humeral fractures. Bone Joint J 2014;96-B(12):1681–7.

25. Scolaro JA, Beingessner D. Treatment of Monteggia and transolecranon fracture-dislocations of the elbow: a critical analysis review. JBJS Rev 2014; 2(1). https://doi.org/10.2106/JBJS.RVW.M.00049.

26. Stein F, Grabias SL, Deffer PA. Nerve injuries complicating Monteggia lesions. J Bone Joint Surg Am 1971;53(7):1432–6.

Elbow Instability
Evaluation and Treatment

Julie E. Adams, MD

KEYWORDS

- Elbow dislocation • Elbow instability • Terrible triad • Coronoid fracture

KEY POINTS

- Elbow dislocations are common.
- Most simple elbow dislocations are readily managed nonoperatively, and most are amenable to early mobilization.
- Attention to important principles in evaluation and management is critical to ensure optimal outcomes.
- Chronic instability may be subtle, but surgical treatment is generally associated with a high rate of satisfactory outcomes with the exception of patients in whom instability is due to chronic bony absence.

INTRODUCTION

Instability of the elbow joint is a subject of much discussion and can present a challenge in evaluation and treatment.

In terms of nomenclature, *simple elbow dislocations* represent those dislocations with soft tissue but not bony injuries, whereas *complex dislocations* are those with concomitant bony injuries. In reality, many dislocations occur with subtle bony injuries, which may represent shear injury or avulsion fracture; some of these may portend a poorer prognosis whereas others may have no bearing on the treatment or prognosis of the injury.

In this article, we consider important points in the evaluation and treatment of elbow instability; fracture dislocations are discussed in detail in Timothy J. Luchetti and colleagues' article, "Elbow Fracture Dislocations: Determining Treatment Strategies," in this issue, whereas rehabilitation is considered in detail in Joey G. Pipicelli and Graham J.W. King's article, "Rehabilitation of Elbow Instability," in this issue. Other portions of this issue of *Hand Clinics* are devoted to instability

of the forearm axis and forearm or elbow fractures in conjunction with instability.

ANATOMIC CONSIDERATIONS

Stability of the elbow is conferred by bony congruence, ligamentous soft tissue stabilizers, and dynamic stability provided by muscles surrounding the elbow.

Although the anterior elbow capsule contributes to stability, in the usual setting it is thin and confers little functional stability to the elbow.

The collateral ligament complexes on the medial and lateral sides of the elbow are the major soft tissue stabilizers of the elbow. Laterally, the lateral collateral ligament complex represents an interplay of various ligamentous tissues. The lateral ulnar collateral ligament (LUCL) represents the coalescence of tissues that provide most of the stability to valgus forces and extends from the lateral epicondyle epicenter to its attachment on the crista supinatoris on the lateral aspect of the ulna. In addition, there is an annular ligament, which is broad, and this capsuloligamentous structure encircles the radial head

University of Tennessee College of Medicine – Chattanooga, Erlanger Orthopaedic Institute, 975 East 3rd Street Suite C 225, Chattanooga, TN 37403, USA

E-mail address: adams.julie.e@gmail.com

Hand Clin 36 (2020) 485–494
https://doi.org/10.1016/j.hcl.2020.07.013

and contributes to the capsule. The radial collateral ligament, which arises from the lateral epicondyle inserts on the annular ligament.

Grossly, it is often difficult to separate these components of the lateral ligament complex and functionally, it is this complex (rather than the individual components) that resists varus forces on the elbow.

On the medial side of the elbow, the medial collateral ligament (MCL) has 2 separate components. The anterior portion is most functionally important in providing resistance to varus forces, and is tensioned when the elbow is extended, whereas the posterior portion is tight in the position of elbow flexion. Both bands of the MCL arise from the anteroinferior aspect of the medial epicondyle; the anterior bundle inserts at the sublime tubercle of the ulna, whereas the posterior band inserts broadly on the posterior medial aspect of the ulna near the joint line.

Functionally, the lateral ligament complex provides resistance to varus forces; these forces are the predominant forces experienced by the elbow joint during activities of daily living, because most functional activities are carried out with the shoulder in some degree of abduction and with a weight carried by the hand. Moreover, the position anatomically of the lateral ligament complex renders it more vulnerable to potential injury. The lateral aspect of the elbow not only experienced heightened forces, but also the anatomic position in which the longer length complex is "draped" over the epicondyle and radial head, which tent the complex and tension it, as well as the position farther away from the axis of the elbow, render it more vulnerable to translational or rotational injuries.

In contrast, the MCL is of relatively short length and of stout construction, and does not see much in the form of stress during most usual activities of daily living. The MCL sees stresses in overhead athletes, such as swimmers, throwers, weight lifters, and in those who load the arm with it in a position of shoulder external rotation with an axial load, such as wrestlers.

Bony constraints, such as the congruence of the radial head and the radiocapitellar joint, the tensioning effect of the radial head on the lateral ligamentous structures, and the axial-based restraint of the radiocapitellar joint, are important stabilizers laterally and axially. The congruent and hingelike joint of the ulnohumeral joint, especially the coronoid process, are important in maintaining joint stability; when traumatically absent, the joint may "collapse" into the defect (such as with anteromedial fracture patterns), leading to rotational and translational instability or,

alternatively, when a substantial portion of the anterior rim of the coronoid is fractured, the distal humerus pushes against it like a battering ram, displacing it, and the joint subluxates.

Mechanism of Injury

Most commonly, elbow dislocations result from a fall on an outstretched hand, although higher-energy trauma is also a common mechanism of injury.

The elbow has been described to have primary stabilizers, including the ulnohumeral joint, the LUCL, and the anterior bundle of the MCL. Stabilizers of secondary importance are the flexor pronator group, the common extensor muscles, and the radiohumeral articulation.[1]

Elbow dislocations most commonly result from an axial load to the elbow through the forearm, which transmits a rotational force. There is ongoing discussion about the involvement of structures injured necessary for dislocation to occur, and the order of failure and which structures are most commonly or uniformly involved; and whether injury proceeds from lateral to medial.[1–5]

It has been suggested that posterolateral dislocation results from an axially loaded arm with the forearm in supination (Fig. 1). An external rotation moment is imparted to the loaded and flexed elbow, causing the soft tissue structures to fail in a sequential circular fashion beginning laterally and progressing anteriorly and posteriorly, with failure of the medial structures last (or not at all) (Figs. 2 and 3).[2]

Although the proposed mechanism of O'Driscoll and colleagues[2] that instability begins with injury of the LUCL and progresses anteriorly and posteriorly has been widely held, there is a body of literature including MRI findings and biomechanics studies that suggest otherwise. One biomechanical study was unable to create posterolateral instability in the setting of an intact MCL; in each case the MCL was injured in order for the dislocation to occur. An MRI study of elbow dislocations noted that the MCL was uniformly torn following posterolateral elbow dislocations, with more variable injury of the LUCL. In addition, clinical studies of examination under anesthesia and surgical treatment with exploration of dislocated elbows in the acute setting indicate a high rate of instability on the medial side in the position of extension, and that the elbow did not dislocate without tearing the MCL.[3–8]

In addition, recent video and MRI evidence presents compelling evidence that elbow dislocations may occur by a different mechanism and with

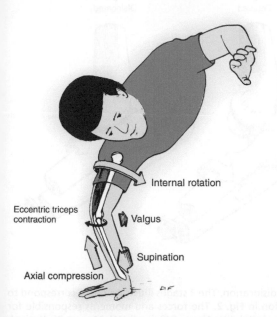

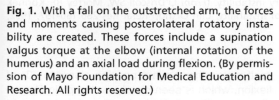

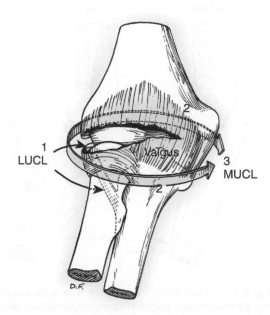

Fig. 1. With a fall on the outstretched arm, the forces and moments causing posterolateral rotatory instability are created. These forces include a supination valgus torque at the elbow (internal rotation of the humerus) and an axial load during flexion. (By permission of Mayo Foundation for Medical Education and Research. All rights reserved.)

Fig. 2. The "Horii circle" soft tissue injury progresses in a "circle" from lateral to medial in 3 stages correlating with those in **Fig. 3**. In stage 1, the ulnar part of the lateral collateral ligament is disrupted. In stage 2, the other lateral ligamentous structures and the anterior and posterior capsule are disrupted. In stage 3, disruption of the medial ulnar collateral ligament (MUCL) can be partial, with disruption of the posterior MUCL only (3A), or complete (3B). The common extensor and flexor origins are often disrupted as well. (*From* O'Driscoll SW, Morrey BF, Korinek S, et al: Elbow subluxation and dislocation: a spectrum of instability, Clin Orthop Relat Res 280:186-197, 1992; with permission.)

injury to different structures as the critical component. An alternative mechanism proposes that the axially loaded elbow, typically in an extended posture with the shoulder abducted and the forearm pronated, experiences a valgus force, causing the MCL to fail in tension first, with or without stripping of the LUCL[3–5,8]

Robinson and colleagues[8] reconcile the differences by postulating that most elbow dislocations include posterolateral and posterior dislocation with most severe and initial involvement on the medial side of the elbow; and a rarer posteromedial dislocation with most severe and initial injury on the lateral side of the elbow.

Fracture dislocation injury patterns are further described in the Timothy J. Luchetti and colleagues' article, "Elbow Fracture Dislocations: Determining Treatment Strategies," elsewhere in this issue.

EVALUATION AND TREATMENT CONSIDERATIONS IN THE ACUTE SETTING

Most elbow dislocations are initially seen in the emergency department, and the usual first evaluator is most commonly not a surgeon. Typically, the patient presents with an acute injury and pain at the

elbow and/or loss of motion. Plain film radiographs are obtained, typically 3-view radiographs, which generally are diagnostic of the dislocation and can help exclude or identify associated fractures.

Clinical examination includes attention to the neurovascular status with particular attention to the sensory and motor function of the radial, ulnar, and median nerves, including the anterior interosseous nerve. The patient is queried and examined for tenderness at the wrist, forearm, elbow, and proximal arm. The skin is inspected for ecchymoses or defects. The presence and location of ecchymoses a few days after injury may (or may not) be a clue to associated injuries; in large part, blood may track along fascial planes as determined by gravity and dependent location, although in some cases location of ecchymoses may be helpful to identify injury.

The skin is examined for open or impending open injury, and palpation reveals any tenderness that might prompt additional workup or

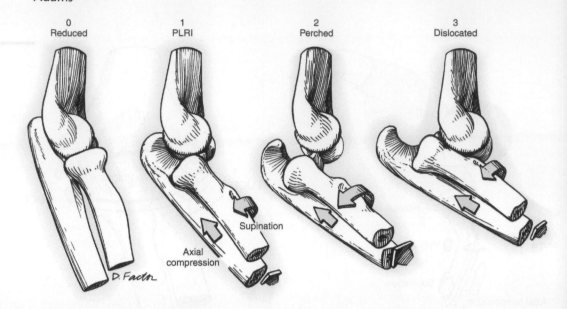

Fig. 3. Elbow instability is a spectrum from subluxation to dislocation. The 3 stages illustrated here correspond to the pathoanatomic stages of capsuloligamentous disruption in **Fig. 2**. The forces and moments responsible for displacements are illustrated. PLRI, posterolateral rotatory instability. (*From* O'Driscoll SW, Morrey BF, Korinek S, et al: Elbow subluxation and dislocation: a spectrum of instability, Clin Orthop Relat Res 280:186-197, 1992; with permission.)

examination. The orthopedic principle to "examine a joint above and a joint below" is a wise one.

In the acute setting, the elbow is reduced. Typically, this is done under general anesthesia or conscious sedation. This may be done in a procedure room, emergency room, or operating room, and is helpful if a fluoroscopy or mini C arm unit is available. The patient is often supine, and adequate analgesia or sedation is provided. It is often helpful to bring the shoulder to a 90° abducted position, supinate the forearm, and have an assistant provide counter traction at the proximal arm. The surgeon or physician may facilitate reduction by using his or her thumbs to push the olecranon tip in a distally and anteriorly directed way, as the elbow is flexed.

After reduction, it is optimal to be able to examine the elbow under anesthesia and sedation and with the fluoroscopy unit. The elbow may be ranged in the flexion-extension arc and it is helpful to determine the point at which the elbow tends to subluxate to determine and document the safe arc of motion. In general, in most cases, the position of elbow instability is extension and supination. Once the examiner identifies the position at which the elbow tends to dislocate, the elbow should be splinted initially in a position approximately 20 to 30° more flexed. One tip is that although the elbow may "appear" to be flexed to, for instance, 90°, in reality, because of the padding under the plaster and patient soft tissue habitus, the elbow joint

itself may rather be in a position closer to 70° of flexion, which is seen clearly on the plain film radiographs. Therefore, the treating surgeon should be aware of this tendency and ensure that the elbow (not the external plaster) is splinted at the appropriate degree of flexion.

Plain film radiographs and/or fluoroscopy can be used to document reduction and assess for any associated fractures.

If there is a concern for, or a documented radial head fracture or substantial coronoid fracture, sometimes a computed tomography (CT) scan with 2-dimensional and 3-dimensional reconstructions and with joint subtraction views (to subtract out the humerus) is helpful to determine fracture size and fragments, comminution, and origin of the fracture fragments. The CT scan is also helpful to assess congruency of the elbow joint. Generally, the CT scan will be obtained after initial reduction and splinting of the elbow in a flexed posture. The challenge is that the best position for obtaining a quality CT scan is with the elbow in an extended posture, but this may put the elbow at risk of dislocation. Likewise, the best position for generation of quality images is with the elbow in the central portion of the scanner and with the arm stretched above the head (rather than at the side or on the abdomen). Suboptimal images are obtained when the elbow is placed at the patient's side or on the abdomen and this position should be avoided when possible, as nondiagnostic images may result. It can be difficult to obtain the images because of patient discomfort and the confines of splinting, as elbow flexion is hard to avoid; however, in some cases, we temporarily splint the elbow in as much extension as possible for the scan, then flex the elbow for final splinting.

An MRI is rarely used in the setting of an acute dislocation or fracture dislocation; rarely, it may be helpful if there is believed to be soft tissue interposition prohibiting reduction.[9]

Although everyone can agree that closed reduction in an expedited fashion is appropriate, the duration (if any) and type of immobilization thereafter and rehabilitation remain a matter of discussion and difference among surgeons.[10–13]

Most surgeons agree that a short or minimal period of immobilization results in improved outcomes and decreased costs for simple dislocation.[10–14]

In one series, 100 adults with simple elbow dislocations were randomized to early active motion within confines of pain immediately after reduction or alternatively to 3 weeks of splint immobilization followed by range of motion as limited by pain. No difference in complications were noted between the 2 groups and it was suggested that early mobilization led to earlier return to work and avocation, and a reduction of approximately 50% in costs. How early should "early mobilization" occur is also a point of discussion. Ross and colleagues[14] reported on 21 young patients with elbow dislocations without known fracture. They performed immediate closed reduction followed by immediate (first day after reduction) supervised mobilization with no use of sling, splint, or immobilizers after the first day. These patients in this series were high-demand individuals in the US Naval Academy, but also had a high level of supervision. The average time to restore full motion was 19 days, and 20 of the 21 patients in this series were successfully treated with nonoperative care, with only 1 patient developing recurrent instability requiring surgical intervention.

One can conclude that likely the great majority of simple elbow dislocations are appropriately managed with splinting for comfort for a short period, followed by early active motion. Typically, this author recommends a week or less of immobilization in a splint following reduction of a simple elbow dislocation, then mobilization within the confines of pain, with clinical and radiographic follow-up to ensure that patients continue to have a congruent located elbow and that range of motion is restored. Rehabilitation is discussed in detail in Joey G. Pipicelli and Graham J.W. King's article, "Rehabilitation of Elbow Instability," in this issue, and this author refers

the interested reader to the detailed excellent protocols described in Joey G. Pipicelli and Graham J.W. King's article, "Rehabilitation of Elbow Instability," in this issue.

Occasionally, one will see a radiographic "drop sign" early on within the first 2 weeks after dislocation. This is also discussed in the excellent Timothy J. Luchetti and colleagues' article, "Elbow Fracture Dislocations: Determining Treatment Strategies"; and Joey G. Pipicelli and Graham J.W. King's article, "Rehabilitation of Elbow Instability," in this issue, but briefly, these patients should be started in active gravity-eliminated elbow flexion exercises. Shoulder abduction and avoidance of varus stress should be used, and close radiographic follow-up weekly is necessary. Most patients will have correction of this radiographic finding with restoration of a congruent stable joint. As discussed in Timothy J. Luchetti and colleagues' article, "Elbow Fracture Dislocations: Determining Treatment Strategies," in this issue, obtaining the lateral plain film radiograph with the arm at the side and with active contraction of the biceps (rather than with the shoulder abducted) can avoid varus forces on a recently dislocated elbow, which result in apparent radiographic instability that may not be clinically problematic.

FRACTURE DISLOCATIONS OF THE ELBOW

Evaluation and treatment of fracture dislocations of the elbow are described in detail in Timothy J. Luchetti and colleagues' article, "Elbow Fracture Dislocations: Determining Treatment Strategies," in this issue. Briefly, the discussion here centers on pattern recognition.

Terrible Triad

Terrible triad injuries occur in the setting of a fracture dislocation of the elbow with injury to the LUCL, a radial head fracture, and a coronoid fracture. The LUCL injury is an avulsion off of the epicondyle, which, during surgical exposure, may be seen as a "bald epicondyle." The radial head fracture is generally a Mason II or III injury in most cases; and the coronoid fracture is most commonly a Regan Morrey type 1 or 2 injury.

Most commonly, terrible triad injuries require operative treatment, although in select cases with careful attention, nonoperative care may be appropriate. Typically, a laterally based surgical incision is used, exploiting the avulsed LUCL to access the joint inevitably through the Kocher interval. The surgeon may palpate the lateral musculature and identify the defect, "using the approach the patient gives you." The radial head is exposed, and assessed for possible open reduction internal fixation (rarely) versus replacement arthroplasty (most commonly). Radial head excision without replacement is contraindicated for this injury. If the radial head is not reconstructable, it is excised in preparation for replacement. The surgeon may use this interval to access the coronoid to consider fixation if indicated. Although placement of fixation from anterior to posterior is difficult with this approach, the surgeon may use a targeting drill guide, such as an anterior cruciate ligament guide to drill and place screws from posterior to anterior to capture fragments. In general, if only 1 screw can be placed because of size of the fragment, the fragment often is insubstantial enough to forego fixation. If, however, 2 or more screws may be placed, it may be worthwhile to fixate the fragment. In this author's opinion, there is little value to the approach of tying down the capsule to the coronoid, and it represents treatment more for the surgeon to "do something" than to provide meaningful stability to the elbow. First, the capsule normally inserts distal to the coronoid tip, not at the tip. If the fracture is a tip fracture with little structural significance, then likely it also confers minimal biomechanical significance; rather, injury occurs "along for the ride" and as a marker of dislocation secondary to the humerus shearing off the tip like a battering ram. Larger coronoid fractures involving the anteromedial facet or in cases in which the radial head is fixated and not replaced may require a separate medial approach or very rarely anterior approach. This is described in the next section.

If the radial head is replaced, the excised radial head fragments are assembled on the back table to provide a guide for sizing. In general, this author prefers smooth-stemmed intentionally loose metallic implants due to their unparalleled track record and a high rate of symptomatic failure of implants with grit blasted stems.[15] In this setting, the size of the radial head arthroplasty is built up to match the thickness of the excised radial head, and the diameter is chosen to match the inner diameter of the eccentric dish of the native radial head; the most common technical error particularly when the elbow is unstable, is to overstuff the radial head to confer stability. The size of the excised radial head, the lack of asymmetry in joint width on the intraoperative postero-anterior or antero-posterior of the elbow, and the position of the head relative to the coronoid and sigmoid notch are all clues to appropriate sizing.

The surgical sequence, therefore, is generally to fixate the radial head versus excision in preparation for replacement, assess ± fixate the coronoid (if indicated and if possible) through the window provided by radial head excision, then replacement of the radial head if it has been excised, repair of the collateral ligament to the humeral origin using bony tunnels or suture anchors with the elbow in a flexed posture, and the forearm in a pronated position. At this point, the surgeon assesses the stability of the elbow in the position of instability (terminal extension and supination) and in positions short of that. If the elbow is stable and congruently located in a posture of reasonable elbow flexion with the forearm pronated, no further surgical treatment is indicated and the elbow is splinted in a position of stability (flexion 20° more than an unstable point, and pronation). If, however, the elbow is unstable, the surgeon considers fixation of the coronoid if not already done, via an anterior or more likely medial incision. The medial incision is done similar to a cubital tunnel approach. The ulnar nerve is identified, and protected. The surgeon retracts the ulnar nerve anteriorly and proceeds from distal to proximal through the "floor of the cubital tunnel," palpating for the sublime tubercle as a clue to the MCL. By doing so, the surgeon can readily identify the sublime tubercle and avoid iatrogenic injury to the MCL. The fracture site is exposed, and consideration of screw versus plate fixation of the coronoid is made. Patients and surgeons should be aware that ulnar nerve irritation following this approach is common. Most cases represent a temporary neurapraxia likely due to traction, but more permanent injury can occur. An anterior incision and approach is an alternative, but care must be taken to avoid injury to the brachial artery, the median nerve, and even the ulnar nerve with this approach.[16,17]

After assessment of the medial side, if the elbow remains unstable, the surgeon should reassess the adequacy of prior repairs, and if no further treatment or adjustments are indicated to restore stability, the patient may be placed in an external fixator device, ensuring with fluoroscopy that the elbow is in a congruently located position. The fixator remains in place for approximately 4 weeks; this is removed in the operating room, and the bars are first removed, leaving the pins in place. The elbow is assessed under anesthesia and fluoroscopy for instability; if the elbow is stable, the pins may be removed. If, however, the elbow is unstable, the bars can easily be reaffixed and the fixator left on for several more weeks. This author prefers a static external fixator device over hinged devices because of simplicity and ease of application, readily available and less expensive implants, and lack of data supporting advantages of hinged fixators over static ones.

VARUS POSTERIOR MEDIAL ROTATORY INSTABILITY

This condition is commonly associated with what often appears to be an isolated coronoid fracture. Commonly the LUCL is concomitantly also injured. The initial plain film radiographs may seem innocuous but this injury portends a poor prognosis if not recognized and appropriately treated. Typically, gravity-assisted varus stress testing is helpful in the clinical examination of these injuries[18] (**Fig. 4**).

Rehabilitation of the elbow following dislocation is beautifully outlined in Joey G. Pipicelli and Graham J.W. King's article, "Rehabilitation of Elbow Instability," in this issue, and the interested reader is referred to that article. In general, however, it has been said that a "stiff stable elbow" is preferable to an unstable elbow; and if there is doubt about the stability of the elbow, concern about joint congruency trumps motion.

CHRONIC INSTABILITY DUE TO LIGAMENTOUS INSUFFICIENCY

Patients may present with instability of the elbow in the chronic setting associated with ligament insufficiency.

On the lateral side, patients may have insufficiency of the LUCL after trauma or iatrogenically. There is concern that excessive corticosteroid injections at the lateral aspect of the elbow may attenuate the lateral ligament structures, or, alternatively, instability may occur after surgical approaches to the elbow, such as for lateral epicondylar debridement. These patients may complain of pain at the lateral side, pain with loading activities such as grasping and lifting, pushing up from a chair, or of frank instability.

Patients may not appreciate instability, and diagnosis may be subtle.

Examination maneuvers include the "lateral pivot shift test" in which the patient lies supine with the arm extended over the head. The examiner holds the patient's forearm at the proximal forearm and at the wrist, with the forearm in supination. An axial and valgus force is applied. As the elbow is extended, patients with posterolateral rotatory instability will complain of pain or apprehension with radial head subluxation. With elbow flexion, a clunk may occur with joint reduction. In the awake setting, patients may exhibit muscular guarding and the examination may be limited because of this.

In the push-up test, a patient is asked to push their body up when rising from a chair, with the forearm in a supinated position. If the patient complains of pain or instability as the elbow extends, the test is deemed positive. The posterolateral rotatory drawer test involves applying an anterior to posterior force to the flexed elbow. If the patient demonstrated subluxation or apprehension, instability is suspected.[19,20] In this author's experience, the lateral pivot shift test and the posterolateral rotatory drawer test are difficult to achieve in the awake patient who may guard the injured arm. For this reason, the most useful test in this author's practice is one described by Steinmann, called the supination rollout test (Scott Steinmann, personal communication, 2010). In this test, the surgeon faces the patient, and places the thumb over the patient's lateral elbow, while the elbow is in a flexed posture (**Fig. 5**). The elbow is gently supinated and extended, and subtle instability and pain/apprehension is sought at the lateral aspect of the elbow; this may be compared with the contralateral side. In this author's experience, this test is 100% sensitive and specific for lateral

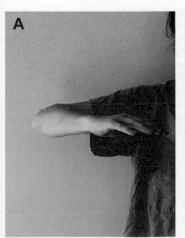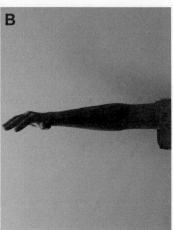

Fig. 4. The varus stress test takes place when the patient abducts the arm to 90° with the forearm in neutral rotation. The elbow is flexed (*A*) and extended (*B*). Patients may experience pain, apprehension, or crepitus, which is indicative of instability. (*Courtesy of* Julie Adams, MD, Chattanooga, TN.)

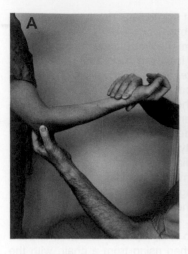 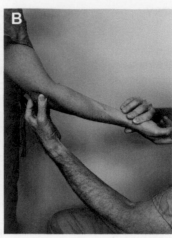

Fig. 5. The supination rollout test, described by Scott Steinmann, MD, involves an awake patient, and may be done in the office. The patient is seated, facing the surgeon, and the surgeon places his or her fingers over the radiocapitellar joint. The elbow is concomitantly supinated as the elbow is moved from a flexed (A) to extended (B) position in an attempt to elicit laxity and/or apprehension, which is suggestive of lateral elbow instability. In our experience, this test is 100% sensitive and specific for lateral elbow instability, and is easily done in the awake patient. (*Courtesy of* Julie Adams, MD, Chattanooga, TN.)

elbow instability even in the apprehensive patient; in a shoulder elbow practice of over 21 years' duration, the supination rollout test is diagnostic and specific for lateral elbow instability (Scott Steinmann, personal communication).

Imaging Studies

Imaging studies include plain film radiographs of the elbow (3 views), and often there is consideration of an MRI. MR arthrogram may be considered to increase the sensitivity and specificity for diagnosis of ligament injuries.[21]

Chronic instability due to lateral ligament insufficiency is generally treated with ligament reconstruction. This has been historically most reliably done with use of an allograft or autogenous tendon graft rather than local tissues if the injury is chronic. However, recently, augmentation techniques with suture tape (both on the medial and lateral aspects of the elbow) have gained popularity and also have demonstrated a high rate of satisfactory outcomes.[22–25]

Injury to the MCL may occur as an isolated injury and can be problematic especially in throwing or overhead athletes, such as baseball pitchers, swimmers, weightlifters, and wrestlers. Patients may present with a flexor pronator mass avulsion and may have a palpable defect; alternatively, they may present with medial-sided elbow discomfort following acute trauma or attritional injury, worse with valgus inducing forces. The great majority of patients do well with nonoperative care, with the exception of athletes who need or desire to return to their sport at a high level. These patients often benefit from repair or reconstruction. Clinical evaluation can include plain film radiographs and usually an MRI, as well as specific provocative maneuvers such as the moving valgus stress test (**Fig. 6**), the valgus stress test (**Fig. 7**), and the milking maneuver (**Fig. 8**).

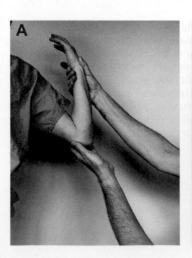 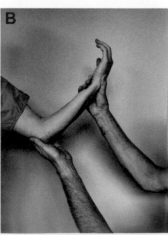

Fig. 6. For the moving valgus stress test, the patient abducts their shoulder to 90°. The fully flexed elbow (A) is quickly extended (B) with application of a valgus torque to the elbow. The test is positive if medial elbow discomfort is present and most painful between 120° and 70°. (*Courtesy of* Julie Adams, MD, Chattanooga, TN.)

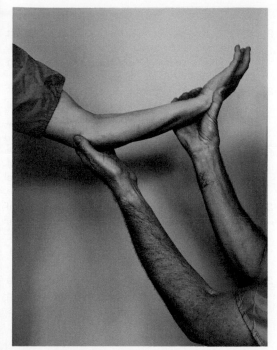

Fig. 7. he valgus stress test involves flexing the elbow to 20° and applying a valgus force to the elbow. Presence of pain or apprehension medially is indicative of MCL pathology. (*Courtesy of* Julie Adams, MD, Chattanooga, TN.)

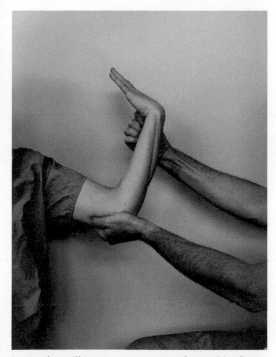

Fig. 8. The milking maneuver is performed by flexing the elbow to 90° or more, with application of a valgus stress to the elbow by traction applied by the examiner to the thumb. Presence of medial-sided pain is indicative of pathology. (*Courtesy of* Julie Adams, MD, Chattanooga, TN.)

In summary, the elbow is a joint that requires attention to evaluate trauma and instability. Close attention to imaging studies, physical examination, and the results of provocative testing is necessary to appropriately diagnose and treat elbow instability.

REFERENCES

1. O'Driscoll SW, Jupiter JB, Cohen MS, et al. Difficult elbow fractures: pearls and pitfalls. Instr Course Lect 2003;52:113–34.
2. O'Driscoll SW, Morrey BF, Korinek S, et al. Elbow subluxation and dislocation. A spectrum of instability. Clin Orthop Relat Res 1992;280:186–97.
3. Schreiber JJ, Potter HG, Warren RF, et al. Magnetic resonance imaging findings in acute elbow dislocation: insight into mechanism. J Hand Surg Am 2014; 39:199–205.
4. Schreiber JJ, Warren RF, Hotchkiss RN, et al. An online video investigation into the mechanism of elbow dislocation. J Hand Surg Am 2013;38:488–94.
5. Schwab GH, Bennett JB, Woods GW, et al. Biomechanics of elbow instability: the role of the medial collateral ligament. Clin Orthop Relat Res 1980; 146:42–52.42.
6. Josefsson PO, Gentz CF, Johnell O, et al. Surgical versus non-surgical treatment of ligamentous injuries following dislocation of the elbow joint. A prospective randomized study. J Bone Joint Surg Am 1987;69:605–8.
7. Josefsson PO, Johnell O, Wendeberg B. Ligamentous injuries in dislocations of the elbow joint. Clin Orthop Relat Res 1987;221:221–5.
8. Ramirez MA, Stein JA, Murthi AM. Varus posteromedial instability. Hand Clinics 2015;31(4):557–63.
9. Cates RA, Steinmann SP, Adams JE. Irreducible anteromedial radial head dislocation caused by the brachialis tendon: a case report. J Shoulder Elbow Surg 2016;25(8):e232–5.
10. de Haan J, den Hartog D, Tuinebreijer WE, et al. Functional treatment versus plaster for simple elbow dislocations (FuncSiE): a randomized trial. BMC Musculoskelet Disord 2010;11:263.
11. Iordens GI, Van Lieshout EM, Schep NW, et al. Early mobilisation versus plaster immobilisation of simple elbow dislocations: results of the FuncSiE multicontre randomised clinical trial. Br J Sports Med 2017;51(6):531–8.
12. Van Lieshout EMM, Iordens GIT, Polinder S, et al. FuncSiE Trial Investigators. Early mobilization versus plaster immobilization of simple elbow dislocations: a cost analysis of the FuncSiE multicenter randomized clinical trial. Arch Orthop Trauma Surg 2019;140(7):877–86.
13. Anakwe RE, Middleton SD, Jenkins PJ, et al. Patient-reported outcomes after simple dislocation of the elbow. J Bone Joint Surg Am 2011;93(13):1220–6.

14. Ross G, McDevitt ER, Chronister R, et al. Treatment of simple elbow dislocation using an immediate motion protocol. Am J Sports Med 1999;27(3):308–11.

15. Marsh JP, Grewal R, Faber KJ, et al. Radial head fractures treated with modular metallic radial head replacement: outcomes at a mean follow-up of eight years. J Bone Joint Surg Am 2016;98(7):527–35.

16. Cheung EV, Steinmann SP. Surgical approaches to the elbow. J Am Acad Orthop Surg 2009;17(5):325–33.

17. Reichel LM, Milam GS, Reitman CA. Anterior approach for operative fixation of coronoid fractures in complex elbow instability. Tech Hand Up Extrem Surg 2012;16(2):98–104.

18. Ramirez, et al. Hand Clin 2015.

19. O'Driscoll SW, Bell DF, Morrey BF. Posterolateral instability of the elbow. J Bone Joint Surg Am 1991;73(3):440–6.

20. Phillips CS, Segalman KA. Diagnosis and treatment of post-traumatic medial and lateral elbow ligament incompetence. Hand Clin 2002;18(1):149–59.

21. Saliman JD, Beaulieu CF, McAdams TR. Ligament and tendon injury to the elbow: clinical, surgical, and imaging features. Top Magn Reson Imaging 2006;17(5):327–36.

22. Sanchez-Sotelo J, Morrey BF, O'Driscoll SW. Ligamentous repair and reconstruction for posterolateral rotatory instability of the elbowslr. J Bone Joint Surg Br 2005;87(1):54–61.

23. Scheiderer B, Imhoff FB, Kia C, et al. LUCL internal bracing restores posterolateral rotatory stability of the elbow. Knee Surg Sports Traumatol Arthrosc 2019. https://doi.org/10.1007/s00167-019-05632-x.

24. Jones CM, Beason DP, Dugas JR. Ulnar collateral ligament reconstruction versus repair with internal bracing: comparison of cyclic fatigue mechanics. Orthop J Sports Med 2018;6(2). 2325967118755991.

25. Wilk KE, Arrigo CA, Bagwell MS, et al. Repair of the ulnar collateral ligament of the elbow: rehabilitation following internal brace surgery. J Orthop Sports Phys Ther 2019;49(4):253–61.

Elbow Fracture-Dislocations
Determining Treatment Strategies

Timothy J. Luchetti, MD[1], Emily E. Abbott, DO[1], Mark E. Baratz, MD*

KEYWORDS

- Elbow • Posteromedial rotatory instability • Posterolateral rotatory instability • PLRI • Olecranon
- Fracture • Dislocation • Radial head

KEY POINTS

- Elbow dislocations are the second most common joint dislocation. Approximately one-quarter of them involve a fracture, and recovery can be fraught with complications.
- There are 3 main patterns of instability in elbow fracture-dislocation; valgus posterolateral rotatory instability, varus posteromedial rotatory instability, and transolecranon fracture-dislocation.
- Each pattern comes with its own soft tissue and bony injuries that determine treatment and rehabilitation strategies.

Elbow dislocations represent the second most common medium to large joint dislocation of the upper extremity after the glenohumeral joint. The incidence has been reported at 5.2 cases per 100,000 person-years.[1] Roughly one-quarter of all elbow dislocations involve a fracture.[2] These injuries can be debilitating for patients, and the sequelae may be fraught with complications, including recurrent instability, posttraumatic arthritis, contracture, and poor functional results.

Although these can be difficult injuries to manage, there are workable algorithms for care. The goal of treatment of these injuries is to achieve stable fixation of the appropriate ligamentous and bony structures in order to achieve a stable, functional, and pain-free elbow.[3] Early determination and appreciation of the magnitude and scope of injury generally leads to a more favorable result.

This article reviews the relevant periarticular anatomy of the elbow and discusses appropriate evaluation and treatment of elbow fracture-dislocations. The 3 mechanism-based classifications of elbow fracture-dislocation are discussed individually because the treatment strategies differ between them.

ANATOMY

The ulnohumeral joint is a ginglymus, or hinge, joint with 1 primary axis of rotation. The ulnohumeral joint allows elbow motion with a typical arc of flexion-extension from 0° to 135°. The ulnohumeral joint is the most important contributor to stability of the elbow.[4–6]

The trochlea is the portion of the distal humerus that matches the proximal ulna. It resembles a spool and forms a highly congruent articulation with the proximal ulna. The other primary stabilizers include the radial head, capitellum, medial and lateral collateral ligaments (LCLs), and the joint capsule. The radial head and capitellum articulate to form the radiocapitellar joint. This articulation allows fluid forearm rotation.[7] If the medial structures of the elbow are compromised, the radiocapitellar articulation does impart some resistance to valgus stress.[8]

The coronoid process is the anterior-most bony prominence of the proximal ulna. The anterior ulnohumeral capsule inserts near the tip of the coronoid.[9] The brachialis muscle inserts roughly 1 cm distal to the tip of the coronoid process.

Orthopaedic Surgery, UPMC, Pittsburgh, PA, USA
[1] Present address: 1300 Oxford Drive Suite 1200, Bethel Park, PA 15102.
* Corresponding author. 1300 Oxford Drive, Suite 1200, Bethel Park, PA 15102.
E-mail address: baratzme@upmc.edu

Hand Clin 36 (2020) 495–510
https://doi.org/10.1016/j.hcl.2020.07.011
0749-0712/20/© 2020 Elsevier Inc. All rights reserved.

This bony prominence serves as a buttress to prevent posterior translation of the ulna in relation to the distal humerus.

The olecranon is the most proximal aspect of the ulna, wrapping around the distal humerus and forming the main articulation with the trochlea. The proximal tip of the olecranon, the olecranon process, is a secondary joint stabilizer in throwing athletes. Otherwise it confers little stability and up to 50% bony resection imparts minimal changes to joint stability.[4]

The medial collateral ligament (MCL) originates from the medial epicondyle of the humerus and serves as the primary restraint for valgus stress. It is made up of the posterior, anterior, and transverse bands.[5,10,11] The anterior band is the most clinically relevant.[12,13] At the base of the coronoid, the anterior band of the MCL inserts onto an area known as the sublime tubercle.[9]

The LCL complex is a ligamentous structure on the lateral aspect of the elbow that includes the radial collateral ligament, the annular ligament, and the lateral ulnar collateral ligament (LUCL).[14] The LUCL is the primary restraint to posterolateral rotatory instability (PRLI).[15–18] It originates on the lateral epicondyle of the humerus. It then fans out and inserts distally on the crista supinatoris, a bony prominence along the lateral edge of the proximal ulna.

The secondary stabilizers to elbow stability include the dynamic muscle-tendon units that cross the joint.[19] The biceps, brachialis, and triceps muscles maintain the relationship between the proximal ulna and the trochlea. The flexor and extensor muscles that originate from the distal humerus provide dynamic resistance to varus, valgus, and rotatory stress.[10,15,20]

CLASSIFICATION BY MECHANISM

There are several structures that can be injured in an elbow fracture-dislocation, and injuries vary based on mechanism and patterns of instability. There are 3 main patterns: valgus posterolateral rotatory instability (PLRI), varus posteromedial rotatory instability (PMRI), and transolecranon fracture-dislocation. The pattern of injury in a given fracture-dislocation is dictated by the position of the arm and the direction of the forces on the elbow at the moment of injury.

Within each of these categories, the involved structures fail in a predictable pattern based on the level of energy imparted on the elbow and position of the arm and direction of the forces. With lower-energy injuries, such as a ground-level fall, only some of the structures may be injured. Most commonly, soft tissue structures are injured during a dislocation but a fracture does not occur.[2] This injury is deemed a simple elbow dislocation and is treated with closed reduction and a short period of immobilization. In any case in which a fracture occurs, the injury is labeled a complex elbow dislocation. These injuries typically require a higher level of energy during the injury event and many represent an operative indication.[19,21]

Valgus Posterolateral Rotatory Instability Pattern

Posterolateral PLRI has been suggested to be the most common mechanism of elbow fracture-dislocation injuries. This injury occurs when the patient falls on an outstretched hand that is planted on the ground with a combination of axial load, valgus force, and relative supination of the forearm with relation to the humerus and trunk.[17,22–24]

As it is classically described, the first structure that fails is the LCL complex at its origin on the lateral epicondyle.[25] This failure occurs because of supination and subluxation of the radial head with respect to the capitellum. The LUCL is the portion that is thought to fail initially and universally in this injury pattern. As the injury proceeds, the radial head can impact the capitellum, resulting in fracture and further destabilization of the joint. Next, the ulna supinates and posteriorly subluxates beneath the trochlea, leading to a shear-type fracture of the coronoid tip. The MCL can then tear as the ulnohumeral joint dislocates completely. This injury is colloquially termed the terrible triad of the elbow. This pattern of energy transmission is sometimes referred to as the Horii circle because of an eponymous article written in the early 1990s.[26]

Despite these postulations, recent video evidence of elbow dislocations in athletes suggests that the MCL is the first structure that is torn and is required to be torn in order for elbow dislocation to occur. The MCL is a primary restraint to valgus loads on the elbow.[27] Future studies may corroborate these findings and solidify the present understanding of the order of soft tissue failure in PLRI fracture-dislocations.

Varus Posteromedial Rotatory Instability Pattern

PMRI is rare compared with PLRI. Typically the articular surface relationships are maintained in this pattern, making it particularly easy for the unwary observer to overlook[28–30] (Fig. 1A). It was not until the mid-2000s that surgeons began writing about this entity in any great detail.[29,31,32] This injury is thought to occur through a backward fall

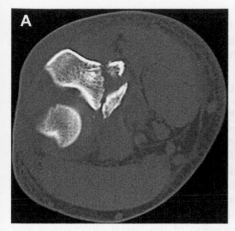
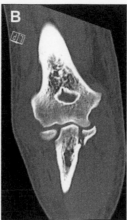

Fig. 1. (*A*) Axial computed tomography (CT) slice shows a comminuted fracture of the coronoid involving the anteromedial facet. (*B*) On this coronal image, a large anteromedial facet fragment is better visualized. This injury is consistent with a PMRI-type fracture-dislocation of the elbow. This fragment must be stabilized in order to ensure a stable elbow.

onto the outstretched arm with the forearm pronated and the shoulder abducted and forward flexed, although other mechanisms have also been described.[27,32]

Because of the varus stress on the elbow, the LCL complex avulses from the lateral epicondyle. The trochlea then acts as a pilon to fracture the anteromedial facet of the coronoid process (**Fig. 1**B). The anteromedial facet is particularly prone to injury in this mechanism because at least 60% of the facet is unsupported by the ulnar metaphysis.[29] As the injury progresses, the unstable coronoid allows the proximal ulna to subluxate posterior to the trochlea.[33] The radial head is not usually fractured in the injury pattern. Although radiographs may appear benign, unrecognized instability can lead to rapid arthritic degradation.[34-36]

Transolecranon (Axial Load) Pattern

The transolecranon pattern of elbow fracture-dislocation is associated with a high level of energy. The injury mechanism typically involves a direct blow to the posterior aspect of the proximal forearm with the elbow flexed. This mechanism drives the distal humerus through the greater sigmoid notch of the ulna, leading to an impaction failure of the olecranon.

The olecranon is the first structure injured and often involves multiple comminuted fragments. The coronoid is often fractured as an independent fragment separate from the rest of the proximal ulna. It may be 1 large piece or alternatively may be comminuted.[28,30] As the injury progresses, the ulna and radial head can be dislocated either anteriorly (most common)[37] or posteriorly.[38] The radial head may or may not be fractured. Both the LCL and MCL complexes fail

in tension by avulsion of their respective origins on the humerus.

This pattern may involve disruption of all osseous stabilizers of the elbow.[19,38-40] The true incidence is likely underappreciated because it is often misclassified as a Monteggia fracture. Unlike the Monteggia injury, the proximal radioulnar joint is spared in the transolecranon fracture-dislocation pattern.[37,41]

EMERGENCY ROOM MANAGEMENT

Most elbow fracture-dislocations occur after a PLRI-type injury mechanism.[2] The elbow dislocation may be reduced by the athletic trainer on the field. A persistent elbow dislocation is unlikely to be missed by the emergency room physician, and a reduction may be achieved before consultation with the orthopedic surgeon. If the joint has not been reduced, elbow radiographs before reduction are helpful to understand the mechanism and likely injured soft tissue structures.

When evaluating a patient with an elbow fracture-dislocation, careful assessment of neurovascular status is paramount. Dysfunction of the ulnar nerve is the most common deficit and is typically a traction neuropraxia.[42,43] Compartment syndrome and floating elbow injuries should be identified early because they represent surgical emergencies.[44] The extent of injury to the soft tissue sleeve should be noted, and open fractures should be identified and treated appropriately. In the event of an open fracture, these patients should have their tetanus immunizations updated and intravenous antibiotics should be instituted based on the Gustilo-Anderson criteria for open injuries.[45,46] Palpation of the wrist, forearm, and humerus can identify areas of tenderness that may suggest concomitant injuries. Tenderness along the distal radioulnar joint or forearm axis may represent interosseous ligament disruption associated with an Essex-Lopresti injury.[24,47]

Once injury films have been obtained, a reduction maneuver should be performed. Conscious sedation is helpful in achieving a relaxed patient and to provide analgesia during the reduction. The maneuver for reduction of a PLRI-type dislocation involves extension of the elbow with the forearm supinated to recreate the position of instability. Axial traction of the hand and direct pressure on the olecranon result in a palpable clunk when successful. Bedside fluoroscopy or standard radiographs can be useful to confirm concentric reduction of the ulnohumeral joint. Once this has been confirmed, the elbow should be taken through a range of motion to identify the stable arc of motion. The elbow should be splinted in flexion and forearm protonation, which is the position of stability. Formal postreduction radiographs should be obtained once the splint has hardened to rule out subluxation or redislocation. If the joint remains subluxated, this represents residual joint laxity. In these cases, and cases of a substantial fracture component, a computed tomography (CT) scan with two-dimensional and three-dimensional reconstructions may be beneficial to better understand the injury.

Transolecranon fracture-dislocations are high-energy injuries that can occur in motor vehicle collisions and severe sports injuries or other such mechanisms.[38] By their nature, they are often associated with concomitant injuries of the ipsilateral upper extremity. Advanced trauma life support fundamentals should be applied in the trauma bay. Evaluation for blunt head and neck trauma as well as chest injuries should be undertaken initially. Radiographic evaluation should include forearm and humerus films as well as standard elbow radiographs in an effort to rule out floating elbow and other ipsilateral injuries. Because these injuries typically involve loss of integrity of the osseous stabilizers of the elbow, a closed reduction should be attempted but may be unsuccessful. If a reduction attempt is unsuccessful, the elbow should be splinted in a position of comfort. These fractures are invariably operative but may be treated on an ambulatory basis barring concomitant injuries.[48]

PMRI-type elbow injuries are subtle and may be missed by the emergency room physician and on-call radiologist. These injuries typically do not present with a persistent overt dislocation of the ulnohumeral joint and therefore may be underappreciated by the patient and evaluating physician, although subtle radiographic signs of instability are typically present.[32] More often than not, the upper extremity specialist is the first to identify this injury in the outpatient setting. The diagnosis is often delayed for weeks or months after the initial injury.

WORK-UP AND DEFINITIVE TREATMENT

Regardless of the injury mechanism, all elbow fracture-dislocations should be initially evaluated with anteroposterior (AP) and lateral elbow radiographs. PLRI-type injuries are typically associated with radial head fracture, lateral and posterior subluxation of the radius with respect to the capitellum, and lateral and posterior dislocation of the ulnohumeral joint. After successful reduction, subtle widening of the lateral ulnohumeral joint on an AP view can be appreciated but may be a normal variant.[49] Radiographs of the contralateral, uninjured elbow can help determine whether or not observed widening represents joint angulation. These injuries are often associated with a coronoid tip fracture that represents less than 10% of the coronoid process; this injury constellation is known as a terrible-triad injury (elbow dislocation, radial head fracture, and coronoid fracture).[7]

Some low-energy PLRI injuries can be treated nonoperatively. If nonoperative treatment is being considered, the elbow should be reevaluated a few days after injury with clinical and radiographic assessment to determine joint stability. In-office fluoroscopy, if available, can be beneficial in this assessment. Otherwise, serial radiographs can be obtained with conventional means or alternatively using the Captain Morgan view. The Captain Morgan view is particularly useful in the setting of elbow instability, and allows the patient to maintain a position of stability while being transported to the radiology suite and while getting plain film radiographs. The patient is instructed to place the hand flat on the abdomen, with the elbow at the side and in a flexed posture. A lateral radiograph is obtained while the patient is standing, with the lateral aspect of the elbow placed against the cassette and the beam directed at the elbow. For the first 1 to 2 weeks, this is done with the elbow in the splint. The lateral view can confirm that the elbow is located and that the radial head fracture has not displaced. It is typical to see an increased space between the trochlea and ulna. The authors refer to this as the sag sign: evidence of residual joint laxity from ligament incompetence and atony of the triceps, biceps, and brachialis. Through the use of a removable splint and overhead exercises, the sag typically resolves in 4 to 6 weeks, as is described in the article on elbow rehabilitation in this issue.

Most elbow fracture-dislocations require operative treatment. When there is uncertainty regarding fracture size, comminution, and origin, high-resolution CT after initial reduction is extremely beneficial for preoperative planning. Large coronoid fractures may require surgical stabilization to restore stability to the elbow,[7] although, in most PLRI injuries, the radial head and LCL process are the only structures that require fixation. The MCL rarely needs to be repaired.[50]

Transolecranon Work-up

Transolecranon fracture-dislocations are not subtle. Radiographs show an obvious olecranon fracture; however, these films should be scrutinized for the presence of articular comminution, coronoid fracture fragments, and associated radial head fractures.[48] These findings have significant implications for the definitive fixation strategy. CT evaluation of these injuries is often recommended to clarify the size of individual fragments and to better evaluate the proximal radioulnar joint, because these injuries are often confused with the adult Monteggia variant.[37,41] Transolecranon injuries require operative treatment with rare exceptions.

Posteromedial Rotatory Instability Work-up

PMRI-type injuries require a high index of suspicion. On the AP radiograph, it is crucial to evaluate the entire ulnohumeral joint. In these injuries, the medial half of the joint may appear narrow. This finding is typically coupled with subtle widening of the radiocapitellar joint. Medial ulnohumeral joint space narrowing is the result of articular impaction of the anteromedial facet of the coronoid and collapse of the joint. Widening of the radiocapitellar joint is the result of LUCL avulsion and the ulnar side of the humerus falling in to the defect created by the coronoid fracture. On the lateral radiograph, a double-crescent sign reflects the depressed anteromedial facet of the coronoid.[32] Three-dimensional reconstructions of the elbow may be of particular benefit in PMRI-type injuries. These injuries are typically operative, although a delay in diagnosis may preclude simple fixation of the involved structures.

Physical examination may be helpful in determining evidence of medial elbow instability. It is assessed by reproducing the varus posteromedial load while the elbow is brought from flexion to extension. Ideally, this is performed during manipulation under anesthesia and with the aid of fluoroscopy. Subluxation or redislocation of the ulnohumeral joint verifies this injury pattern.

FIXATION STRATEGIES
Radial Head Fractures

In isolation, most radial head fractures can be treated nonoperatively. The classification system most often applied to these fractures is the Mason classification.[51] By this system, nondisplaced or minimally displaced fractures are deemed Mason type I. These fractures are almost always treated with early active motion. Mason type II fractures are partial articular fractures with a minimum of 2 mm of displacement, and can often be treated nonsurgically as well.[52] If surgery is necessary, these fractures can typically be treated with 1 or several buried headless or headed screws to reconstitute the articular surface. In the setting of a fracture-dislocation, there generally is a lower threshold for operative treatment of radial head fractures.[21]

Mason type III fractures represent complete articular fractures in which no portion of the radial head is in continuity with the shaft (Fig. 2A–D). These fractures rarely can be treated with open reduction and internal fixation in the form of multiple screws and/or a precontoured plate that stabilizes the head fragments to the shaft. The plate should be placed in the anatomic safe zone, which represents the nonarticulating arc of the radial head that is directly opposite the proximal radioulnar joint with the forearm in neutral[53] (Fig. 2E–H). This zone can be identified clinically by palpating Lister tubercle and the radial styloid. By extrapolating the plane that is created by these 2 landmarks, the anatomic safe zone is determined. It is visible as the area on the head with a paucity of articular cartilage.

More commonly, significant articular comminution and multiple fragments preclude stable fixation of Mason III radial head fractures. If the radial head is in more than 3 pieces, fixation is not likely to be successful. In these situations, a radial head arthroplasty is preferable (Fig. 3). In the setting of a fracture-dislocation, the radial head is generally not excised without replacement with an arthroplasty prosthesis.[54] The radial head is an integral osseous stabilizer to valgus stress and its removal precludes a stable elbow joint if both collateral ligaments are also torn.

When performing a radial head arthroplasty, a modular design allows easier adjustment of the height of the prosthesis in relation to the ulna. The prosthesis should be positioned roughly 2 mm distal to the coronoid tip on the AP view. This position recreates the appropriate relationship with the proximal radioulnar joint, and also ensures that the ulnohumeral joint is even from medial to lateral. Overstuffing the joint causes

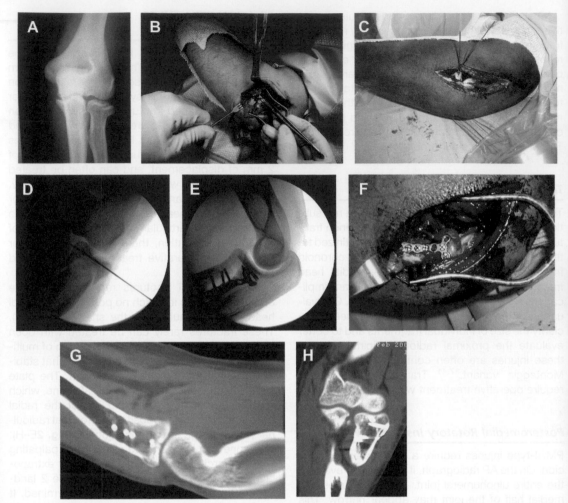

Fig. 2. (A) Anteroposterior (AP) radiograph shows a Mason type III radial head fracture. The fracture is comminuted. There is an articular step-off. (B) Lateral approach to the elbow. A rotated articular radial head fracture is visualized before fixation. (C) Fracture fragments are provisionally fixed with Kirschner wires. (D) Mason type 3 fracture. Fluoroscopic AP image shows the articular segment with provisional pinning. Note that the articular surface appears reduced, but the fragments are still splayed along the metaphysis. This image better shows the fracture through the radial neck. (E) Lateral fluoroscopic image shows a well-reduced articular surface. (F) Plate/screw construct. The plate was placed in the anatomic safe zone, which represents the nonarticulating portion of the head. (G) Sagittal CT image 2 months after a radial head open reduction with internal fixation (ORIF). (H) Coronal CT scan 2 months after a radial head ORIF. Note the concentrically reduced ulnohumeral joint.

the lateral ulnohumeral joint to be widened, which places undue stress on the medial aspect of the joint and may preclude normal elbow motion. Intraoperative fluoroscopy can help confirm appropriate positioning.

Several studies have shown equivalent range of motion and patient-reported outcomes in elbow fracture-dislocations treated with either open reduction and internal fixation or radial head arthroplasty.[55,56] These studies were not randomized-controlled trials and therefore a significant selection bias likely affects their results.

What is clear is that restoration of osseous stability, whether by open reduction with internal fixation or replacement, leads to the best results for all patients.

Coronoid Fractures

Coronoid fractures were originally classified by Regan and Morrey[57] based on the lateral plain film radiographs; however, this system failed to recognize obliquity in fracture patterns. O'Driscoll described an anteromedial facet fracture as its own category with 3 subsets for a total of 7

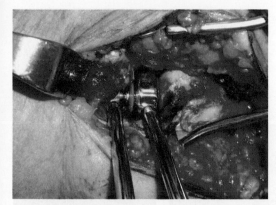

Fig. 3. Final seating of a radial head arthroplasty implant. Note the bipolar nature of this particular design. This case featured a comminuted radial head fracture that was not amenable to repair.

fracture types. Another classification expands the Regan and Morrey classification types, but adds fractures with anteromedial and anterolateral obliquity, and is based on CT scans with reported high interobserver and intraobserver reliability.[32]

Coronoid tip fractures, most commonly seen in PLRI-type injuries, often do not need to be addressed surgically. Tip fractures that include greater than 10% of the height of the coronoid may be considered for surgical stabilization (**Fig. 4**). If the radial head fracture is being treated by radial head replacement, the coronoid fracture can be approached through the lateral incision once the head fragments have been removed.

These fractures can be treated by cannulated screw fixation if the fragment is large enough. An over-the-top anterior cruciate ligament tibial reaming guide can be used to capture the tip fragment and triangulate a drill tunnel for antegrade screw placement.

The spin move is possible when there is complete disruption of the lateral ulnar collateral (LUCL) origin and the common extensor origin. Absence of these soft tissue restraints allows increased access via a supination moment to the elbow. This technique facilitates visualization, reduction, and fixation of the fractured coronoid, and is easier in slender individuals with less soft tissue.

When the tip fragment is too small for screw purchase or when there is comminution, the suture lasso method has been proposed. This technique involves grabbing the anterior capsule just proximal to its insertion on the tip fragment with a heavy nonabsorbable suture. The limbs of the suture are then brought down through drill holes in the ulna and tied over the posterior cortex of the ulna. Often a suture button is used. In a study by

Garrigues and colleagues,[31] this technique led to better clinical results than screw/plate constructs or suture anchors regardless of the fracture pattern. However, the amount of stability that these procedures confer is questionable. If the fracture fragment is so small that it cannot accept a screw or plate, it is often left alone. Moreover, the anterior capsule does not attach to the coronoid tip; it attaches to a point distal to the tip, so capsulorrhaphy procedures such as these do not reconstruct normal anatomy.

Anteromedial facet fractures are typically seen with PMRI-type injuries. These fractures are typically operative and are commonly suited to a medial approach. The Hotchkiss over-the-top approach uses the interval between the flexor carpi ulnaris (FCU) and the palmaris longus. This approach is helpful for treating coronoid tip fractures and MCL tears simultaneously, but it is not the best approach for visualizing anteromedial facet fractures.[58] The FCU approach is an intramuscular approach that involves releasing the humeral origin of the FCU while maintaining the ulnar origin. The capsule is then approached directly beneath the FCU origin and the anteromedial facet can be visualized. The third option is to approach the coronoid through the floor of the cubital tunnel. In situations where the ulnar nerve is being transposed, this becomes a more inviting choice.[59] Other approaches to the coronoid include anterior exposures, but these leave the median nerve vulnerable to traction injury and may make it difficult to achieve fixation for more anteromedial fracture fragments.[31]

Most anteromedial facet fractures are amenable to fixation. These fractures are typically treated with 1 or several cortical screws and an overlying anteromedial buttress plate (**Fig. 5**). When the fragments are too small or are comminuted, the suture lasso technique can be considered if stability is not restored by fixation of other injured structures. The MCL insertion on the sublime tubercle is rarely avulsed in PMRI injuries, and this insertion should be preserved during approach and fixation of the coronoid fracture.

Olecranon Fractures

When fixing olecranon fractures, the authors prefer lateral patient positioning with the upper arm suspended over a radiolucent bolster. This position allows a direct posterior approach to the elbow and maintains freedom of motion of the elbow during reduction and fixation. The triceps tendon insertion should be spared and subperiosteal dissection of the fracture fragments allows adequate visualization of the joint surface. The medial and

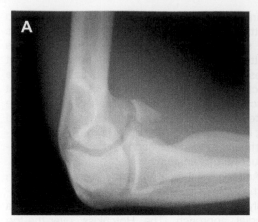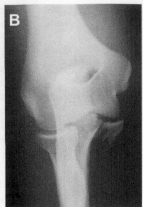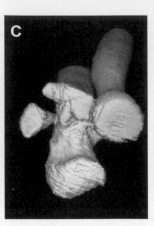

Fig. 4. (*A*) Lateral radiograph of the elbow shows a large, displaced coronoid fracture. (*B*) In the AP view, the coronoid fracture clearly involves the anteromedial facet, which in this place maintains its articulation with the medial trochlea. The remainder of the ulnohumeral joint is difficult to visualize. This injury is a classic PMRI. (*C*) CT three-dimensional reconstruction obtained at the time of injury can be useful to determine the extent of comminution and articular relationships.

lateral joint lines can be exposed via extension of the subperiosteal dissection up and around the ulnohumeral joint, which may be necessary if a coronoid fragment or the radial head needs to be addressed. With this technique, it is paramount to preserve the underlying insertion of the anterior band of the MCL onto the sublime tubercle and the LUCL insertion on the crista supinatoris, respectively.

The articular surface must be reconstituted by careful identification and provisional fixation of individual osteoarticular fragments. Buried Kirschner wires (K-wires) and/or unicortical 2.0-mm minifragment plates can help for provisional fixation. In severely comminuted fractures, a transarticular K-wire can be used to capture and hold the olecranon tip to the distal humerus to maintain that relationship while the remainder of the reduction is performed.

Tension band wire fixation can be used for the definitive fixation construct for isolated olecranon fractures, but this strategy has led to early failures and high complication rates in the setting of transolecranon fracture-dislocations.[37,38,60] This method should be limited to simple fracture patterns, including transverse and short oblique fracture morphologies in the setting of isolated olecranon fractures. Because transolecranon fracture-dislocations are high-energy injuries, they are typically associated with significant comminution, which precludes stable fixation with tension band wires alone; plate and screw fixation is the treatment of choice for these injuries.

Locking plate technology can be applied to any olecranon fracture pattern and should be considered in these injuries. After provisional fixation has been achieved, a plate can be placed directly over the posterior ulnar shaft and fixed initially with

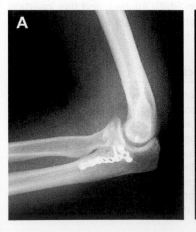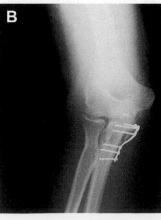

Fig. 5. (*A*) Lateral radiograph view of an anteromedial facet fracture treated with a buttress plate. (*B*) AP radiograph view of anteromedial facet fracture treated with a buttress plate.

a cortical shaft screw distal to the fracture bed. Next, proximal fixation should be achieved with locking screw technology in order to prevent escape of the olecranon tip. One or several so-called home-run screws are often used, which are directed to capture the proximal olecranon tip and subchondral bone of the articular surface.

In cases of medial wall comminution, failure to capture the medial wall can lead to elbow instability if the MCL is attached to the medial wall fragment. Dual-plate fixation can stabilize the medial wall fragment, restoring stability to the elbow.

Lateral Collateral Ligament Complex

The LCL complex is almost always avulsed from its origin on the lateral epicondyle. Intraoperatively, the bony origin is devoid of any soft tissue attachment, a finding that has been described as the naked capitellum sign.[61] Regardless of the injury pattern, the LCL should be repaired to its origin. The authors recommend a running, locking stitch be passed through the bulk of the LUCL with a stout #2 or #5 Ethibond, which is then secured to the origin as described next.

A drill hole is made at the isometric origin of the LCL that visually matches the center of the capitellum profile. This drill hole can then perforate the lateral column of the distal humerus either on the posterior or anterior surface. One limb of the suture can be passed through the tunnel and the limbs can be tied over a bone bridge.[61] Alternatively, a suture button can be used by passing both strands through the tunnel. Likewise, another alternative is use of a suture anchor at the LUCL origin and repairing the injured ligament back to this structure.[62]

It is of utmost importance that the ulnohumeral joint and radiocapitellar joints are reduced before tying the sutures. This step can be achieved by placing the elbow in a position of flexion and pronation in order to close down the lateral ulnohumeral joint and remove any PLRI forces from the joint. Intraoperative fluoroscopy and range of motion should be used to confirm concentric reduction after the sutures have been tied.[31,36]

Medial Collateral Ligament

The MCL is often torn in elbow fracture-dislocations, but it rarely needs to be fixed. It has been shown that repair of a structurally significant coronoid fracture is more important than fixing the MCL.[36] In PLRI-type injuries, the stability of the joint should be assessed intraoperatively after the LUCL has been repaired and any necessary bony fixation has been accomplished. If there is persistent laxity to valgus stress, the MCL can be repaired through a separate medial approach to the elbow.

There are 2 approaches that have been described. The FCU-splitting approach is the classic approach to this ligament, but the over-the-top approach described by Hotchkiss[63] allows better access to a concomitant coronoid fracture if fixation is necessary. The Hotchkiss approach uses the interval between the palmaris longus and the FCU so that the surgical window is slightly more radial and anterior in order to view both the ligament and the coronoid process.

Unlike the LCL complex, which is typically avulsed off the humerus, the MCL can be torn proximally off the humerus, distally off the sublime tubercle, or it can be an intrasubstance tear. Repair of the ligament depends on the location of the tear. Proximal tears can be treated similarly to the LCL with either a bone tunnel, a suture button, or a suture anchor. Distal avulsions can be repaired to the sublime tubercle with a #2 nonabsorbable suture passed through drill holes in the tubercle.

The first priority in managing elbow fracture-dislocations is achieving a concentric joint. Clinicians are good at managing elbow stiffness. It is more challenging to manage chronic joint instability. Persistent instability despite treatment of the radial head, coronoid, and collateral ligaments is fortunately uncommon. In our experience, it is more common in higher-energy injuries in patients with higher body mass index, particularly perimenopausal women.[64] If there is persistent instability in the operating room, there are several strategies:

1. Immobilize in flexion and pronation (provided a concentric reduction can be obtained)
2. Augmented ligament repair/reconstruction
3. Application of an internal joint stabilizer
4. Application of an external fixator

Flexion of the elbow with pronation of the forearm is often sufficient to achieve a concentric joint, particularly with an intact MCL. This position counteracts the posterolateral subluxation that accompanies PLRI as pronation moves the radial head into a position that is anterior and medial on the capitellum,[65] If the posterior capsule is intact, flexion uses the capsule as a hinge to help reduce the ulnohumeral joint.

If midsubstance rupture of ligaments precludes repair, nonabsorbable suture or suture tape can be used to supplement or substitute for ligament repair (**Fig. 6**).

The internal joint stabilizer (Skeletal Dynamics, Miami, FL) is a hinged device with an axis pin through the humerus and plate fixation to the

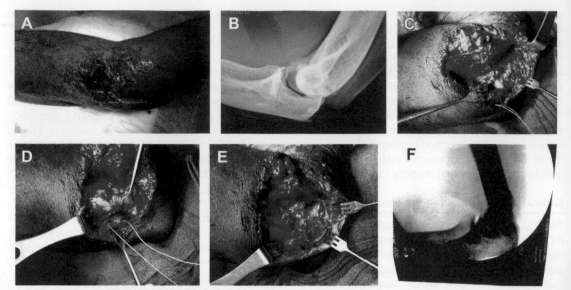

Fig. 6. (*A*) Lateral degloving injury from a rollover motor vehicle crash. (*B*) Lateral view of the elbow sag sign and resulting incompetent LUCL. (*C*) Absent lateral tissue from degloving injury. (*D*) Number 5 braided nonabsorbable suture passed through the ulna at the proximal and distal margins of the lateral crista. (*E*) Suture spanning the defect in the lateral soft tissues. (*F*) Lateral view of the elbow showing a concentric reduction following suture stabilization of the lateral side of the elbow.

ulna. Our indication for this device is the unstable elbow that defies the methods discussed earlier to achieve a concentric joint reduction (**Fig. 7**A). The implant is typically placed on the lateral side of the elbow. It remains in place for a minimum of 8 to 12 weeks but can remain in place for longer intervals (**Fig. 7**B, C).

External fixators can be applied in lieu of the internal joint stabilizer. There are both hinged and static fixators. Hinged fixators require great precision to place the hinge along the flexion-extension axis of the elbow. If the hinge is off axis, a concentric reduction cannot be maintained. Static fixators are easier and quicker to apply. Again, a concentric joint reduction trumps early elbow motion. The authors recommended an incision on the lateral aspect of the humerus to ensure safe placement of proximal pins to protect the radial nerve. Distal pin placement can be performed percutaneously. The fixator is generally kept in place for 4 to 6 weeks. Although a stiff elbow is expected, this is generally manageable with therapy, static progressive splinting, and, if necessary, contracture release.

AFTERCARE AND REHABILITATION PRINCIPLES

The goal in treating complex elbow fracture-dislocations is to repair the injury so as to allow early postoperative motion.[66,67] Early motion

must be accomplished without jeopardizing joint stability. Conditions that may preclude early motion include hematoma formation, hardware with marginal soft tissue coverage, and marginal fixation of bone, or a construct where a concentrically reduced joint is only possible with elbow flexion.

The authors use isometric exercises and the overhead motion protocol for rehabilitation of elbow fracture-dislocations.[68] If the MCL is intact and an LCL repair has been performed, the elbow should be stable. We would typically immobilize in 90° of flexion in a neutral forearm rotation for 5 to 7 days.[69] If the LCL was repaired but the MCL was not, we immobilize in 90° of flexion and in full supination, because supination helps close the medial joint line.[69]

We typically see patients in the clinic at 5 to 7 days postsurgery. A standing lateral view is obtained with the patient's hand on the stomach and lateral aspect of the elbow against the cassette. This position is used to confirm the elbow is not subluxated. It also determines whether there is a sag sign: separation between the trochlea and olecranon fossa. Isometric exercises are initiated to restore resting tone to the triceps, brachialis, and biceps. Overhead exercises are performed with the patient supine and the shoulder flexed to 90°. Active-assisted flexion and extension exercises are performed with assistance of the good arm. With the elbow at 90°, the forearm is rotated into pronation and supination.

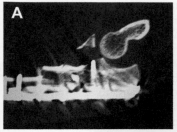
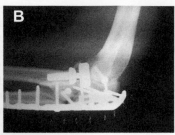
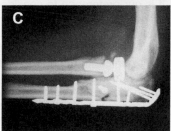

Fig. 7. (A) Sagittal CT of a nonconcentric joint after fixation of a comminuted ulnar shaft fracture. In this case, the treating physician did not achieve a stable elbow. (B) Lateral radiograph view of the ulnohumeral joint reduced and an internal joint stabilizer in place. (C) Lateral radiograph of the joint reduced 3 months after the internal joint stabilizer was removed. A concentric joint has been maintained.

Between exercises, the elbow is maintained in a removable posterior elbow splint.

Follow-up is each week or every other week depending on the degree of residual laxity. In uncomplicated injuries, immobilization is typically discontinued after 4 weeks. In more complex injuries, immobilization and overhead exercises are continued until a concentric reduction of the elbow is confirmed on a lateral view with elbow in flexion and extension. Once active motion has been initiated, patients are typically given 3 to 4 weeks to regain motion. If restoration of motion seems to stall, consideration is given to static progressive splinting. Patients are typically given 6 months to regain acceptable motion. If a residual deficit remains, consideration is given to surgical release.

COMPLICATIONS
Recurrent Instability

Recurrent subluxation or dislocation is preferably identified intraoperatively or in the early postoperative period. The causes include an undersized radial head, failure to stabilize the coronoid, failure to recognize ligament insufficiency, failure of the ligament repair, malreduction of the ulna in a trans-olecranon fracture-dislocation, or global laxity that does not respond to other measures.

Recurrent instability in the early postoperative period can be managed according to the techniques described earlier. Late instability is more challenging for 5 reasons:

1. Nonunited or malunited fracture
2. Oversized or undersized radial head implant
3. Coexisting contracture with scar interposed in the joint

4. Scarring of the ulnar nerve
5. Unrepairable ligaments

Approaching these injuries is often facilitated by advanced imaging, specifically CT scan. The scan allows the clinician to assess the size and position of the coronoid, radial head, and contour of the olecranon fossa. It also may help identify intra-articular hardware or bone fragments.

Any dislocation or subluxation that has been present for several weeks will have some degree of contracture and scar within the joint. In most cases, both can be addressed via a lateral, extensor splitting approach to the elbow. Elevating the anterior half of the common extensor off the lateral epicondyle and the capsule off the anterior aspect of the humerus provides a wide view of 75% to 80% of the joint. If a radial head implant was placed and appears too large, it can be removed. If the native head is nonunited or malunited, it can be resected. Interposed soft tissue is removed and the joint reduced. Intraoperative valgus stress can define whether the MCL is competent. Placing traction on the proximal radius via a towel clip and checking ulnar variance with and without traction identifies longitudinal instability of the forearm if the variance changes by 3 mm or more. If there is valgus laxity or longitudinal instability, it has been our practice to place a radial head implant in those instances where the native head is removed or the previously placed head is inappropriately sized.

In most cases of chronic elbow subluxation, there is a loss of elbow flexion. In this instance, the ulnar nerve is typically scarred to the medial joint capsule. Preoperative evaluation of ulnar nerve function identifies ulnar nerve compression. Even without preoperative symptoms, it is our practice to routinely decompress the ulnar nerve in cases where there is a significant extension contracture.[59]

If the native ligaments are not of sufficient quality to repair, we reconstruct with palmaris longus or split flexor carpi radialis autograft. These reconstructions may need to be protected with simultaneous placement of an internal joint stabilizer or external fixator.

Heterotopic Ossification

Heterotopic ossification is common following elbow fracture-dislocation. It typically forms adjacent to the site of ligament disruption. In these cases, it usually is a radiographic finding that does not adversely affect elbow motion. When there is a high-energy injury, delayed treatment, a head injury, or a concurrent burn, heterotopic ossification can form in the surrounding muscle and ligaments. In the past, it was suggested that this bone not be removed until the edges had corticated on plain radiographs and a bone scan was cold. This process could take up to 2 years. It is our practice to wait 4 to 6 months until fractures have healed and the adjacent soft tissues and scars have softened. There is some controversy regarding the use of radiation[70] or indomethacin[71] in conjunction with resection of heterotopic ossification.[72] It has been our practice to not use either modality unless we are treating recurrent heterotopic ossification.

Elbow Stiffness

Patients appreciate when their physician can provide realistic expectations following surgical treatment. It is a given that elbow stiffness of some degree will accompany an elbow fracture-dislocation. Each individual acclimates to elbow stiffness to a different degree. In general, people have an easier time dealing with a loss of extension than a loss of flexion. Loss of flexion that impedes patients' ability to feed themselves or perform basic grooming can be incapacitating. Similarly, loss of pronation is typically easier to accommodate than loss of supination. In an uncomplicated elbow fracture-dislocation in a young, healthy individual, it is often possible to start overhead exercises in 5 to 7 days. Disabling stiffness in this setting is rarely an issue.

In those patients who fail the rehabilitation measures described earlier, we generally give them 6 months of therapy and static progressive splinting before offering surgery.

Elbow contracture release surgery can be performed open or arthroscopically. Surgeons should remember that, in higher-energy injuries, the anterior joint capsule and, perhaps, the brachialis has been violated, which disrupts the soft tissue planes surrounding the radial nerve. It is our approach to treat contractures from lower-energy injuries with flexion contracture less than 60° by arthroscopic means.

It is our preference to consider operative treatment with open approaches for contractures of greater magnitude or where there is motion-limiting heterotopic bone or hardware to remove. Pure flexion contractures we treat through a lateral approach as described earlier.

When there is a loss of both flexion and extension, particularly with associated ulnar nerve symptoms, we use a combined medial and lateral approach. On the medial side, we release the ulnar nerve and posteromedial capsule. On the lateral side, we do the same release and go between the triceps and lateral column to release the posterolateral capsule.

If there is primarily a loss of flexion, we use a medial approach and release the ulnar nerve and the posteromedial and posterior capsule. An osteophyte on the coronoid or heterotopic ossification in the coronoid fossa, creating a bony block to flexion, can be excised through a medial over-the-top approach. The proximal half of the flexor-pronator mass is released from the medial epicondyle leaving a small cuff of tissue. The exposed anterior capsule is resected, exposing the coronoid and coronoid fossa. The excess bone is removed, and the flexor-pronator mass is repaired.

The same releases can be performed through a single posterior incision. With large medial and/or lateral flaps, we have been unhappy with this approach because it seems more prone to seroma formation that impedes early postoperative motion.

Posttraumatic Arthritis

Joint space narrowing is a common sequela of elbow fracture-dislocation. In most cases, it is observed without symptoms or loss of motion. Symptomatic arthritis is more likely to occur in higher-energy injuries, with residual subluxation, intra-articular hardware, and malunions. There are 2 scenarios:

1. Arthritis with pain isolated to the extremes of motion
2. Arthritis with pain throughout the arc of motion

Establishing the extent of arthritis is best defined with a CT scan. End-arc pain is more typically seen in the setting of idiopathic osteoarthritis with marginal osteophytes, whereas patients experiencing pain throughout the arc of motion are more likely to have widespread articular changes throughout the joint. CT scans of osteoarthritic patients or occasional patients with posttraumatic changes who may benefit from debridement show prominent osteophytes on the coronoid and coronoid fossa as well as olecranon process and olecranon fossa. Open or arthroscopic resection of the offending osteophytes combined with contracture release generally improves motion and reduces discomfort.

Arthritis with pain throughout the arc of motion is typically accompanied by a CT scan that reveals a joint devoid of healthy articular cartilage. There a few options for patients with posttraumatic arthritis, and this is compounded by the fact that patients with posttraumatic arthritis from an elbow fracture-dislocation are generally younger. Options include:

1. Elbow arthrodesis
2. Interposition arthroplasty
3. Elbow hemiarthroplasty (limited availability in the United States)
4. Total elbow arthroplasty

Perretta and colleagues[73] examined risk factors for repeat surgery following elbow arthroplasty. The rate of elbow revision was highest (57%) in patients for trauma-related arthroplasty. Our own experience has been similar.

Clinical experience with hemiarthroplasty for posttraumatic elbow arthritis is exceptionally limited. Werthel and colleagues[74] reviewed 16 patients with an average age of 45 years who underwent hemiarthroplasty for posttrauma arthritis. With an average follow-up of 51 months, 5 of 16 patients required revision surgery. Of the surviving implants, only 57% had a good to excellent clinical outcome.[74]

Elbow arthrodesis has been described for salvage of severe upper limb trauma. It is rarely considered a viable option in patients with posttraumatic arthritis because of the associated limitations in activities of daily living.[76]

As a result of the limited options, it is our preference to consider interposition arthroplasty. It requires a concentric ulnohumeral joint with intact primary and secondary stabilizers, namely intact collateral ligaments and a radiocapitellar joint. We have used arthroscopic assistance to debride the joint and insert the graft so as to preserve the MCL. This procedure is facilitated by releasing and then repairing the lateral complex. No hinged fixator is necessary. Motion is initiated at 2 weeks.

In a small series with 3.6 years of follow-up, 75% of patients had improved clinical outcomes.[76]

In summary, this article describes evaluation and treatment strategies for patients with elbow fracture-dislocation. Attention to initial evaluation and treatment principles can improve outcomes; expected outcomes and complications (and treatment) following these injuries are also described.

DISCLOSURE

The authors have nothing to disclose.

REFERENCES

1. Stoneback JW, Owens BD, Sykes J, et al. Incidence of elbow dislocations in the United States population. J Bone Joint Surg Am 2012. https://doi.org/10.2106/JBJS.J.01663.
2. Josefsson PO, Nilsson BE. Incidence of elbow dislocation. Acta Orthop 1986. https://doi.org/10.3109/17453678609014788.
3. Buijze G, Kloen P. Clinical evaluation of locking compression plate fixation for comminuted olecranon fractures. J Bone Joint Surg Am 2009. https://doi.org/10.2106/JBJS.H.01419.
4. An KN, Morrey BF, Chao EYS. The effect of partial removal of proximal ulna on elbow constraint. Clin Orthop Relat Res 1986. https://doi.org/10.1097/00003086-198608000-00041.
5. Morrey BF, An KN. Functional anatomy of the ligaments of the elbow. Clin Orthop Relat Res 1985. https://doi.org/10.1097/00003086-198512000-00015.
6. Morrey BF, An KN. Stability of the elbow: Osseous constraints. J Shoulder Elbow Surg 2005;S174–8. https://doi.org/10.1016/j.jse.2004.09.031.
7. Schneeberger AG, Sadowski MM, Jacob HAC. Coronoid process and radial head as posterolateral rotatory stabilizers of the elbow. J Bone Joint Surg Am 2004. https://doi.org/10.2106/00004623-200405000-00013.
8. Morrey BF, Tanaka S, An KN. Valgus stability of the elbow. A definition of primary and secondary constraints. Clin Orthop Relat Res 1991. https://doi.org/10.1097/00003086-199104000-00021.
9. Cage DJN, Abrams RA, Callahan JJ, et al. Soft tissue attachments of the ulnar coronoid process: An anatomic study with radiographic correlation. Clin Orthop Relat Res 1995. https://doi.org/10.1097/00003086-199511000-00026.
10. Fuss FK. The ulnar collateral ligament of the human elbow joint. Anatomy, function and biomechanics. J Anat 1991;175:203–12.
11. Sojbjerg JO, Ovesen J, Nielsen S. Experimental elbow instability after transection of the medial

collateral ligament. Clin Orthop Relat Res 1987. https://doi.org/10.1097/00003086-198705000-00026.

12. Floris S, Olsen BS, Dalstra M, et al. The medial collateral ligament of the elbow joint: Anatomy and kinematics. J Shoulder Elbow Surg 1998. https://doi.org/10.1016/S1058-2746(98)90021-0.

13. O'Driscoll SW, Jaloszynski R, Morrey BF, et al. Origin of the medial ulnar collateral ligament. J Hand Surg Am 1992. https://doi.org/10.1016/0363-5023(92)90135-C.

14. Seki A, Olsen BS, Jensen SL, et al. Functional anatomy of the lateral collateral ligament complex of the elbow: Configuration of Y and its role. J Shoulder Elbow Surg 2002. https://doi.org/10.1067/mse.2002.119389.

15. Dunning CE, Zarzour ZDS, Patterson SD, et al. Ligamentous stabilizers against posterolateral rotatory instability of the elbow. J Bone Joint Surg Am 2001. https://doi.org/10.2106/00004623-200112000-00009.

16. Nestor BJ, O'Driscoll SW, Morrey BF. Ligamentous reconstruction for posterolateral rotatory instability of the elbow. J Bone Joint Surg Am 1992. https://doi.org/10.2106/00004623-199274080-00014.

17. O'Driscoll SW, Bell DF, Morrey BF. Posterolateral rotatory instability of the elbow. J Bone Joint Surg Am 1991. https://doi.org/10.1016/b978-1-4160-5650-8.00330-7.

18. Olsen BS, Vaesel MT, Søjbjerg JO, et al. Lateral collateral ligament of the elbow joint: anatomy and kinematics. J Shoulder Elbow Surg 1996. https://doi.org/10.1016/s1058-2746(96)80004-8.

19. Ring D, Jupiter JB. Current concepts review: Fracture-dislocation of the elbow. J Bone Joint Surg Am 1998. https://doi.org/10.2106/00004623-199804000-00014.

20. Cohen MS, Hastings H. Rotatory instability of the elbow: The anatomy and role of the lateral stabilizers. J Bone Joint Surg Am 1997. https://doi.org/10.2106/00004623-199702000-00010.

21. Broberg MA, Morrey BF. Results of treatment of fracture-dislocations of the elbow. Clin Orthop Relat Res 1987. https://doi.org/10.12671/jksf.2000.13.1.178.

22. Deutch SR, Jensen SL, Olsen BS, et al. Elbow joint stability in relation to forced external rotation: An experimental study of the osseous constraint. J Shoulder Elbow Surg 2003. https://doi.org/10.1016/S1058-2746(02)86814-8.

23. O'Driscoll SWM. Elbow instability. Acta Orthop Belg 1999. https://doi.org/10.5005/jp/books/12787_101.

24. Sotereanos DG, Darlis NA, Wright TW, et al. Unstable fracture-dislocations of the elbow. Instr Course Lect 2007;56:369–76.

25. Josefsson PO, Gentz CF, Wenderberg B. Surgical versus non-surgical treatment of ligamentous injuries following dislocation of the elbow joint. A prospective randomized study. J Bone Joint Surg Am 1987. https://doi.org/10.2106/00004623-198769040-00018.

26. Horii E, Nakamura R, Watanabe K, et al. Posterolateral rotatory instability of the elbow - A case report and anatomical study of the lateral collateral ligament. Nihon Seikeigeka Gakkai Zasshi 1993;67(1):34–9.

27. Schreiber JJ, Warren RF, Hotchkiss RN, et al. An online video investigation into the mechanism of elbow dislocation. J Hand Surg Am 2013. https://doi.org/10.1016/j.jhsa.2012.12.017.

28. Doornberg JN, Ring D. Coronoid fracture patterns. J Hand Surg Am 2006. https://doi.org/10.1016/j.jhsa.2005.08.014.

29. Doornberg JN, Ring DC. Fracture of the anteromedial facet of the coronoid process. J Bone Joint Surg Am 2006. https://doi.org/10.2106/JBJS.E.01127.

30. Ring D. Fractures of the coronoid process of the ulna. J Hand Surg Am 2006. https://doi.org/10.1016/j.jhsa.2006.08.020.

31. Garrigues GE, Wray WH, Lindenhovius ALC, et al. Fixation of the coronoid process in elbow fracture-dislocations. J Bone Joint Surg Am 2011. https://doi.org/10.2106/JBJS.I.01673.

32. Sanchez-Sotelo J, O'Driscoll SW, Morrey BF. Medial oblique compression fracture of the coronoid process of the ulna. J Shoulder Elbow Surg 2005. https://doi.org/10.1016/j.jse.2004.04.012.

33. O'Driscoll SW, Jupiter JB, Cohen MS, et al. Difficult elbow fractures: pearls and pitfalls. Instr Course Lect 2003;52:113–4.

34. Beingessner DM, Dunning CE, Stacpoole RA, et al. The effect of coronoid fractures on elbow kinematics and stability. Clin Biomech 2007. https://doi.org/10.1016/j.clinbiomech.2006.09.007.

35. Beingessner DM, Stacpoole RA, Dunning CE, et al. The effect of suture fixation of type I coronoid fractures on the kinematics and stability of the elbow with and without medial collateral ligament repair. J Shoulder Elbow Surg 2007. https://doi.org/10.1016/j.jse.2006.06.015.

36. Forthman C, Henket M, Ring DC. Elbow dislocation with intra-articular fracture: the results of operative treatment without repair of the medial collateral ligament. J Hand Surg Am 2007. https://doi.org/10.1016/j.jhsa.2007.06.019.

37. Mouhsine E, Akiki A, Castagna A, et al. Transolecranon anterior fracture dislocation. J Shoulder Elbow Surg 2007. https://doi.org/10.1016/j.jse.2006.07.005.

38. Ring D, Jupiter JB, Sanders RW, et al. Transolecranon fracture-dislocation of the elbow. J Orthop Trauma 1997. https://doi.org/10.1097/00005131-199711000-00001.

39. Jupiter JB, Leibovic SJ, Ribbans W, et al. The posterior monteggia lesion. J Orthop Trauma 1991.

https://doi.org/10.1097/00005131-199112000-00003.

40. Teasdall R, Savoie FH, Hughes JL. Comminuted fractures of the proximal radius and ulna. Clin Orthop Relat Res 1993. https://doi.org/10.1097/00003086-199307000-00007.

41. Ring D, Jupiter JB, Simpson NS. Monteggia fractures in adults. J Bone Joint Surg Am 1998. https://doi.org/10.2106/00004623-199812000-00003.

42. Malkawi H. Recurrent dislocation of the elbow accompanied by ulnar neuropathy: A case report and review of the literature. Clin Orthop Relat Res 1981. https://doi.org/10.1097/00003086-198111000-00034.

43. Shin R, Ring D. The ulnar nerve in elbow trauma. J Bone Joint Surg Am 2007. https://doi.org/10.2106/JBJS.F.00594.

44. Hwang RW, De Witte PB, Ring D. Compartment syndrome associated with distal radial fracture and ipsilateral elbow injury. J Bone Joint Surg Am 2009. https://doi.org/10.2106/JBJS.H.00377.

45. Gustilo RB, Anderson JT. Prevention of infection in the treatment of one thousand and twenty five open fractures of long bones: retrospective and prospective analyses. J Bone Joint Surg Am 1976. https://doi.org/10.2106/00004623-197658040-00004.

46. Minhas SV, Catalano LW. Comparison of open and closed hand fractures and the effect of urgent operative intervention. J Hand Surg Am 2018;1–7. https://doi.org/10.1016/j.jhsa.2018.04.032.

47. Szabo RM, Hotchkiss RN, Slater J. The use of frozen-allograft radial head replacement for treatment of established symptomatic proximal translation of the radius: Preliminary experience In five cases. J Hand Surg Am 1997. https://doi.org/10.1016/S0363-5023(97)80163-3.

48. Doornberg J, Ring D, Jupiter JB. Effective treatment of fracture-dislocations of the olecranon requires a stable trochlear notch. Clin Orthop Relat Res 2004. https://doi.org/10.1097/01.blo.0000142627.28396.cb.

49. Rowland AS, Athwal GS, MacDermid JC, et al. Lateral ulnohumeral joint space widening is not diagnostic of radial head arthroplasty overstuffing. J Hand Surg Am 2007. https://doi.org/10.1016/j.jhsa.2007.02.024.

50. Duerig M, Mueller W, Ruedi TP, et al. The operative treatment of elbow dislocation in the adult. J Bone Joint Surg Am 1979. https://doi.org/10.2106/00004623-197961020-00012.

51. Mason ML. Some observations on fractures of the radial head with a review of one hundred cases. Br J Surg 1954;42(172):123–32.

52. Åkesson T, Herbertsson P, Josefsson PO, et al. Primary nonoperative treatment of moderately displaced two-part fractures of the radial head. J Bone Joint Surg Am 2006;88(9):1909–14.

53. Kuhn S, Burkhart KJ, Schneider J, et al. The anatomy of the proximal radius: Implications on fracture implant design. J Shoulder Elbow Surg 2012. https://doi.org/10.1016/j.jse.2011.11.008.

54. Ring D, Jupiter JB, Zilberfarb J. Posterior dislocation of the elbow with fractures of the radial head and coronoid. J Bone Joint Surg Am 2002. https://doi.org/10.2106/00004623-200204000-00006.

55. Leigh WB, Ball CM. Radial head reconstruction versus replacement in the treatment of terrible triad injuries of the elbow. J Shoulder Elbow Surg 2012. https://doi.org/10.1016/j.jse.2012.03.005.

56. Watters TS, Garrigues GE, Ring D, et al. Fixation versus replacement of radial head in terrible triad: Is there a difference in elbow stability and prognosis? Clin Orthop Relat Res 2014. https://doi.org/10.1007/s11999-013-3331-x.

57. Regan W, Morrey B. Fractures of the coronoid process of the ulna. J Bone Joint Surg Am 1989;71:1348–54.

58. Huh J, Krueger CA, Medvecky MJ, et al. Medial elbow exposure for coronoid fractures: FCU-split versus over-the-top. J Orthop Trauma 2013. https://doi.org/10.1097/BOT.0b013e31828ba91c.

59. Williams BG, Sotereanos DG, Baratz ME, et al. The contracted elbow: Is ulnar nerve release necessary? J Shoulder Elbow Surg 2012. https://doi.org/10.1016/j.jse.2012.04.007.

60. Mortazavi SMJ, Asadollahi S, Tahririan MA. Functional outcome following treatment of transolecranon fracture-dislocation of the elbow. Injury 2006. https://doi.org/10.1016/j.injury.2005.10.028.

61. Guss MS, Hess LK, Baratz ME. The naked capitellum: a surgeon's guide to intraoperative identification of posterolateral rotatory instability. J Shoulder Elbow Surg 2019;28(5):e150–5.

62. Duckworth AD, Kulijdian A, McKee MD, et al. Residual subluxation of the elbow after dislocation or fracture-dislocation: Treatment with active elbow exercises and avoidance of varus stress. J Shoulder Elbow Surg 2008. https://doi.org/10.1016/j.jse.2007.06.006.

63. Hotchkiss RN, Kasparyan NG. The medial "over the top" approach to the elbow. Tech Orthop 2000;15:105–12.

64. Zhang D, Tarabochia M, Janssen S, et al. Risk of subluxation or dislocation after operative treatment of terrible triad injuries. J Orthop Trauma 2016. https://doi.org/10.1097/BOT.0000000000000674.

65. Galik K, Baratz ME, Butler AL, et al. The effect of the annular ligament on kinematics of the radial head. J Hand Surg Am 2007. https://doi.org/10.1016/j.jhsa.2007.06.008.

66. Iordens GIT, Den Hartog D, Van Lieshout EMM, et al. Good functional recovery of complex elbow dislocations treated with hinged external fixation: a

multicenter prospective study. Clin Orthop Relat Res 2015. https://doi.org/10.1007/s11999-014-3959-1.

67. McKee MD, Pugh DMW, Wild LM, et al. Standard surgical protocol to treat elbow dislocations with radial head and coronoid fractures. JBJS Essent Surg Tech 2005. https://doi.org/10.2106/jbjs.d.02933.

68. Schreiber JJ, Paul S, Hotchkiss RN, et al. Conservative management of elbow dislocations with an overhead motion protocol. J Hand Surg Am 2015. https://doi.org/10.1016/j.jhsa.2014.11.016.

69. Mathew PK, Athwal GS, King GJW. Terrible triad injury of the elbow: Current concepts. J Am Acad Orthop Surg 2009. https://doi.org/10.5435/00124635-200903000-00003.

70. Hamid N, Ashraf N, Bosse MJ, et al. Radiation therapy for heterotopic ossification prophylaxis acutely after elbow trauma: A prospective randomized study. J Bone Joint Surg Am 2010. https://doi.org/10.2106/JBJS.I.01435.

71. Burd TA, Hughes MS, Anglen JO. Heterotopic ossification prophylaxis with indomethacin increases the risk of long-bone nonunion. J Bone Joint Surg

Br 2003. https://doi.org/10.1302/0301-620x.85b5.13970.

72. Moore KD, Goss K, Anglen JO. Indomethacin versus radiation therapy for prophylaxis against heterotopic ossification in acetabular fractures. J Bone Joint Surg Br 1998. https://doi.org/10.1302/0301-620X.80B2.8157.

73. Perretta D, van Leeuwen WF, Dyer G, et al. Risk factors for reoperation after total elbow arthroplasty. J Shoulder Elbow Surg 2017;26(5):824–9.

74. Werthel JD, Schoch B, Adams J, et al. Outcomes after hemiarthroplasty of the elbow for the management of posttraumatic arthritis: minimum 2-year follow-up. J Am Acad Orthop Surg 2019. https://doi.org/10.5435/JAAOS-D-18-00055.

75. Reichel LM, Wiater BP, Friedrich J, et al. Arthrodesis of the Elbow. Hand Clin 2011. https://doi.org/10.1016/j.hcl.2011.02.002.

76. Chauhan A, Palmer BA, Baratz ME. Arthroscopically assisted elbow interposition arthroplasty without hinged external fixation: surgical technique and patient outcomes. J Shoulder Elbow Surg 2015. https://doi.org/10.1016/j.jse.2015.02.003.

Rehabilitation of Elbow Instability

Joey G. Pipicelli, MScOT, CHT[a,b], Graham J.W. King, MD, MSc, FRSC[a,c,*]

KEYWORDS

• Elbow instability • Rehabilitation • Splinting • Dislocation

KEY POINTS

- The primary elbow stabilizers are the ulnohumeral articulation, the anterior bundle of the medial collateral ligament, and the lateral collateral ligament.
- Elbow stability is enhanced with activation of the dynamic muscular stabilizers which cross the joint.
- Overhead range of motion exercise uses gravity to compress the elbow improving joint tracking and stability.
- Injury of the medial or lateral collateral ligaments requires forearm positioning in supination or pronation, respectively, to provide optimal elbow congruity during rehabilitation.
- Application of static-progressive orthoses are of benefit when managing persistent stiffness to the elbow and forearm.

The elbow is the second most commonly dislocated major joint in adults with an estimated incidence of 5.2 dislocations per 100,000 persons per year.[1,2] To optimize outcomes, close communication between the surgeon and therapist is necessary to allow for the implementation of an individualized rehabilitation program. By doing so, one can balance the competing demands of soft tissue and bony healing with those of mobility. This article reviews key concepts that enable the clinician to apply an evidence-informed approach when managing elbow instability.

ANATOMY AND KINEMATIC REVIEW

Bony Anatomy

The distal humerus, proximal ulna, and the radial head together form three articulations: (1) the ulnohumeral joint, (2) the radiocapitellar joint, and (3) the proximal radioulnar joint. The radial head is

an important valgus stabilizer of the elbow, whereas the coronoid process provides an important varus buttress.

Soft Tissue Anatomy

The medial collateral ligament

The medial collateral ligament (MCL) is a primary elbow stabilizer providing restraint to valgus and posteromedial rotatory instability.[3,4] The MCL is not isometric because it inserts posterior to the axis of ulnohumeral rotation. The MCL consists of three components: (1) the anterior bundle, (2) posterior bundle, and (3) the transverse bundle.

The anterior bundle of the MCL arises from the inferior aspect of the medial epicondyle and inserts into the sublime tubercle of the ulna.[5] This structure is taut when the elbow is extended.[5,6]

The posterior bundle of the MCL inserts posterior to the anterior bundle. This orientation makes

Dr. King receives royalties and is a consultant for Wright Medical. Dr. Joey Pipicelli has no conflict of interests.
[a] Roth | McFarlane Hand & Upper Limb Centre, 268 Grosvenor Street, London, Ontario N6A 4V2, Canada; [b] Division of Hand Therapy, St. Joseph's Health Care, London, Ontario, Canada; [c] Division of Orthopaedics, Western University, St. Joseph's Health Care, London, Ontario, Canada
* Corresponding author. Roth | McFarlane Hand and Upper Limb Centre, St. Joseph's Health Care – London, 268 Grosvenor Street, London, Ontario N6A 4V2, Canada.
E-mail address: gking@uwo.ca

Hand Clin 36 (2020) 511–522
https://doi.org/10.1016/j.hcl.2020.07.003
0749-0712/20/© 2020 Elsevier Inc. All rights reserved.

the posterior bundle lax in extension and taut in flexion.[5,6] The posterior bundle is a secondary elbow stabilizer and important in preventing posteromedial rotatory instability. The transverse bundle is of little significance.[5]

Lateral collateral ligament

The lateral collateral ligament (LCL) consists of the lateral ulnar collateral ligament (LUCL), the annular ligament, and the radial collateral ligament (RCL).[7] The LCL stabilizes the elbow against varus and posterolateral rotational loads.[8–10] Both the LUCL and RCL contribute to posterolateral stability.[10–13] Cadaveric studies demonstrate that posterolateral rotatory instability results when the LUCL and RCL are sectioned and the overlying extensor musculature.[12,13] The annular ligament stabilizes the radial head to the ulna during forearm rotation.[14]

Dynamic stabilizers The muscles that cross the elbow provide dynamic stability. The elbow flexors and extensors do not provide significant passive varus-valgus stability.[15,16] The flexor-pronator group of muscles resist dynamic valgus forces.[15,17–19] The extensor-supinator group of muscles provides dynamic secondary stability to varus forces when the arm is in pronation.[20] Josefsson and colleagues[21] confirmed the important impact of the elbow musculature on dynamic stability by observing after simple dislocation that elbow instability increased when patients were examined under anesthesia, that is, when voluntary muscle tone was minimal.

Elbow Stability

The bones, ligaments, capsule, and muscles around the elbow contribute to overall stability. The contribution of each structure depends on muscle activation, arm, and forearm position.[22] Elbow stability is provided by static and dynamic constraints. This has been described as the "fortress of elbow stability" by O'Driscoll and colleagues.[23] The three primary static constraints include the ulnohumeral articulation, the MCL, and the LCL. If these three structures are intact, the elbow should be stable. The secondary stabilizers include the radiocapitellar articulation, the flexor-pronator, and extension-supinator musculature. Because these muscles cross the elbow, they provide a compressive load to the articulation thereby creating dynamic stability.[19]

The LCL, MCL, and anterior joint capsule are typically disrupted in simple dislocations. The extent of injury to the common flexor and extensor origins likely has an important influence on postdislocation stability. In the setting of dislocations with associated fractures, injury to the radial head and coronoid are most common. Shearing fractures of the capitellum and trochlea can also occur.

The classic mechanism for a typical posterolateral elbow dislocation is an axial load in a valgus position with the forearm supinated. O'Driscoll and colleagues[11] postulated that the injury progresses from lateral to medial. In stage 1 there is a complete tear of the LUCL. Stage 2 involves disruption of the remaining RCL and the anterior and posterior joint capsule, which can cause a perched dislocation. Stage 3 injuries tear the MCL, resulting in a complete dislocation.

More recently other mechanisms of dislocation have been described.[24] Schreiber and colleagues[25] analyzed video evidence of deforming forces and upper extremity position and found that the typical dislocation occurs through an extended elbow with a combined axial load, external rotation, and deforming valgus moment. This suggests that the anterior bundle of the MCL may also be the initial site of soft tissue disruption. MRI studies of acute elbow dislocations report complete tears involving the anterior band of the MCL were significantly more common than complete tears involving the LUCL.[26] This implies that some elbow dislocations may be as a result of acute valgus instability and distinct in nature and mechanism from posterolateral rotatory instability as described by O'Driscoll and colleagues.[11] It is important for clinicians to understand that the location and magnitude of soft tissue disruption varies depending on the mechanism of injury, which should alter the management approach.[27]

REHABILITATION GUIDELINES TO OPTIMIZE OUTCOMES

The elbow is notoriously unforgiving following trauma, with stiffness a common reported complication. To optimize outcomes close communication between the surgeon and therapist is necessary to allow for the implementation of an individualized rehabilitation program. In order for this to occur, the therapist and treating physician should be aware of the following details:

- The mechanism of injury and the various structures involved, if known.
- If a closed reduction was performed, which most often occurs in isolated dislocations without concomitant fractures, the therapist must be made aware of the status of the MCL and LCL and the arc of motion in which the elbow remains congruously reduced (the safe arc of motion).

This is ideally evaluated and documented by the physician who performs the elbow reduction under anesthesia or sedation. The stable arc of motion is determined by gradually extending the elbow from the stable flexed position (with the forearm in supination, neutral, and pronation). The angle at which the elbow starts to subluxate is documented. This information is crucial to allow for the implementation of early motion within the safe arc and appropriate positioning within a protective orthoses. If this information is not available, then extension should be limited to 60° initially and progressively increased by 10° on a weekly basis.

- The status of the ligamentous and osseous injuries in operative cases should be communicated to the therapist. For instance, was the fixation stable or tenuous? Which ligaments were fixed? What was the stable arc of motion during surgery?
- The surgeon should advise the therapist if a radiographic "drop sign" is present. A drop sign is a measurable increase in ulnohumeral joint distance, which is evident on lateral radiograph (**Fig. 1**).[28] The typical distance is 2 to 3 mm and a positive sign is a distance greater than 4 mm.[28] A drop sign can be present after simple and complex dislocations treated with or without surgery and is indicative of persistent elbow instability.

After communicating these important details to the therapist, a custom treatment program is created. We believe that most patients should

begin controlled mobilization and protective orthotic positioning under the supervision of a therapist within a week following an elbow dislocation or fracture-dislocation.

Pain and Edema Control

Acute pain and edema are common following elbow trauma and can become a substantial obstacle during early rehabilitation. Effective management is patient-specific and can include multimodal techniques including elevation, heat, ice, compressive dressings, and pharmacologic means. It is imperative that analgesics be taken as prescribed at frequent intervals during the first 2 to 4 weeks as needed. This allows the patient to be an active participant in rehabilitation and assist with implementation of early motion.

It is common for moderate to severe swelling to develop during the first few days post-trauma. Instruction should be provided to elevate the elbow above the heart whenever possible, especially when sleeping. During the inflammatory phase ice or cold packs are effective at reducing inflammation and controlling bleeding. We recommend ice be applied at frequent intervals for 20 minutes throughout the day especially after exercise sessions to minimize edema and muscle spasm. Manual edema mobilization, soft tissue mobilization, and retrograde message is implemented to facilitate edema reduction.[29] Compressive bandaging, such as a tensor or Tubi-grip (Mölnlycke Health Care, Gothenburg, Sweden), is applied after retrograde message to prevent edema

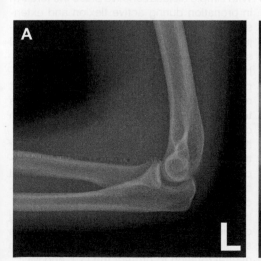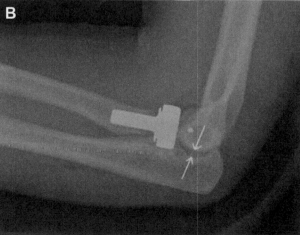

Fig. 1. Radiographic drop sign is a measurable increase in ulnohumeral joint distance evident on lateral radiograph. It is a sign of persistent elbow instability, which can occur after simple (*A*) and complex dislocations (*B*) managed with or without surgery. ([*B*] *From* Pipicelli JG, Chinchalkar S J, Grewal R, Athwal GS. Techniques in Hand & Upper Extremity Surgery 2011;15(4):198–208; with permission.

reaccumulation. Tubi-grip is applied while sleeping; however, careful attention must be placed to ensure that edema does not accumulate in the hand. If this occurs, an edema glove is helpful.

Protective Orthotic Application

All patients should be placed in a posterior elbow resting orthosis positioning the elbow at 90° of flexion. The forearm should be included within the orthosis in a position specific to the injury pattern to provide optimal ligamentous protection.

- LCL-deficient elbow: In this case, the forearm should be positioned in pronation.[12,30,31] This tensions the extensor/supinator group of muscles, which contribute to lateral-sided stability by pivoting the forearm around the intact medial structures.
- MCL-deficient elbow: The elbow should be positioned in supination because this pivots the forearm around the intact lateral structures and tension the flexor/pronator group of muscles, which contributes to medial-sided stability.[30,32,33]
- Combined LCL and MCL deficiencies: The forearm should be positioned in neutral rotation to protect the medial and lateral ligaments.[30]

Some clinicians use a locking hinged elbow brace postreduction.[31,34–36] This brace is worn at all times as a protective device and can be locked at 90° of flexion (or some other angle of flexion) in the desired position of forearm rotation. The hinge is unlocked to allow motion to be performed within the safe arc defined by the clinician within the confines of the brace. Some devices have adjustable mechanical stops to assist patients in understanding the limits of motion. We are not advocates of hinged protective orthoses. Biomechanical studies have demonstrated that such devices may increase elbow instability during passive motion.[37–39] It is difficult to place and maintain the hinge at the anatomic axis of motion; this may cause joint maltracking leading to pain and impaired ligamentous healing.[39] Furthermore, their weight and high cost further leads us to avoid hinged brace use in most patients. In select cases, however, these braces may be useful to provide a mechanical block to extension if the patient has difficulty complying with instructions regarding the safe arc of motion.

Initial Exercise Regime

The optimal rehabilitation for patients with ligament injuries about the elbow remains unclear. Traditionally, therapists prescribe active motion exercises with the position of forearm rotation based on the status of the ligaments. More recently, overhead exercises have become commonly recommended. The intention is to have the arm overhead using gravity to compress the ulnohumeral joint and thereby improve joint tracking and stability.[30,31,37,40–42]

In an ideal situation, the elbow reduction for a dislocation includes assessment of the safe arc of ulnohumeral motion, meaning that the person reducing the elbow can range the elbow and determine at what point the elbow joint tends to subluxate or dislocate. The elbow is immobilized in a degree of flexion in excess of the point at which the elbow dislocates. However, in simple dislocations, meaning those without associated fractures, the safe arc of ulnohumeral joint motion may not be assessed at time of injury, because these injuries are often reduced in the emergency room and no assessment of the angle at which the elbow subluxates is made. Furthermore, in such instances, the severity of injury to the medial and lateral ligaments and surrounding musculature is unknown. In such cases, overhead motion is our preferred method of rehabilitation because this has been shown to enhance joint stability regardless of the forearm position. It is also safe with combined ligament and common flexor origin/common extensor origin deficiency.[30,37,40,41,43] The overhead position helps to maintain the collateral ligaments concentrically optimizing healing.

Forearm position during active flexion and extension should be based on the status of the ligaments:

- With simple dislocations we place the forearm in pronation during active flexion and extension exercises because lateral soft tissue injuries tend to be more severe than medial soft tissue injuries.
- In the postsurgical setting, if the LCL was repaired and the MCL was intact (ie, did not require repair and was stable on stress testing), the forearm is positioned in pronation during flexion and extension exercise.
- If the LCL repair is stable but the integrity of the MCL is in question (ie, instability postrepair or not repaired), full supination should be considered because this protects the deficient MCL.[43]
- If the LCL repair is not robust and the MCL is deficient, then flexion and extension exercises should be performed with the forearm in neutral rotation to protect the LCL and MCL.

Forearm rotation exercises are performed with the elbow maintained at 90° of flexion or greater.

We recommend that patients perform active flexion and extension exercises in the overhead position every 2 hours for 10 to 15 repititions (**Fig** 2A,B). This exercise is progressed to 15 to 20 repetitions hourly. If this increase in exercise frequency causes inflammation, pain, or muscle fatigue progression should be slower and based on the patient's tissue response.

Forearm rotation exercises are performed with the elbow maintained at 90 degrees of flexion or greater. This position places minimal tension on the MCL and LCL during motion. Forearm rotation exercises can be performed in the overhead position (**Fig** 2C,D) or at the patient's side in the traditional gravity dependent position.

In addition to elbow and forearm exercise we also instruct patients in hand, wrist, and shoulder motion to prevent secondary stiffness. Emphasis is placed on avoiding gravity-loaded varus and valgus elbow positions while performing shoulder motion exercises. For instance, internal rotation of the shoulder by placing the hand behind the back is never advised. Typical shoulder exercises prescribed are pendular, and internal and external rotation performed with the arm at the side.

Radiographic Drop Sign

In the presence of a radiographic drop sign (see **Fig. 1**) we also prescribe isometric exercise of the triceps, biceps, and brachialis in addition to overhead motion.[30] Isometric exercises are performed while in the resting orthosis. We advise patients to perform five repetitions, holding each repetition for 5 to 10 seconds, five times per day. Isometric exercise enhances the compressive forces acting across the elbow reducing the joint subluxation. This exercise also assists to retrain the muscles crossing the ulnohumeral articulation to fire appropriately ultimately reducing the joint.[30,44] It is also important to perform frequent active wrist and finger flexor and extensor motion. These muscles cross the elbow providing a compressive load when activated further enhancing stability.

Patients should be followed weekly with serial radiographs to monitor their status. If the drop sign is not improving, the resting orthosis is modified to place the elbow in 110° of flexion to further enhance stability while continuing with isometric and overhead exercises. It is our experience that with the implementation of isometric exercises and active overhead motion, the drop sign

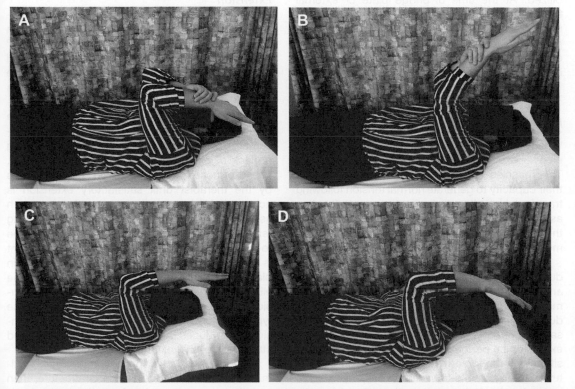

Fig. 2. (*A, B*) Overhead elbow flexion and extension following elbow dislocation with medial-sided instability. Note the position of the forearm in supination. (*C, D*) Forearm rotation exercises performed in the overhead position with the elbow positioned in 90° of flexion to protect the medial and lateral ligamentous structures.

spontaneously reduces within the first 3 weeks following initiation. Discontinuation of isometric exercises occurs once correction of the drop sign is confirmed radiographically.

If a drop sign does not reduce by 3 weeks, then surgical intervention should be considered. A closed reduction and application of an external fixator with the elbow reduced is considered if the ligaments have already been repaired yet the elbow remains unstable. If the patient has not had repair of the injured structures, repair of the LCL should be performed and stability reassessed. If the elbow is still unstable, repair of the MCL should be considered. If elbow instability persists despite ligament repairs, a static bridging external fixator or plate should be applied to maintain concentric reduction of the elbow.[45] The bridging fixation is typically maintained for 6 weeks. Although the elbow is fixated by the plate or external fixator device, patients are instructed to continue with isometric exercises. By activating the muscles around the elbow, which act as dynamic stabilizers, the process assists with muscular reeducation to ensure these dynamic elbow stabilizers function appropriately on fixator removal. Forearm rotation, shoulder, wrist, and hand exercises are also continued while the elbow is immobilized. At the time of bridge plate or external fixator removal the stability of the elbow is rechecked. If it is stable, a gentle manipulation is performed to assist in recovery of motion. If the elbow is still unstable, the bridging fixation is left in place or reapplied for an additional month, which is uncommonly required.

Range of Motion Exercises and Progression

When initiating rehabilitation for the unstable elbow, exercise should always begin actively. The muscles surrounding the elbow often lose their capacity to generate normal tension following trauma, which alters their effectiveness to function as dynamic stabilizers. Frequent active motion of the elbow and forearm assist with retraining the muscles to activate more efficiently and normally.

Gentle passive motion should be introduced during the late fibroplasia phase at 3 to 4 weeks and continue into the remodeling phase. Passive motion should be gentle, graded in nature, produce minimal pain, and stay within the established safe arc of motion. We prefer passive flexion and extension be performed while in the overhead position with the forearm position based on the status of the ligaments to maximize stability.[37,41] We instruct patients to use the other hand to gently push the elbow in flexion only holding for 5 to 10 seconds then perform the same for extension.

Once passive flexion and extension has been completed, active overhead exercises should be performed. The therapist educates the patient to ensure that no varus or valgus forces are placed on the elbow during exercise to protect the collateral ligaments.

Passive forearm rotation exercises should not begin until 4 to 6 weeks postinjury. These exercises must be performed gently to prevent any tilting of the ulnohumeral joint, which would cause stress to the LCL in supination and MCL in pronation. Passive rotation must be performed with the elbow at greater than 90° of flexion. Passive force should be applied by the therapist and patient at the midforearm level to ensure even force distribution to the proximal and distal radioulnar joints.

The patient should be able to demonstrate proper execution of passive motion exercises before inclusion into their home exercise program. The amount of force applied during passive exercise should be low; however, each position should be held for a minimum of 5 to 10 seconds ensuring a low load prolonged stretch.

Orthotic Considerations Following Elbow Instability

Extension

Lacking up to 30° of terminal extension is considered functional as most activities of daily living can be accomplished despite such a deficit 30°.[46] Some occupations and athletes need more or full extension to allow a full return to activities.[47] The intention of progressive static extension orthoses worn at night is to maintain any extension achievements made during the day. We begin nighttime extension splinting 4 to 6 weeks postinjury or postsurgery depending on joint stability and depending on lack of expected gains with therapy (**Fig. 3**). These orthoses are adjusted on a weekly basis by the therapist until satisfactory extension is achieved. Under selected circumstances, such as development of a firm contracture prohibiting terminal extension, this device also is worn three to four times per day for 30 minutes. The patient is advised to be sedentary with the orthosis in place to avoid varus and valgus loads on the elbow. The iplentation of profressive static extension orthoses during the early remodelling phase typically allows good recovery of terminal extension and reduces the need for more costly hinged static progressive extension devices.

If extension orthotic application produces minimal improvement in the flexion contracture, then a static-progressive extension orthosis should be added to the rehabilitation program. These devices are not instituted until the physician believes

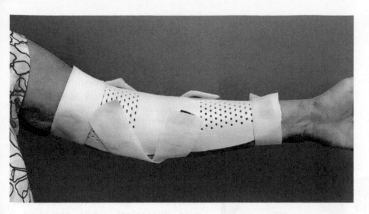

Fig. 3. Progressive static night elbow extension orthosis. Forearm position is directly related to ligamentous stability. In this photograph the forearm is positioned in neutral rotation to protect the LCL and MCL complex.

sufficient osseous and soft tissue healing has occurred. This is typically at 8 weeks postreduction or postsurgery. Static progressive devices have been shown to be effective at making improvement in motion.[48–51] These turnbuckle devices are custom fabricated by elbow therapists and are also available commercially in a prefabricated form (**Figs. 4**A,B respectively) We typically recommend these devices be used two to four times per day for up to 1 to 2 hours per session.

Elbow flexion

Classically, 130° of flexion has been reported to be the flexion required for most functional activities; however, more recent studies suggest that greater elbow flexion is needed for some activities, such as using a cellular phone.[46,52] This amount of flexion is difficult to regain after trauma and may require the use of flexion orthoses to achieve it. Such devices are used only after sufficient osseous and ligamentous healing has occurred, which is typically 6 weeks postreduction. Use of such devices too early in the rehabilitation process can lead to inflammation, injury, and possibly heterotopic bone formation.[53]

Several elbow flexion orthotic designs exist in the literature.[49,50,54,55] We most often use static progressive elbow flexion cuffs or hinged static-progressive turnbuckle orthoses. Decision-making is critical when choosing the type of flexion device to apply. When a patient can achieve 110° of flexion or greater, a flexion cuff is an appropriate option to apply an effective rotational force to the ulnohumeral joint to enhance flexion (**Fig. 5**A).[55] However, for the patient who has difficulty to attain 110°, a hinged turnbuckle orthosis is preferred because this design minimizes the compressive load placed onto the ulnohumeral joint while maximizing the rotational force (**Fig. 5**B).[55] We recommend flexion orthoses to be worn three to four times per day up to 30 minutes per session while monitoring for signs of ulnar nerve irritation. During elbow flexion the ulnar nerve elongates and can become compressed in the cubital tunnel by fibrosis or edema. Some patients develop medial elbow pain or numbness in the ulnar nerve distribution, which can limit recovery of elbow flexion. Surgical release of the ulnar nerve may be required in selected cases if flexion remains limited.[56]

If difficulty regaining flexion and extension exists, patients are instructed to interchange static-progressive flexion and extension devices during the day. Typically, we recommend wearing both devices three to four times per day for up to

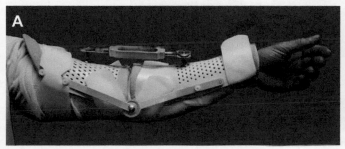

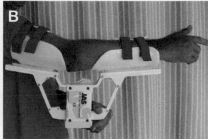

Fig. 4. (*A*) Custom-made static progressive turnbuckle elbow extension orthosis. (*B*) Commercially available static-progressive elbow extension-flexion orthosis from Joint Active Systems (Effingham, IL).

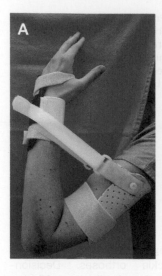

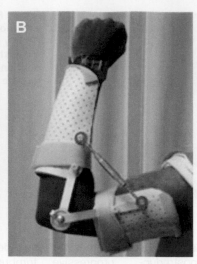

Fig. 5. (A) Custom-made static progressive elbow flexion cuff. Such orthotic designs should be used with elbows that can achieve 110° of flexion or greater. In such cases no hinge is required to the orthosis because the rotational force is high and the compressive load is small through the ulnohumeral joint. (B) Custom-made static progressive elbow flexion turn-buckle orthosis. The hinge in these devices absorbs the compressive forces through the elbow for patients with less than 110° of elbow flexion to minimize joint compressive forces and minimize discomfort, while providing a low-load long-duration stretch. (From Chinchalkar SJ, Szekeres M. Rehabilitation of elbow trauma. Hand Clinics 2004;20(4):363-74; with permission.)

30 minutes per session. In addition to this, patients are advised to wear the nighttime extension orthosis to maintain extension gains achieved with daytime orthosis use and exercises. We do not recommend flexion devices be worn at night because of concerns about development of ulnar neuropathy or circulatory compromise.

Forearm-rotational splinting

Forearm rotation may also be limited following an elbow dislocation; this occurs more commonly if there is a concomitant radial head fracture. An arc of 100° of forearm rotation with 50° in pronation and 50° in supination has been published as a guideline for what patients require to complete most activities of daily living.[46] More recent studies suggest that greater pronation, however, is needed for keyboarding activities.[52] Various types of dynamic and static progressive designs have been found to be successful at improving rotation.[57–62] In general, rotational orthoses should

not be used until at least 8 weeks postreduction to ensure sufficient osseous and ligamentous healing has occurred. At our facility we usually use custom molded dynamic orthoses initially (**Fig. 6**A). If improvement is limited, we transition into a commercially available static-progressive design (**Fig. 6**B). We find the stress-relaxation principle of static-progressive splinting to be beneficial at improving rotation when dynamic splinting produces minimal improvement.[49]

OTHER USEFUL THERAPEUTIC TECHNIQUES
Superficial Thermal Modalities

Heat is a common adjunctive therapy, which is applied during therapy sessions and encouraged for home use. Heat is used with the intent to precondition the soft tissues to allow for adequate muscle relaxation and increase tissue extensibility. Heating agents that are effective for soft tissues include hot packs, whirlpools, or fluidotherapy. If

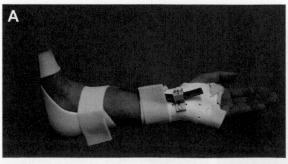

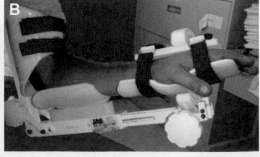

Fig. 6. (A) Custom fabricated dynamic pronation-supination orthosis. (B) Commercially available static progressive pronation/supination orthosis. ([B] from Pipicelli JG, Chinchalkar S J, Grewal R, Athwal GS. Techniques in Hand & Upper Extremity Surgery 2011;15(4):198–208; with permission.)

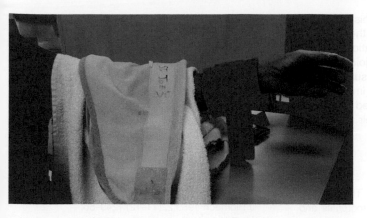

Fig. 7. Hot packs are a common heating agent application that is effective to precondition the tissues before range of motion exercises to enhance motion. An effective method of increasing extension is to position the elbow at tolerable end range while applying a light load (1–2 lb) for the duration of heating application.

stretching is desired, an effective method of increasing elbow extension is to position the elbow at a tolerable end-range for the duration of the heating application, which is typically 20 minutes (**Fig. 7**). Once bone and soft tissue healing are deemed adequate, the same technique is used for elbow flexion while applying a light load for the duration of the heating application.

Manual Joint Mobilizations

Progressive manual joint mobilization therapy is used to assist with pain reduction, decrease muscle spasm, and to regain motion if immediately followed by active and passive motion exercises.[63,64] However, these treatment maneuvers are performed with caution to minimize stress to the healing bony structures, ligaments, and surrounding soft tissues. Maitland[63] described five joint mobilization grades with higher grades indicating mobilizations are performed closer to or at end range. Grade V represents a joint manipulation that should not be part of the rehabilitation program following elbow trauma. Grade I mobilizations are applied beginning at 2 weeks postreduction. This technique includes small oscillatory movements of the elbow, which are effective in simulating tendon and proprioceptive end organs. This can assist in minimizing muscle spasm and cocontraction. Such mobilizations are performed at the comfortable resting position of the ulnohumeral joint, which is typically midrange. Beginning at Week 4, grade II and III joint mobilizations are applied, which are slightly more forceful near or at the end of available joint motion. These maneuvers should be performed only by experienced clinicians, and with caution, to minimize stress to the healing bony structures, ligaments, and surrounding soft tissues. At 6 to 8 weeks, grades III and IV mobilizations are applied. These mobilizations are performed at the end of available motion to stretch the joint capsule.

Progression of Strengthening and Functional Retraining

Strengthening of the dynamic stabilizers of the ulnohumeral joint can begin 4 to 6 weeks postreduction, depending on the status of the ligament and osseous injuries. If persistent pain and swelling is contributing to minimal improvement in joint motion stabilizer strengthening should be gradual and graded to prevent an inflammatory reaction, which can contribute to further stiffness. The purpose of early dynamic elbow strengthening is to reduce atrophy and improve the muscles' ability to generate normal tension. This should enhance their ability to function as dynamic stabilizers. The patient is instructed to perform 15 to 30 repetitions using a 1- to 2-lb weight for two to three sets once daily to strengthen the wrist flexors and extensors. Digital flexors and extensors are strengthened using a "stress ball" or therapeutic putty. These exercises are performed with the elbow at 90°, resting on a table and with the forearm in neutral rotation. At 6 weeks and beyond isotonic strengthening can progress as tolerated.

At 8 weeks, isotonic strengthening of the elbow flexors and extensors and the shoulder girdle can begin. Light weights or resistive elastic bands are used. Emphasis should be placed on strengthening the triceps because this may aid in minimizing flexion contracture. We prefer exercises be performed in the dependent plane minimizing varus and valgus load to the elbow until patients are 12 weeks postinjury. Thereafter, strengthening can incorporate job- or sport-specific exercises that focus on muscle performance. Strengthening continues until the patient is satisfied with overall upper extremity function.

SUMMARY

A comprehensive understanding of elbow anatomy and biomechanics is essential to optimize the rehabilitation of elbow injuries. This allows for the implementation of a systematic therapy program that encourages early mobilization within a safe arc of motion while maintaining joint stability. Close communication between the surgeon and therapist is necessary to allow for the implementation of an individualized program based on the patient's specific injury pattern and their surgical or nonsurgical management.

REFERENCES

1. Capo JT, Collins C, Beutel BG, et al. Three-dimensional analysis of elbow soft tissue footprints and anatomy. J Shoulder Elbow Surg 2014;23:1618–23.
2. Stoneback JW, Owens BD, Sykes J, et al. Incidence of elbow dislocations in the United States population. J Bone Joint Surg Am 2012;94(3):240–5.
3. Pichora JE, Fraser GS, Ferreira LF, et al. The effect of medial collateral ligament repair tension on elbow joint kinematics and stability. J Hand Surg Am 2007;32(8):1210–7.
4. Armstrong AD, Dunning CE, Faber KJ, et al. Single-strand ligament reconstruction of the medial collateral ligament restores valgus elbow stability. J Shoulder Elbow Surg 2002;11(1):65–71.
5. Callaway GH, Field LD, Deng XH, et al. Biomechanical evaluation of the medial collateral ligament of the elbow. J Bone Joint Surg Am 1997;79(8):1223–31.
6. Tyrdal S, Olsen BS. Combined hyperextension and supination of the elbow joint induces lateral ligament lesions. An experimental study of the pathoanatomy and kinematics in elbow ligament injuries. Knee Surg Sports Traumatol Arthrosc 1998;6(1):36–43.
7. Mehta JA, Bain GI. Posterolateral rotatory instability of the elbow. J Am Acad Orthop Surg 2004;12:405–15. 10.
8. King G, Dunning C, Zarzour Z, et al. Single-strand reconstruction of the lateral ulnar collateral ligament restores varus and posterolateral rotatory stability of the elbow. J Shoulder Elbow Surg 2002;11(1):60–4.
9. Morrey BF, An K-N. Articular and ligamentous contributions to the stability of the elbow joint. Am J Sports Med 1983;11(5):315–9.
10. Olsen BS, Søjbjerg JO, Helmig P, et al. Lateral collateral ligament of the elbow joint: anatomy and kinematics. J Shoulder Elbow Surg 1996;5(2):103–12.
11. O'Driscoll SW, Morrey BF, Korinek S, et al. Elbow subluxation and dislocation. A spectrum of instability. Clin Orthop Relat Res 1992;(280):186–97.
12. Dunning CE, Zarzour ZDS, Patterson SD, et al. Ligamentous stabilizers against posterolateral rotatory instability of the elbow. J Bone Joint Surg Am 2001;83(12):1823–8.

13. McAdams TR, Masters GW, Srivastava S. The effect of arthroscopic sectioning of the lateral ligament complex of the elbow on posterolateral rotatory stability. J Shoulder Elbow Surg 2005;14(3):298–301.
14. Søjbjerg JO, Ovesen J, Gundorf CE. The stability of the elbow following excision of the radial head and transection of the annular ligament. Arch Orthop Trauma Surg 1987;106(4):248–50.
15. An KN, Hui FC, Morrey BF, et al. Muscles across the elbow joint: a biomechanical analysis. J Biomech 1981;14(10):659–69.
16. An KN, Kaufman RK, Chao EY. Physiological considerations of muscle force through the elbow joint. J Biomech 1989;22(11–12):1249–56.
17. Lin F, Kohli N, Perimutter S, et al. Muscle contribution to elbow joint valgus stability. J Shoulder Elbow Surg 2007;16(6):795–802.
18. Park MC, Ahmad CS. Dynamic contributions of the flexor-pronatory mass to elbow valgus stability. J Bone Joint surg Am 2004;86(10):2268–74.
19. Udall JH, Fitzpatrick MJ, McGarry MH, et al. Effects of flexor-pronator muscle loading on valgus stability of the elbow with an intact, stretched, and resected medial ulnar collateral ligament. J Shoulder Elbow Surg 2009;18(5):773–8.
20. Cohen MS, Hastings H. Rotatory instability of the elbow. The anatomy and role of the lateral stabilizers. J Bone Joint Surg Am 1997;79(2):225–33.
21. Josefsson PO, Johnell O, Wendeberg B. Ligamentous injuries in dislocations of the elbow joint. Clin Orthop Relat Res 1987;221:221–5.
22. King GJW, Morrey BF, An KN. Stabilizers of the elbow. J Shoulder Elbow Surg 1993;2(3):165–74.
23. O'Driscoll SW, Jupiter JB, King GJ, et al. The unstable elbow. Instr Course Lect 2001;50:89–102.
24. Deutch SR, Jensen SL, Olsen BS, et al. Elbow joint stability in relation to forced external rotation: an experimental study of the osseous constraint. J Shoulder Elbow Surg 2003;12(3):287–92.
25. Schreiber JJ, Warren RF, Hotchkiss RN, et al. An online video investigation into the mechanism of elbow dislocation. J Hand Surg Am 2013;38(3):488–94.
26. Schreiber JJ, Potter HG, Warren RF, et al. Magnetic resonance imaging findings in acute elbow dislocations: insight into mechanism. J Hand Surg Am 2014;39(2):199–205.
27. Armstrong A. Simple elbow dislocation. Hand Clin 2015;31(4):521–31.
28. Coonrad RW, Roush TF, Major NM, et al. The drop sign, a radiographic warning sign of elbow instability. J Shoulder Elbow Surg 2005;14(3):312–7.
29. Artzberger SM, Prignac VW. Manual edema mobilization: an edema reduction technique for the orthopedic patient. In: Mackin EJ, Hunter JM, Callahan AD, et al, editors. Rehabilitation of the hand and upper extremity. 6th edition. St Louis (MO): Mosby; 2011. p. 868–81.

30. Pipicelli JG, Chinchalkar SJ, Grewal R, et al. Therapeutic implications of the radiographic "drop sign" following elbow dislocation. J Hand Ther 2012; 25(3):346–53 [quiz: 354].

31. Szekeres M, Chinchalkar SJ, King GJW. Optimizing elbow rehabilitation after instability. Hand Clin 2008;24(1):27–38.

32. Safran MR, McGarry MH, Shin S, et al. Effects of elbow flexion and forearm rotation on valgus laxity of the elbow. J Bone Joint Surg Am 2005;87(9 I): 2065–74.

33. Armstrong AD, Dunning CE, Faber KJ, et al. Rehabilitation of the medial collateral ligament-deficient elbow: an in vitro biomechanical study. J Hand Surg Am 2000;25(6):1051–7.

34. Reichel LM, Milam GS, Sitton SE, et al. Elbow lateral collateral ligament injuries. J Hand Surg Am 2013; 38(1):184–201.

35. Cohen MS, Hastings H. Acute elbow dislocation: evaluation and management. J Am Acad Orthop Surg 1998;6(1):15–23.

36. Wolff AL, Hotchkiss RN. Lateral elbow instability: nonoperative, operative, and postoperative management. J Hand Ther 2006;19(2):238–43.

37. Lee AT, Schrumpf MA, Choi D, et al. The influence of gravity on the unstable elbow. J Shoulder Elbow Surg 2013;22(1):81–7.

38. Manocha RHK, Johnson JA, King GJW. The effectiveness of a hinged elbow orthosis in medial collateral ligament injuries: an in vitro biomechanical study. Am J Sports Med 2019; 47(12):2827–35.

39. Manocha RH, King GJW, Johnson JA. In vitro kinematic assessment of a hinged elbow orthosis following lateral collateral ligament injury. J Hand Surg 2018;43(2):123–32.

40. Alolabi B, Gray A, Ferreira LM, et al. Rehabilitation of the medial- and lateral collateral ligament-deficient elbow: an in vitro biomechanical study. J Hand Ther 2012;25(4):363–73.

41. Manocha RHK, Kusins JR, Johnson JA, et al. Optimizing the rehabilitation of elbow lateral collateral ligament injuries: a biomechanical study. J Shoulder Elbow Surg 2017;26(4):596–603.

42. Schreiber JJ, Paul S, Hotchkiss RN, et al. Conservative management of elbow dislocations with an overhead motion protocol. J Hand Surg 2015;40(3): 515–9.

43. Pipicelli JG, Chinchalkar SJ, Grewal R, et al. Rehabilitation considerations in the management of terrible triad injury to the elbow. Tech Hand Up Extrem Surg 2011;15(4):198–208.

44. Amis AA, Dowson D, Wright V. Elbow joint force predictions for some strenuous isometric actions. J Biomech 1980;13(9):765–75.

45. McKee MD, Bowden SH, King GJ, et al. Management of recurrent, complex instability of the elbow

with a hinged external fixator. J Bone Joint Surg Br 1998;80(6):1031–6.

46. Morrey BF, Askew LJ, Chao EY. A biomechanical study of normal functional elbow motion. J Bone Joint Surg Am 1981;63:872–7.

47. Blonna D, Lee GC, O'Driscoll SW. Arthroscopic restoration of terminal elbow extension in high-level athletes. Am J Sports Med 2010;38(12):2509–15.

48. Chen B, Lin J, Liu L, et al. Static progressive orthoses for elbow contracture: a systematic review. J Healthc Eng 2017;2017:7498094.

49. Bonutti M, Windau JE, Ables BA, et al. Static progressive stretch to reestablish elbow range of motion. Clin Orthop 1994;303:128–34.

50. Green DP, McCoy H. Turnbuckle orthotic correction of elbow-flexion contractures after acute injuries. J Bone Joint Surg Am 1979;61:1092–5.

51. Gelinas JJ, Faber KJ, Patterson SD, et al. The effectiveness of turnbuckle splinting for elbow contractures. J Bone Joint Surg Br 2000;82:74–8.

52. Sardelli M, Tashjian RZ, MacWilliams BA. Functional elbow range of motion for contemporary tasks. J Bone Joint Surg Am 2011;93:471–7.

53. Michelsson JE, Rauschning W. Pathogenesis of experimental heterotopic bone formation following temporary forcible exercising of immobilized limbs. Clin Orthop 1983;176:265–72.

54. Altman E. Therapist's management of the stiff elbow.. In: Mackin EJ, Hunter JM, Callahan AD, et al, editors. Rehabilitation of the hand and upper extremity. 6th edition. St Louis (MO): Mosby; 2011. p. 1075–88.

55. Szekeres M. A biomechanical analysis of static progressive elbow flexion splinting. J Hand Ther 2006; 19:34–8, 33.

56. Blonna D, O'Driscoll SW. Delayed-onset ulnar neuritis after release of elbow contracture: preventive strategies derived from a study of 563 cases. Arthroscopy 2014;30(8):947–56.

57. Muramatsu K, Ihara K, Shigetomi M, et al. Posttraumatic radioulnar synostosis treated with a free vascularized fat transplant and dynamic splint: a report of two cases. J Orthop Trauma 2004;18: 48–52.

58. Bell SN, Benger D. Management of radioulnar synostosis with mobilization, anconeus interposition, and a forearm rotation assist splint. J Shoulder Elbow Surg 1999;8:621 1.

59. Colello-Abraham K. Dynamic pronation-supination splint. In: Hunter JM, Schneider LH, Mackin EJ, et al, editors. Rehabilitation of the hand: surgery and therapy. 3rd edition. St Louis (MO): Mosby; 1990. p. 1134–9.

60. Lee MJ, LaStayo PC, vonKersburg AE. A supination splint worn distal to the elbow: a radiographic, electromyographic, and retrospective report. J Hand Ther 2003;16:190–8.

61. Shah MA, Lopez JK, Escalante AS, et al. Dynamic splinting of forearm rotational contracture after distal radius fracture. J Hand Surg Am 2002;27: 456–63.

62. McGrath MS, Ulrich SD, Bonutti PM, et al. Static progressive splinting for restoration of rotational motion of the forearm. Hand Ther 2009;22:3–8.

63. Maitland GD. Treatment. In: Peripheral manipulation. London: Butterworth Heinemann; 1993. p. 64–106.

64. Kaltenborn FM. Manual mobilization of the extremity joints: basic examination and treatment techniques. 4th edition. Oslo, Norway: Olaf Norlis Bokhandel; 1989.

Solutions for the Unstable and Arthritic Distal Radioulnar Joint

Juan Manuel Breyer, MD[a,b,*], Pamela Vergara, MD[a,c]

KEYWORDS

- Distal radioulnar joint • Arthritis • Instability • Arthroplasty • Resection arthroplasty
- Ulnar head replacement

KEY POINTS

- A severely damaged and painful distal radioulnar joint can be reconstructed by resection arthroplasty or by hemi- or total arthroplasty.
- Resection arthroplasties as Darrach and Sauvé-Kapandji procedure have good overall outcomes, with limitations in more active patients related to potential symptomatic radio ulnar impingement.
- Hemi- and total arthroplasties have shown increased function, better patient-rated outcome measures, reduced pain, and high satisfaction that persist over time.

An unstable and arthritic distal radioulnar joint (DRUJ) is a challenge for surgeons, because it represents broad joint involvement of both the articular cartilage and also the soft tissue structures, manifesting as joint dysfunction and pain. Biomechanically, the DRUJ has 2 functions—forearm rotation and force transmission—and acts as a weight-bearing joint with lifting and gripping from carpus to forearm.[1] This latter function is less recognized in the literature; when an object is raised with the hand and forearm in a neutral position, the brachial muscle pulls and flexes the ulna, which pushes the radius through the DRUJ, and the radius raises the hand and the object (**Fig. 1**), expressing its role as a weight-bearing joint. Given this, osteoarthritis (OA) and chronic instability of the DRUJ presents with considerable function impairment, pain, and even weakness in gripping and raising an object.

Nonoperative treatment is useful in cases of mild OA and instability. In this setting, nonsteroidal anti-inflammatory drugs, physical therapy, and steroid injection may improve the secondary DRUJ stabilizers, resulted in improved motion and pain control.[2] In the same context of early OA and mild instability, ulna shortening (US) has been described as an alternative. This works to stabilize the DRUJ by increasing the tension in the triangular fibrocartilage complex (TFCC)[3,4] and ulnocarpal ligaments, as well as changing the contact area between the sigmoid notch and the ulnar head to a place in the distal ulnar head where healthy articular cartilage remains. US is contraindicated in advanced OA or when there is an oblique, distally orientated sigmoid notch, type 3, according to the De Smet classification,[5] due to an increased incidence of degenerative changes in this scenario. In the same way, some biomechanical studies warn about increased contact area and pressure at the DRUJ after US, which could be sufficient to induce degenerative changes in the cartilage.[6,7]

Scheker and colleagues[8] describe an ulnar shortening osteotomy in 32 patients with early

---

[a] Orthopedic Department, Hospital del Trabajador, 185 Ramon Carnicer 185, Santiago, Providencia, Chile; [b] Orthopedic Department, Clinica Alemana-Universidad del Desarrollo, Santiago, Chile; [c] Orthopedic Department, Clinica Las Condes, Santiago, Chile
* Corresponding author.
E-mail address: jbreyer@alemana.cl

Hand Clin 36 (2020) 523–530
https://doi.org/10.1016/j.hcl.2020.07.008

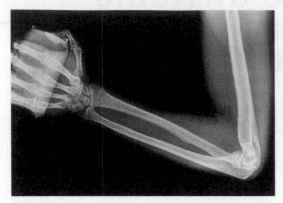

Fig. 1. The distal radioulnar joint is as weight-bearing joint, to grip and raise object with the hand.

OA of the DRUJ. From self-assessments, 50% of patients were very satisfied with the procedure and had complete pain relief. The same lead investigator also described 124 patients with an ulnar shortening osteotomy, in which 69 (55.6%) had OA as part of the indication for US; 13 of 124 patients required a semiconstrained arthroplasty (conversion rate 10.4%). There was no statistical difference in this subgroup, although there was a slight trend toward association of sigmoid notch type 3 with conversion to DRUJ arthroplasty.[9]

In more severe OA and instability, a wide variety of surgical alternatives have been described, including fusions, resection arthroplasties, and prostheses. The following sections provide a more in-depth review of resection arthroplasty and prostheses for addressing more severe cases of OA and instability.

The fusion of radius and ulna to create a one-bone forearm is a salvage procedure that involves sacrificing forearm rotation, with poor reported outcomes due to insufficient pain relief and high rates of complications.[10]

Resection arthroplasties include different types of distal ulna resection in association with arthrodesis or other and soft tissue procedures. Although good overall results have been described for these types of procedures, they have shown some limitations in achieving pain relief and stability of the DRUJ, especially in more active patients.

Hemi- and total arthroplasties are a good option for patients with unstable and arthritic DRUJ, due to good outcomes, high patient satisfaction, and a high implant survival rate.

RESECTION ARTHROPLASTY
Darrach Procedure

Ulnar head resection was first described by Malgaigne in 1855[11] and Moore in 1880,[12] but it was later popularized by Darrach in 1912[13] as a distal ulnar resection with preservation of supporting soft-tissue structures. It was initially described to treat symptomatic DRUJ conditions following distal radius fractures and then extended as a treatment option for conditions that result in DRUJ incongruity or arthritis.

Reported outcomes after distal ulnar excision for posttraumatic arthritis have generally been favorable in low-demand patients, demonstrating improved pain, grip strength, and motion in 80% to 91% of them.[14–17] In young active patients, the results are different in terms of the long-term complications, including pain, instability of the residual ulnar stump, and impingement.[14,18,19]

Af Ekenstam and colleagues[20] report 24 patients treated with the Darrach procedure after a fracture of the distal radius; 12 (50%) rated themselves as unimproved, even though range of motion improved in 75% of patients and none of them had a worse range of motion postoperatively. Grawe and colleagues[21] evaluated 27 patients who received the Darrach procedure for posttraumatic DRUJ pathology over a 13-year follow-up period. Although nearly one-third of patients had signs of residual ulnar stump instability under stress radiographies, this did not influence either the good forearm range of motion accomplished or the subjective results reported (Quick Disabilities of the Shoulder, Arm, and Hand [DASH] score of 17 and a Patient-Rated Wrist Evaluation score of 14).

Sauvé-Kapandji Procedure

The Sauvé-Kapandji (S-K) procedure has been described under several eponyms but most commonly is attributed to Sauvé and Kapandji (1936). It is an arthrodesis of the distal radio ulnar joint with the creation of a proximal ulnar pseudarthrosis to maintain rotation.[14] It is indicated as part of the treatment of a distal radioulnar instability, ulnocarpal pathology, and arthrosis or incongruency after a distal radius fracture.[22]

The main difference with the Darrach procedure is that by preserving the head of the ulna, the S-K procedure preserves ulnar support of the carpus, distal radioulnar ligaments, and ulnocarpal ligaments, which results in better postoperative appearance.[22,23] It has been suggested that S-K may also prevent ulnar translation of the carpus, although supporting evidence is mixed.[24,25]

Millroy and colleagues[26] report 71 patients with a 6-month follow-up in which only 7 patients (9.8%) referred pain with overuse. All patients improved the range of wrist and forearm motion, and all but 3 agreed that the surgery had been beneficial and they would elect to undergo it again. Nakamura and colleagues[27] described 15 non-rheumatoid patients with chronic DRUJ. After the S-K procedure, wrist pain improved in all patients, wrist flexion-extension increased in 9 patients, and grip strength was at least 80% of the contralateral wrist in 11 patients. Static and dynamic radiographic examination revealed an unstable proximal ulnar stump in all patients.

Unfortunately, this procedure is fallible, more so in posttraumatic and high wrist demand settings.[28] The complication rate is around 50%,[29] and the causes included heterotopic ossification, hardware irritation, nonunion/delayed union of the arthrodesis, and painful instability of the proximal ulna stump, among others.

One common complication seen following a Darrach or S-K procedure is radioulnar convergence, first described by Bell and colleagues[30] as "ulnar impingement syndrome," which represents an instability of the residual ulnar stump (**Fig. 2**). It might present as a painful lifting, snapping on rotation, limited range of motion, loss of strength, or occasional, bony scalloping of the radius as seen in radiograph.[19] Many techniques have been described to prevent these complications. There are reports using the extensor carpi ulnaris (ECU), flexor carpi ulnaris, and pronator quadratus to control the unstable distal ulna and to increase forearm motion.[31–35] Although most studies report radioulnar convergence as common, it seems that it is not necessarily due to poor functional results[21,27] but rather an indication that prior studies lacked an adequate method to evaluate the role of the DRUJ as a load-bearing joint through its lifting capacity, thus underestimating the real impact of proximal ulnar stump impingement.

Hemiresection Procedures

In 1985, Bowers[36] first described the distal ulnar resection with an interposition technique (hemiresection interposition technique [HIT]); since then, many variations have been described. It consists in an oblique resection of the articular region of the ulnar head, leaving a conical distal end, and preserving the attachments of an intact TFCC. Soft tissue as capsule or an anchovy of surrounding tendons can be inserted to create an interposition arthroplasty in attempts to prophylactically prevent radioulnar convergence through soft-tissue interposition.

There are some studies that report the long-term results of HIT arthroplasty, with most in patients with rheumatoid arthritis.[37,38] Nawijn and colleagues[39] report the results of 31 patients treated with an HIT due to inflammatory, degenerative, or posttraumatic arthritis. Patients expressed satisfaction with HIT arthroplasty, despite a mean QuickDASH score of 31. Patients with inflammatory arthritis had higher satisfaction and lower pain scores, whereas patients with prior trauma, prior surgery, or DRUJ subluxation were generally less satisfied.

Faithfull and Kwa[40] described 15 patients treated with a Bowers procedure as a treatment of ulnocarpal impingement, primary OA, or posttraumatic disruption of the DRUJ. After the procedure, all patients had improved pain conditions, but the best results were in patients with OA or traumatic disruption. Patients with reduction in preoperative forearm rotation all improved, with increases ranging from 40° to 140°.

Comparative results between the 3 resection procedures have been made. Minami and colleagues[19] describe a comparative study in 61 patients with OA of the DRUJ and an average 10-year follow-up: Darrach procedure on 20 wrists, the S-K procedure on 25, and the HIA (Bowers) on 16. Pain relief from Darrach had a statistically nonsignificant trend of being inferior to the other 2 procedures. The S-K procedure and HIT showed significant postoperative improvements in flexion, extension, and grip strength. Distal ulnar instability was frequent (60% of patients for Darrach, 50% for S-K, and 20% for HIT) after all procedures. The investigators concluded that the Darrach procedure is better indicated for severe osteoarthritic changes of the DRUJ in elderly patients.

Verhiel and colleagues[29] assessed differences in long-term patient-reported outcomes on physical function, pain, and satisfaction in patients with posttraumatic DRUJ, treated with Darrach (57 patients) and S-K procedures (28 patients). There were no significant differences in Patient-Reported Outcomes Measurement Information System Upper Extremity Function score, pain, or satisfaction scores between the 2 groups. Complication rates were relatively high, at 30% (Darrach) and 50% (S-K), with no significant differences. The most common complication was instability of the ulnar stump (14% in Darrach, 7% S-K); the percentage is low in both cases compared with other studies, which could be caused by the ulnar stump frequently being stabilized in this study cohort.

George and colleagues[41] evaluated the Darrach and S-K procedures following radio-distal ulnar fractures in 48 patients younger than 50-years. The Darrach (n = 30) and the S-K procedure (n = 18) yielded comparable and unpredictable results with respect to both subjective and objective parameters. The mean DASH scores were 23 in the Darrach group (range, 4–61) and 23 in the

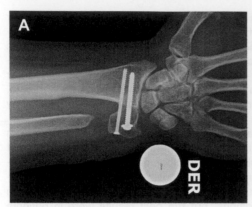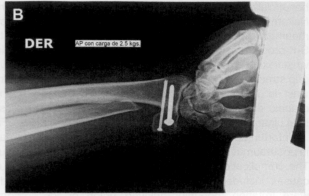

Fig. 2. A resection arthroplasty can produce an ulnar impingement syndrome (radioulnar convergence). (*A*) Static posteroanterior (PA) wrist radiograph after an S-K procedure. (*B*) Dynamic PA radiograph of the same patient, under load of 2.5 kg that shows the ulnar impingement on the radius.

S-K group (range, 0–60). The complication rate was 33% in the Darrach group and 50% in S-K group and included hardware irritation and symptoms of the dorsal sensory branch of the ulnar.

ARTHROPLASTY

The aim of performing a DRUJ arthroplasty is to achieve pain relief, preserving forearm rotation and the ability to raise an object without pain. The first DRUJ prosthesis emerged in the late 1980s, with the Whebe (1988) and Kapandji (1989) prostheses. The Whebe prosthesis is a custom-made partial implant with a titanium alloy and a plasma spray stem (Mark 1, Biomet, Warsaw, IN, USA). Two subsequent custom designs have also been made: Mark 2 (1992) and Mark 3 (2004).[42] The Kapandji implant was a total arthroplasty with minor improvement and success.[43] One of the first prosthesis to be patented in the United State was Scheker's total prosthesis in 1990 followed by Cooney's partial prosthesis in 2001.[42] Currently, several implants have been developed, with most being hemiarthroplasties.

Hemiarthroplasty

Partial joint prostheses have had the greatest development and number of designs. Some of the more commonly used implants are the Herbert, Avanta, and Ascension prostheses. In 1995, Herbert and van Schoonhoven designed a partial prosthesis widely used in Europe, comprising a ceramic head and a titanium stem (KLS Martin, Freiberg, Germany).[44] The prosthesis designed by Berger and Cooney, the Avanta U-Head (uHead, Small Bone Innovation, Morrisville, PA, USA), was one of the first to be widely used in the United States, originally designed in 2000

and redesigned in 2007. It has a cobalt chrome implant with a plasma-coated stem and a metal head, with space to reattach the soft tissue and ligaments to the prosthesis.[45] A different design is the Ascension prosthesis (Ascension Orthopedics, Austin, TX, USA), designed to reduce the resection of the ulnar head, preserving the ulnar styloid and the insertion of the DRUJ ligaments, thus reducing joint instability.[46]

Total Arthroplasty

There are only 3 total DRUJ arthroplasties: Kapandji (1989), Scheker (1997), and Schuurman (2013). The Aptis prosthesis (Aptis Medical, Louisville, KY, USA) was designed by Scheker in 1997 and is the only total prosthesis with major development and use (**Fig. 3**). It is a semiconstrained implant, completely stable, obviating the needs of ligaments stabilizers. The interface is an ultra-high molecular polyethylene sphere that allows the proximal-distal migration of the radius during pronosupination, which is why it is considered a semiconstrained implant.[47]

Outcomes and Complications of Arthroplasty

Overall, there have been good results for partial and total arthroplasties, even though the number and quality of evaluations comprise small series and short follow-ups (eg, 4 years[48]), and many studies are funded and/or performed by the implants' designers or manufacturers. Generally, following a DRUJ prosthesis, all reports shows increased function, better patient-rated outcome measures, reduced pain, and high satisfaction that persist over time, summarized in systematic reviews.[48,49]

Van Schoonhoven reported the long-term outcomes of 16 Herbert prostheses, evaluated at

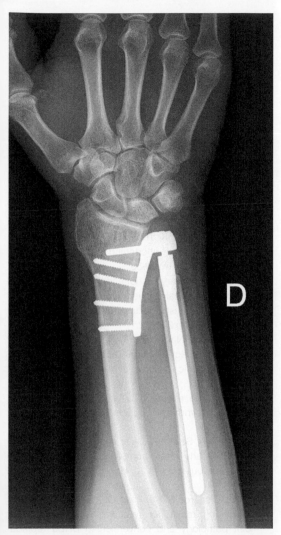

Fig. 3. Total arthroplasty, the Aptis prosthesis.

28 months and 11 years. All clinical parameters improved significantly at the short-term follow-up, with no statistically significant change at the long-term follow-up. Average pain improved from 3.7 before surgery to 1.7 at both follow-ups, and grip strength improved from 42% to 72% and 81%, compared with the unaffected side.[50]

Kakar and colleagues[51] reviewed 47 patients with the Avanta prosthesis, with a follow-up of 56 months. Although there was no significant improvement in forearm rotation and wrist function, there was a significant decrease in pain scores from 4.6 to 2.2 and improvement in the mean Mayo wrist score from 14 to 69 points after surgery.

Savvidou and colleagues[52] reported the first series of Scheker prostheses, with 35 patients at 5 years follow-up. These patients had a significant improvement in pain at rest (5.11–1.02) and pain

with activity (8.25–2.71). The investigators also evaluated and reported lifting capacity, describing similar lifting capacities of the prothesis arm compared with the nonprothesis arm.

All reports across series describe patients with different diagnoses and indications for their prostheses. Although posttraumatic and degenerative arthritis is by far the main cause for the arthroplasty, there are some cases with secondary DRUJ injury from rheumatoid arthritis, Madelung deformity, rescue of resection arthroplasties (Darrach, S-K, Bowers), etc.

In terms of complications, instability seems to be the main concern of partial prosthesis. It is common to see instability in radiographs without a perfect match of the ulnar head at the sigmoid notch, but this is not always symptomatic, so secondary surgery for prosthesis stability is probably close to 10%.[48,49] Van Schoohoven[44] described 2 recurrent instabilities out of 23 cases, with one treated with a radial osteotomy for a deformity and the other with a soft tissue procedure. In their report on the Herbert implant, Axelsson and colleagues[53] found 15 of 22 radiographic signs of unstable prostheses, but surgery (capsuloplasty) was required in only one case and without correlations to worse outcomes. Similar reports are with the U-Head prosthesis; Shipley and colleagues[54] reported 4 out of 22 recurrent instabilities, but only 2 were symptomatic that required surgery, and Willis and colleagues[55] reported just 1 surgery in 19 prostheses for recurrent instability.

Another common complication after partial implant is osteolysis or radiolucency at the distal ulna stump, which may be as common as 90% to 100%. This distal ulna lysis could be a type of stress shielding and is not apparently related to prosthesis loosening. It used to appear in the first year and apparently does not progress with years.[53,56,57] Distal ulna lysis is not common for the total prostheses, is reported only in 30% of cases, and is mild.

One special concern of partial implants is the progression of cartilage damage at the sigmoid fossa, which is commonly seen in radiographs in addition to the remodeling of the fossa, but it used to benign and usually does not need a surgical treatment.[50,53] Among 47 patients, Kakar and colleagues[51] described one case of sigmoid notch replacement for notch erosion for a patient with the Avanta prosthesis.

The Aptis total prosthesis does not have the sigmoid notch erosion or instability issues of the partial implants, but it does have some complications related to soft tissue, with cases of synovitis of the ECU, ossifications, and irritation of the superficial radial nerve and synovitis of the tendons of the first dorsal compartment due to excessive length of the radial screws. Late secondary surgery is common (21%), but most of them use simple soft tissue procedures that resolve the problem and with good long-term results.[49,52,58] DeGeorge and colleagues[59] describe a large series with a 35.8-month follow-up, with major complications in 8 of 50 wrists (16.0%) and minor ones in 20 of 50 wrists (40.0%). Soft tissue (wound problems and tenosynovitis) and nerve-related complications were most common. Three patients had a periprosthetic fracture (6%) and 2 underwent implant removal due to infection.

Despite the short follow-up of most series, the global implant survival rate is good, with 90% to 100% at 5 years reported in most series. Calcagni and colleagues[49] report a longevity of 95% for the Herbert and Avanta implants, but Kakar and colleagues[51] report 86% survival at 6 years with the Avanta prosthesis (8 of 47 patients, 5 aseptic loosening, 1 revision for sigmoid notch erosion, and 2 for conversion to the total Aptis prosthesis for persistent instability). The survival rate of Aptis prostheses is high in the Calcagni and colleagues[49] review (98%), and this has been confirmed by Bellevue and colleagues.[58]

It is difficult to conclude if hemi- or total arthroplasty is better or which partial prosthesis is best. Hemiarthroplasties have the advantage of being a simpler procedure than total, but with some risk of instability and pain, and long-term bone issues (sigmoid notch erosion and distal ulna absorption). Constrained total arthroplasty has the advantage of replacing the entire joint and being stable in itself, with a greater potential to improve function and pain (considering an unstable DRUJ). However, total implants are more complex and have minor soft-tissue complications.

SUMMARY

Unstable and arthritic DRUJ management presents a surgical challenge, because there is no perfect solution, so each treatment must be evaluated according to the needs and expectations of the patient. In cases of an early OA and mild instability, ulnar shortening osteotomy seems a reasonable alternative to save time before considering more radical treatments. Resection arthroplasties provide good results in low-demand patients. In younger or active patients, hemi- and total arthroplasties would be a better option, considering good short- to medium-term outcomes and low implant failure rates. Still, their use and indication must be made cautiously, considering that these results are based on a small number of patients.

DISCLOSURE

The authors have nothing to disclose.

REFERENCES

1. Shaaban H, Giakas G, Bolton M, et al. The distal radioulnar joint as a load-bearing mechanism - a biomechanical study. J Hand Surg Am 2004;29(1): 85–95.
2. Kakar S, Carlsen BT, Moran SL, et al. The management of chronic distal radioulnar instability. Hand Clin 2010;26(4):517–28.
3. Friedman SL, Palmer AK. The ulnar impaction syndrome. Hand Clin 1991;(7):295–310.
4. Chun S, Palmer AK. The ulnar impaction syndrome: follow-up of ulnar shortening osteotomy. J Hand Surg Am 1993;18A:46–53.
5. De Smet L, Fabry G. Orientation of the sigmoid notch of the distal radius: determination of different types of the distal radioulnar joint. Acta Orthop Belg 1993;59(3):269–72.
6. Nishiwaki M, Nakamura T, Nakao Y, et al. Ulnar shortening effect on distal radioulnar joint stability: A biomechanical study. J Hand Surg Am 2005; 30(4):719–26.
7. Loh YC. The results of ulnar shortening for ulnar impaction syndrome. J Hand Surg Am 1999;24B: 316–20.
8. Scheker LR, Severo A. Ulnar shortening for the treatment of early post-traumatic osteoarthritis at the distal radioulnar joint. J Hand Surg Am 2001;26 B(1):41–4.
9. Farías-Cisneros E, Kaufman CL, Scheker LR. Ulnar shortening: results for treatment of distal radioulnar joint pathology and conversion to DRUJ replacement arthroplasty. Acta Ortop Mex 2018;32(5): 245–50. Available at: http://www.ncbi.nlm.nih.gov/pubmed/30726583.
10. Peterson CA, Maki S, Wood MB. Clinical results of the one-bone forearm. J Hand Surg Am 1995; 20(4):609–18.
11. Malgaigne J, Brailliere J. Traité des fractures et des luxations. Paris: 1855.
12. Moore EM. Three cases illustrating luxation of the ulna in connection with Colles'fracture. Med Rec 1880;17:305–8.
13. Darrach W. Anterior dislocation of the head of the ulna. Ann Surg 1912;56:802–3.
14. Zimmerman RM, Kim JM, Jupiter JB. Arthritis of the distal radioulnar joint: From darrach to total joint arthroplasty. J Am Acad Orthop Surg 2012;20(10): 623–32.
15. Tulipan DJ, Eaton RG, Eberhart RE. The Darrach procedure defended: Technique redefined and long-term follow-up. J Hand Surg Am 1991;16(3): 438–44.

16. Charles R, Hartz RDB. Long term results of resection of the Distal ulnar for posttraumatic condicitions.pdf 1979. p. 219–25.

17. McKee MD, Richards RR. Dynamic radio-ulnar convergence after the Darrach procedure. J Bone Joint Surg Br 1996;78(3):413–8.

18. Bieber EJ, Linscheid RL, Dobyns JH, et al. Failed distal ulna resections. J Hand Surg Am 1988;13(2): 193–200.

19. Minami A, Iwasaki N, Ishikawa JI, et al. Treatments of osteoarthritis of the distal radioulnar joint: long-term results of three procedures. Hand Surg 2005;10(2–3):243–8.

20. Af Ekenstam F, Engkvist O, Wadin K. Results from resection of the distal end of the ulna after fractures of the lower end of the radius. Scand J Plast Reconstr Surg Hand Surg 1982;16(2):177–81.

21. Grawe B, Heincelman C, Stern P. Functional results of the Darrach procedure: A long-term outcome study. J Hand Surg Am 2012;37(12):2475–80.e2.

22. Lluch A. The Sauvé-Kapandji procedure 2013.

23. Slater RR. The Sauvé-Kapandji Procedure. J Hand Surg Am 2008;33(9):1632–8.

24. Nakagawa N, Abe S, Kimura H, et al. Comparison of the Sauvé-Kapandji procedure and the Darrach procedure for the treatment of rheumatoid wrists. Mod Rheumatol 2003;13(3):239–42.

25. Kobayashi A, Futami T, Tadano I, et al. Radiographic comparative evaluation of the Sauve-Kapandji procedure and the Darrach procedure for rheumatoid wrist reconstruction. Mod Rheumatol 2005;15(3):187–90.

26. Millroy P, Coleman S, Ivers R. The Sauvé-Kapandji operation technique and results. J Hand Surg Br 1992;17(B):411–4.

27. Nakamura R, Tsunoda K, Watanabe K, et al. The Sauvé-Kapandji procedure for chronic dislocation of the distal radio-ulnar joint with destruction of the articular surface. J Hand Surg Br 1992;17(2): 127–32.

28. Carter PB, Stuart PR. The Sauve-Kapandji procedure for post-traumatic disorders of the distal radio-ulnar joint. J Bone Joint Surg 2000;82(7):1013–8.

29. Verhiel SHWL, Özkan S, Ritt MJPF, et al. A comparative study between Darrach and Sauvé-Kapandji procedures for post-traumatic distal radio-ulnar joint dysfunction. Hand 2019. https://doi.org/10.1177/1558944719855447.

30. Bell MJ, Hill RJ, McMurtry RY. Ulnar impingement syndrome. J Bone Joint Surg Br 1985;67(1):126–9.

31. Breen TF, Jupiter JB. Extensor carpi ulnaris and flexor carpi ulnaris tenodesis of the unstable distal ulna. J Hand Surg Am 1989;14(4):612–7.

32. Syed AA, Lam WL, Agarwal M, et al. Stabilization of the ulna stump after Darrach's procedure at the wrist. Int Orthop 2003;27(4):235–9.

33. Minami A, Iwasaki N, Ishikawa J, et al. Stabilization of the Proximal Ulnar Stump in the Sauvé-Kapandji Procedure by Using the Extensor Carpi Ulnaris Tendon: Long-Term Follow-Up Studies. Hand 2006; 31A:440–4.

34. Minami A, Kato H, Iwasaki N. Modification of the Sauve-Kapandji procedure with extensor carpi ulnaris tenodesis. J Hand Surg Am 2000;25(6):1080–4.

35. Kleinman WB, Greenberg JA. Salvage of the failed Darrach procedure. J Hand Surg Am 1995;20(6): 951–8.

36. Bowers WH. Distal radioulnar joint arthroplasty: the hemiresection-interposition technique. J Hand Surg Am 1985;10(2):169–78.

37. Lee CH, Chung US, Lee BG, et al. Long-term results of simple hemiresection arthroplasty in the rheumatoid distal radio-ulnar joint. J Hand Surg Eur Vol 2013;38(7):719–26.

38. Ahmed SK, Cheung JPY, Fung BKK, et al. Long term results of matched hemiresection interposition arthroplasty for DRUJ arthritis in rheumatoid patients. Hand Surg 2011;16(2):119–25.

39. Nawijn F, Verhiel S, Jupiter JB, et al. Hemiresection interposition arthroplasty of the distal radioulnar joint: a long-term outcome study. Hand 2019. https://doi.org/10.1177/1558944719873430.

40. Faithfull DK, Kwa S. A review of Distal Ulnar Hemi-Resection Arthroplasty. J Hand Surg Br 1992; 17(B):408–10.

41. George MS, Kiefhaber TR, Stern PJ. The Sauve-Kapandji procedure and the Darrach procedure for distal radio-ulnar joint dysfunction after Colles' fracture. J Hand Surg Am 2004;29(6):608–13.

42. Wehbé MA. Prosthetic Arthroplasty of the Distal Radioulnar Joint. Historical Perspective and 24-Year Follow-Up. Hand Clin 2013;29(1):91–101.

43. Kapandji A. Distal radio-ulnar prosthesis. Ann Chir Main Memb Super 1992;11:320–32.

44. Van Schoonhoven J, Fernandez DL, Bowers WH, et al. Salvage of failed resection arthroplasties of the distal radioulnar joint using a new ulnar head prosthesis. J Hand Surg Am 2000;25(3):438–46.

45. Berger RA, Cooney WP. Use of an ulnar head endoprosthesis for treatment of an unstable distal ulnar resection: Review of mechanics, indications, and surgical technique. Hand Clin 2005;21(4): 603–20.

46. Kopylov P, Tägil M. Distal radioulnar joint replacement. Tech Hand Up Extrem Surg 2007;11(1): 109–14.

47. Scheker LR, Babb BK, Killion PE. Distal ulnar prosthetic replacement. Orthop Clin North Am 2001;32: 365–76.

48. Moulton LS, Giddins GEB. Distal radio-ulnar implant arthroplasty: A systematic review. J Hand Surg Eur Vol 2017;42(8):827–38.

49. Calcagni M, Giesen T. Distal radioulnar joint arthroplasty with implants: A systematic review. EFORT Open Rev 2016;1(5):191–6.

50. Van Schoonhoven J, Mühldorfer-Fodor M, Fernandez DL, et al. Salvage of failed resection arthroplasties of the distal radioulnar joint using an ulnar head prosthesis: Long-term results. J Hand Surg Am 2012;37(7):1372–80.

51. Kakar S, Swann RP, Perry KI, et al. Functional and radiographic outcomes following distal ulna implant arthroplasty. J Hand Surg Am 2012;37(7):1364–71.

52. Savvidou C, Murphy E, Mailhot E, et al. Semiconstrained distal radioulnar joint prosthesis. J Wrist Surg 2013;02(01):041–8.

53. Axelsson P, Sollerman C, Kärrholm J. Ulnar head replacement: 21 cases; mean follow-up, 7.5 years. J Hand Surg Am 2015;40(9):1731–8.

54. Shipley NY, Dion GR, Bowers WH. Ulnar head implant arthroplasty: An intermediate term review of 1 surgeons experience. Tech Hand Up Extrem Surg 2009;13(3):160–4.

55. Willis AA, Berger RA, Cooney WP. Arthroplasty of the distal radioulnar joint using a new ulnar head endoprosthesis: preliminary report. J Hand Surg Am 2007;32(2):177–89.

56. Herzberg G. Periprosthetic bone resorption and sigmoid notch erosion around ulnar head implants: A concern? Hand Clin 2010;26(4):573–7.

57. Sauerbier M, Arsalan-Werner A, Enderle E, et al. Ulnar head replacement and related biomechanics. J Wrist Surg 2013;02(01):027–32.

58. Bellevue KD, Thayer MK, Pouliot M, et al. Complications of semiconstrained distal radioulnar joint arthroplasty. J Hand Surg Am 2018;43(6):566.e1-9.

59. DeGeorge BR, Berger RA, Shin AY. Constrained implant arthroplasty for distal radioulnar joint arthrosis: evaluation and management of soft tissue complications. J Hand Surg Am 2019;44(7): 614.e1-9.

The One Bone Forearm

Brett Schiffman, MD, Douglas Hanel, MD*

KEYWORDS

- One bone forearm • Proximal radioulnar joint • Distal radioulnar joint • Axial instability • Ulnius
- Synostosis

KEY POINTS

- The one bone forearm is a reliable salvage procedure for axial instability of the forearm.
- The choice of technique should be dictated by adjacent bone loss with the simplest procedure being PRUJ and DRUJ synostosis when available.
- We present our series of 11 patients treated with synostosis procedures along with description of the procedure, outcomes, and complications.

INTRODUCTION

The one bone forearm (OBF) is a salvage procedure for instability of the forearm, which may result from trauma, congenital deformity, previous surgery, tumor, or infection.[1–10] The procedure is performed with the intent of creating an osseous bridge between the radius and ulna, to correct symptomatic angular, axial, or rotatory radioulnar joint instability. Thus, OBF maintains the forearm's articulation in the elbow, via the ulna; and the wrist, with the radius.[1] By creating a stable osseous bridge between the ulnohumeral and radiocarpal joints, OBF can address defects in the bony architecture of the radius and ulna, their articulations, or their associated ligamentous complexes. Although there are alternative procedures that may address arthrosis or instability of the proximal radioulnar joint (PRUJ) or the distal radioulnar joint (DRUJ), global instability of the forearm is a complex clinical pathology without many available operative interventions.

The OBF procedure was first described by Hey-Groves in 1921.[2] There have been multiple operative techniques published; however, there is no clear consensus on optimal technique, indications, or contraindications.[1,3–7,11] Generally, osseous bridge of the forearm is obtained by one of two techniques: through creating a radioulnar

synostosis or alternatively by creating an "ulnius."[3] In the radioulnar synostosis procedure, the articulations of the DRUJ and PRUJ are obliterated and a synostosis is created with appropriate osteosynthesis. In contrast, in the ulnius procedure the distal portion of the radius is translocated to the proximal portion of the ulna, generating one contiguous forearm bone that articulates with the humerus and carpus.

HISTORICAL PERSPECTIVE

Case series of the OBF procedures have been published, but literature on outcomes is sparse.[1,3,8–10] Peterson and colleagues[1] published a series of 19 patients with seven patients obtaining excellent, six good, five fair, and one poor outcome. They reported complications in 10 patients, and a 32% nonunion rate. A worse outcome was associated with traumatic cause of pathology, two or more reconstructive surgeries before OBF, history of nerve injury, or infection.

Kim[9] published a retrospective cohort of eight patients treated with all patients achieving bony union and a mean QuickDash score of 39 (7–75). Using a Peterson score, four patients had good/excellent result, two fair results, and two poor result. Complications were related to severity of initial trauma with five of eight patients having

Department of Orthopaedics and Sports Medicine, University of Washington, Box 359798, 908 Jefferson Street, Seattle, WA 98104, USA
* Corresponding author.
E-mail address: dhanel@uw.edu

Hand Clin 36 (2020) 531–538
https://doi.org/10.1016/j.hcl.2020.07.007

complication; three soft tissue complications requiring flap or local coverage after the OBF operation, one fracture after OBF, and one postoperative infection.

Allende and Allende[8] published a case series of seven patients with average Peterson score of 7.7 (good). They reported no complications of nonunion, fracture, hardware failure, or infection.

Agraharam and colleagues[10] reported results of 38 patients with excellent outcome in 12 patients, good in six patients, fair in two patients, and poor in two patients on Peterson score with four patients developing nonunion (10.5%). The patient population was stratified into two cohorts with the traumatic group having a mean DASH score of 12.8 (1.7–33) and the elective group having mean DASH score of 10.9 (0.8–50.8).

SURGICAL TECHNIQUE: PROXIMAL AND DISTAL RADIOULNAR SYNOSTOSIS

The patient-specific position of the forearm rotation is determined with splints preoperatively. The optimal position takes into account occupation, activities of interest, necessary activities of daily living, but most importantly the patient's preference.

After initiation of anesthesia, the patient is positioned supine with the operative limb on a hand table. Our preference is to proceed without a tourniquet. Doing so allows immediate identification and control of vascular structures, such as the anterior and posterior interosseus vessels that are difficult to access once osteosynthesis is complete.

Two-incisions are used, one for exposure of the DRUJ and the second for exposure of the PRUJ. The distal incision runs along the volar aspect of the subcutaneous border of the ulna, and at the neck of ulna the incision curves dorsally toward the dorsal articular surface of the ulna with the radius (**Fig. 1.**) The dissection is performed from proximal to distal to identify and protect the dorsal cutaneous branches of the ulnar nerve. Dissection of the subcutaneous tissue reveals the dorsal capsule of the DRUJ. The retinaculum of the fifth dorsal compartment is incised and the extensor digiti quinti tendon retracted radially. Cutting the floor of fifth compartment exposes the articulation between the radius and ulna. Retractors are passed between subcutaneous tissue and the dorsal retinaculum of the radius to assist with exposure. The articular cartilage and subchondral cortical bone of the radius sigmoid notch and the ulnar head are removed with osteotomes, curettes, and high-speed burrs. In those patients who have an abnormal DRUJ, a previously resected distal ulna, or a dysplastic distal ulna as demonstrated in (**Fig. 2**), the procedure may still be performed; but in this case the distal synostosis site is prepared between the ulna metadiaphysis and the area of the radius adjacent to it.

The PRUJ is exposed with a Boyd-Anderson approach. The skin incision is placed along the dorsal radial aspect of the proximal ulna. The incision is extended proximally to the lateral epicondyle in cases of chronic radial head dislocations. The anconeus muscle is elevated from the lateral face of the ulna and the dissection proceeds radially over the dorsal surface of the interosseus membrane. The lateral collateral ligament attachment to ulna is left intact. When the radial head is encountered a retractor is placed over the neck of the radius, and the anterior capsule and orbicular ligament incised. The dissection continues distally until the radial tuberosity and biceps tendon are encountered and kept intact. The exposure is completed by elevating the entire anconeus insertion and supinator origin off of the lateral face of the ulna. By staying in the plain

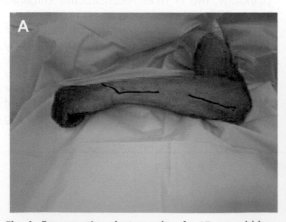 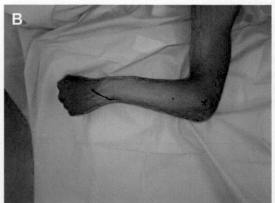

Fig. 1. Preoperative photographs of a 17-year-old boy with multiple hereditary exostosis of left forearm.

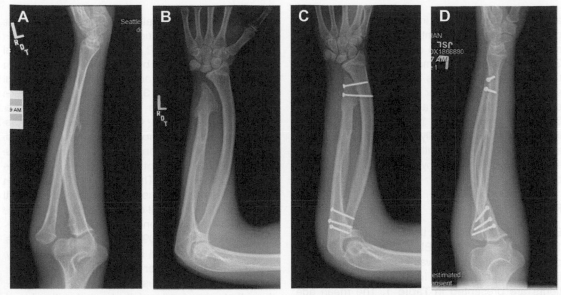

Fig. 2. Preoperative and postoperative radiographs of a 17-year-old boy with multiple hereditary exostosis of left forearm.

between the ulna volarly and all of the soft tissues of posterior compartment of the proximal forearm dorsally the posterior interosseus nerve is protected in the supinator muscle. Gentle retraction is provided with broad retractors placed around the radial neck. Gentle pressure maintains exposure and allows appropriate preparation of the PRUJ. In cases of congenital deformity, there may be chronic dislocation of the radial head that requires excision. Curettes, osteotomes, and a high-speed burr are used to remove cartilage and subchondral cortical bone. The dissection ends when bleeding cancellous bone is exposed.

Once both the PRUJ and DRUJ have been prepared, the rotation of the forearm is placed into the position of pronosupination determined with the patient preoperatively. Rotation is provisionally

secured with 0.062 Kirschner wires applied while digital compression is directed at the synostosis sites. Each site is packed with allograft cancellous chips and native bone, such as the remnants of an excised radial or ulnar head. Definitive fixation is obtained by placing a combination of 3.5-mm and 2.7-mm cortical lag screws under image intensification (**Fig. 3**). Two or three screws are placed at each articulation engaging six cortices proximally and four to six cortices distally (see **Fig. 2**).

Fascia that approximates easily is closed with 3–0 absorbable suture and skin is closed with simple interrupted 3–0 nylon sutures. Wounds are dressed with nonadherent gauze, sterile 4 × 4 gauze, and Dacron batting. The limb is protected in a long arm splint. The elbow is flexed 90°, the forearm position is dictated by the synostosis,

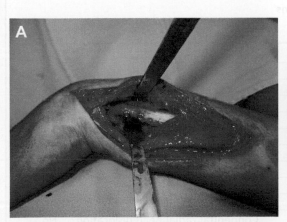
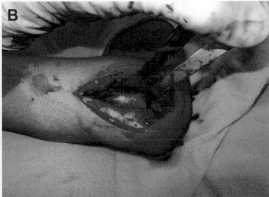

Fig. 3. Intraoperative photographs of a 17-year-old boy with multiple hereditary exostosis of left forearm.

and the wrist is placed in 10° of extension. The digits are left free. Patients begin digital range of motion immediately and remain in the splint for 2 weeks. Sutures are removed after 2 weeks and the operative extremity is fitted with an orthoplast splint that is removed for simple range of motion exercises. Radiographs are obtained at 6-week, 3-month, 6-month, and 12-month postoperative intervals. Union is usually obtained by 6 weeks and certainly by 3 months. Limb strengthening and use is determined by radiographic evidence of union.

RESULTS

Between 1998 and 2018, the senior author treated 12 patients with the OBF procedure described previously. One patient was lost to follow-up after 6 weeks. Demographics for the remaining 11 patients are presented in **Table 1**. The mean age was 36.5 years (9–70 years). Indications for OBF were post-traumatic arthritis in four patients, failed DRUJ arthroplasty in three patients, congenital radial head dislocation in two patients, multiple hereditary exostosis in one patient, and ulnar shaft fibrous nonunion secondary to neurofibromatosis in one patient. The mean number of operations before creation of an OBF were 2.2 (0–10).

All patients elected to have the forearm placed in pronation, ranging from 5° to 60° with a mean of 35° (**Table 2**). Ten of the 11 patients had synostosis at both the PRUJ and DRUJ. One patient was missing the distal third of the ulna and only the PRUJ was fused. All synostoses were secured with compression screws and allograft cancellous bone was packed adjacent to the fusion sites. The child with neurofibromatosis was augmented with

a fibular strut allograft that bridged the ulna nonunion site. One patient with a history of an ulnar nonunion had BMP applied to the fusion sites in addition to allograft bone.

Patients were followed for a mean of 18 months (1–110 months) (**Table 3**). There were no postoperative infections. One patient (9.09%) had a nonunion at one site. One patient (9.09%) was dissatisfied with the position of the forearm and is listed as a malunion (**Table 4**). Four patients (36.36%) required a total of eight additional procedures (range, 0–4). Three patients (27.27%) underwent hardware removal because of prominent screw heads for a total of five operations. The patient with the malunion (9.09%) underwent revision. One patient (9.09%) with a nonunion was treated with additional bone grafting followed by dome osteotomy after developing a malunion. One patient (9.09%) sustained a peri-implant fracture that was successfully treated with closed management.

The mean pain score on the Numeric Rating Scale at last follow-up was 2.11 (2–7; standard deviation [SD] = 2.31). Mean elbow range of motion arc was 110.2° (50°–135°; SD = 27.11); mean wrist flexion-extension arc was 71.67° (20°–115°; SD = 34.45).

QuickDASH scores were obtained in 3 of 11 patients, with mean score 39.4 (0–72.7). Mean Peterson score was 6.3 (good outcome) with one patient having excellent, one patient good, and one patient poor outcome.

DISCUSSION

Overall, the creation of an OBF was successful in this series, achieving the goals of the operation,

Table 1
Patient demographics

Case	Gender	Age	Side Affected/ Dominance	Operations Before OBF (n)	Indication	Tobacco
1	F	53	R/R	1	Post-traumatic arthritis	No
2	M	38	L/R	1	Post-traumatic arthritis	No
3	M	31	R/R	0	Failed DRUJ arthroplasty	No
4	M	9	L/R	2	Neurofibromatosis, ulna nonunion	No
5	M	45	R/R	4	Failed DRUJ arthroplasty	Yes
6	M	47	R/R	4	Failed DRUJ arthroplasty	Yes
7	M	70	L/R	1	Post-traumatic arthritis	No
8	F	52	R/R	10	Post-traumatic arthritis	No
9	F	17	R/R	1	Multiple hereditary exostosis	No
10	M	22	L/R	0	Congenital radial head dislocation	No
11	M	17	L/R	0	Congenital radial head dislocation	No

Table 2
Surgical description

Case	Approach	Location of Synostosis	Screw Fixation (Proximal/ Distal)	Bone Graft	Position (Degrees)
1	Kocher	PRUJ/DRUJ	2.7 mm × 3/2.7 mm × 2	Allograft cancellous chips	20 pronation
2	Kocher	PRUJ/DRUJ	3.5 mm × 3/3.5 mm × 3	Allograft cancellous chips	45 pronation
3	Boyd Anderson	PRUJ/DRUJ	2.7 mm × 4/2.7 × 2	Allograft cancellous chips, BMP	15 pronation
4	Boyd Anderson	PRUJ/DRUJ	2.7 mm × 2 and 2.4 mm × 1/2.7 mm × 2	Allograft cancellous chips, fibular strut	5 pronation
5	Boyd Anderson	PRUJ/DRUJ	2.7 mm × 3/3.5 mm × 4	Allograft cancellous chips	30 pronation
6	Boyd Anderson	PRUJ/DRUJ	3.5 mm × 3/3.5 mm × 3	Allograft cancellous chips	20 pronation
7	Boyd Anderson	PRUJ/DRUJ	2.7 mm × 3/2.7 mm × 3	Allograft cancellous chips	45 pronation
8	Boyd Anderson	PRUJ	2.7 mm × 2 and 3.5 mm × 2.7 mm × 2 / 3.5mm × 2	Allograft cancellous chips	45 pronation
9	Boyd Anderson	PRUJ/DRUJ	3.5 mm × 2 and 2.5 × 1/3.5 mm × 1	Allograft cancellous chips	45 pronation
10	Boyd Anderson	PRUJ/DRUJ	3.5 mm × 3/2.7 mm × 3	Allograft cancellous chips	60 pronation
11	Boyd Anderson	PRUJ/DRUJ	2.7 mm × 3/2.7 mm × 3	Allograft cancellous chips, radial head autograft	45 pronation

Abbreviation: BMP, bone morphogenic protein.

which were correction of symptomatic angular deformity and securing a stable radioulnar joint. The union rate, the functional arc of elbow and wrist motion, the Numeric Rating Pain Scale score, and patient-reported outcomes were similar to those reported in contemporary literature.[8–10] QuickDASH and Peterson score of 39.4 and 6.3 are consistent with those found by Kim[9] (39) and Allende and Allende[8] (7.7). Complication rates reported in the literature range from 0% to 63%. Although our complication rate was higher and Peterson scores less than that reported by Allende and Allende,[8] this likely is attributed to the pathology and history of our study population. Peterson reported that worse outcomes after OBF were associated with traumatic cause of pathology, two or more reconstructive surgeries before OBF, a history of nerve injury, or infection. In our study 7 of 11 patients, had a history of forearm trauma and 2.2 previous procedures before OBF.

The complications in our series deserve special attention. The most common complication was prominent screw heads that became symptomatic as wounds matured and swelling subsided. When we made sure that all screw heads were deeply countersunk this problem was avoided.

The child with neurofibromatosis required four additional operations to address a nonunion, a distal radius deformity that was treated with a dome osteotomy of the radius, followed by two procedures for hardware removal. This patient initially underwent the OBF procedure for ulnar fibrodysplastic nonunion secondary to neurofibromatosis type 1 (NF1). At follow-up of 110 months, a pain score of 0 on the Numeric Rating Score was reported with an arc of motion at the elbow of 130° and 80° at the wrist. Fibrodysplastic nonunion secondary to neurofibromatosis in the forearm is rare and is a clinical challenge to treat. Success of treatment has been shown to be related to timing of intervention and presence or absence of the NF1 gene.[12–15] Nonunion rate in patients with NF1 with conventional graft have been reported to be between 44% and 73%, with rates decreasing to 0% to 45% in patients without the NF1 gene. Although this patient was at increased risk for nonunion, it is possible that risk could have been decreased by using autograft or vascularized bone graft rather than conventional allograft chips.[12,16]

One patient required revision OBF because of forearm position. In the revision procedure, the

Table 3
Outcomes of OBF

Case	Pain Score (0-10)	Wrist Motion (Degrees) Flexion/Extension	Elbow Motion	Return to OR (n)	Complication	QuickDASH	Peterson Score	Length of Follow-up (mo)
1	4	65/50	0-127	0	No	N/A	N/A	35
2	2	N/A	45-135	0	No	N/A	N/A	1
3	7	N/A	10-135	1	Symptomatic hardware	N/A	N/A	5
4	0	50/30	0-130	4	Nonunion, malunion, fracture, symptomatic hardware	N/A	N/A	110
5	2	40/60	5-130	2	Symptomatic hardware	45.5	7	18
6	3	N/A	15-110	0	No	N/A	N/A	6
7	0	20/45	40-135	1	Malunion	N/A	N/A	4
8	N/A	10/10	N/A	0	No	72.7	2	13
9	N/A	20/30	50-100	0	No	N/A	N/A	3
10	1	N/A	0-130	0	No	N/A	N/A	3
11	0	N/A	0-135	0	No	0	10	5

Abbreviations: N/A, not applicable; OR, operating room.

Table 4
Complications

Case	Complication	Return to OR (n)	Procedure
3	Symptomatic hardware	1	Removal of hardware
4	Nonunion	4	Nonunion repair
4	Malunion		Corrective osteotomy
4	Symptomatic hardware		Hardware removal
4	Symptomatic hardware		Hardware removal
4	Fracture		N/A
5	Symptomatic hardware	2	Hardware removal (wrist)
5	Symptomatic hardware		Hardware removal (elbow)
7	Forearm malposition	1	Revision OBF

Abbreviation: N/A, not applicable.

forearm was changed from a position of 45° of pronation to neutral rotation. At the time of initial evaluation and discussion of the procedure, the patient preferred the pronated position that would allow more effective keyboard use. However, after the procedure the patient had disability related to position of the forearm because it limited or eliminated many activities. At 4 months after revision his pain score was 0, elbow motion 0° to 135°, and combined wrist motion 65°.

Although there exist numerous surgical procedures that can be used to treat the diverse set of pathology resulting in symptomatic angular, axial, or rotatory radioulnar joint stability, the OBF procedure is a reliable and predictable salvage procedure. It effectively and simultaneously addresses instability, pain, and arthrosis involving the PRUJ and DRUJ. The procedure does not rely on inherent ligamentous or bony stability of the forearm. Good results have been demonstrated with arthroplasty and stabilization procedures of the radioulnar joints; however, they are at high risk for failure in the setting of angular, axial, or rotatory instability of the forearm. Care should be taken to avoid OBF in the setting of ulnohumeral or radiocarpal arthritis and active infection. Additionally, careful investigation of the cause of the radioulnar pathology should be performed to identify risk factors for failure including post-traumatic cause, NF1 gene, number of surgeries performed before OBF, and history of nerve injury or infection. Patients should be counseled that the technique described here has a high rate of union, while maintaining functional elbow and wrist motion. Secondary procedures, such as removal of hardware, were encountered in 30% of cases.

SUMMARY

The OBF procedure is a viable salvage procedure for traumatic or congenital bone loss with axial instability of the forearm. In this case series, there was a 9% incidence of nonunion and 36% required additional surgery. Overall, there was a high union rate, functional range of motion, and low functional pain score.

DISCLOSURE

The authors have nothing to disclose.

REFERENCES

1. Peterson CA II, Maki S, Wood MB. Clinical results of the one-bone forearm. J Hand Surg Am 1995;20: 609–18.
2. Hey-Groves EW. Modern methods of treating fractures. In: Fractures of the upper limb. 2nd edition. Bristol (United Kingdom): John Wright; 1921. p. 203–5.
3. Peterson HA. The ulnius: a one-bone forearm in children. J Pediatr Orthop B 2008;17(2):95–101.
4. Castle ME. One bone forearm. J Bone Joint Surg Am 1974;56:1223–7.
5. Lowe HG. Radioulnar fusion for defects in the forearm bones. J Bone Joint Surg Br 1963;45:351–9.
6. Murray RA. The one bone forearm. J Bone Joint Surg Am 1955;37:366–70.
7. Reid RL, Baker GI. The single-bone forearm: a reconstructive technique. Hand 1973;5:214–9.
8. Allende C, Allende BT. Posttraumatic one-bone forearm reconstruction: a report of seven cases. J Bone Joint Surg Am 2004;86(2):364–9.
9. Kim SY, Chim H, Bishop AT, et al. Complications and Outcomes of One-Bone Forearm Reconstruction. Hand (N Y) 2017;12(2):140–144.
10. Agraharam D, Velmurugesan P, Dheenadhayalan J, et al. One-bone forearm reconstruction a salvage solution for the forearm with massive bone loss. J Bone Joint Surg Am 2019;101(15):e74.

11. Vitale CC. Reconstructive surgery for defects in the shaft of the ulna in children. J Bone Joint Surg Am 1952;34:804–9.

12. Solla F, Lemoine J, Musoff C, et al. Surgical treatment of congenital pseudoarthrosis of the forearm: review and quantitative analysis of individual patient data. Hand Surg Rehabil 2019;38(4):233–41.

13. Kohler R, Solla F, Pinson S, et al. Congenital pseudarthrosis of the forearm in a neurofibromatosis patient: case report and review of the literature. Rev Chir Orthop Reparatrice Appar Mot 2005;91: 773–81.

14. Bell DF. Congenital forearm pseudarthrosis: report of six cases and review of the literature. J Pediatr Orthop 1989;9:438–43.

15. Kaempffe FA, Gillespie R. Pseudarthrosis of the radius after fracture through normal bone in a child who had neurofibromatosis. A case report. J Bone Joint Surg Am 1989;71:1419–21.

16. Allende V, Masquijo JJ. Congenital forearm pseudarthrosis associated with dislocation of the radial head: surgical treatment with one-bone forearm. Rev Asoc Argent Ortop Traumatol 2017;82:242–8.

Solutions for the Unstable and Arthritic Elbow Joint

Danil A. Rybalko, MD*, Michael R. Hausman, MD

KEYWORDS

- Elbow arthritis • Elbow instability • Interposition arthroplasty • Internal joint stabilizer

KEY POINTS

- Chronic elbow pain due to an unstable, arthritic joint is a problem with no perfect solution.
- Interposition arthroplasty in conjunction with ligament reconstruction may offer a reasonably durable solution for select patients with painful, unstable, and arthritic elbows.
- Adequate bone stock is a prerequisite for interposition arthroplasty.
- Elbow stability and congruent range of motion must be maintained or restored with ligament reconstruction, and if needed, use of an internal joint stabilizer.
- Patients should understand that they may achieve good, but not complete, pain relief and will have functional but not full range of motion of the elbow.

INTRODUCTION

An arthritic, unstable, and painful elbow, especially in a young, active patient, presents a challenging problem to the treating surgeon. The pathophysiology may be posttraumatic, degenerative or of rheumatologic origin. Although total elbow arthroplasty (TEA) may be an option, postoperative activity limitations and concern for implant survival[1,2] limit the patient population that can benefit from this procedure. Furthermore, salvage options for a failed TEA are fraught with complications and are limited.[3,4] Interposition arthroplasty may offer a more appropriate solution for the younger patients, but a critical prerequisite is normal bone anatomy and stability of the elbow (or ability to restore stability), which may preclude this procedure in some patients.[5]

OVERVIEW OF TREATMENT OPTIONS

An unstable, arthritic elbow resulting in significant limitation of motion and pain results in substantial functional implications. Chronic elbow instability and arthritis often result from direct traumatic injury to the elbow, forearm, or the structures responsible for maintaining longitudinal stability of the forearm.[6–8] However, other etiologies such as inflammatory arthritis and degenerative pathology play a role as well.[9]

Primary osteoarthritis of the elbow is somewhat unusual in that it often presents with osteophyte formation and a significant loss of motion. However, the osteophytes form around the periphery of the articular surface and the central portion of the joint is usually preserved, with acceptable cartilage present. Pain at the terminal extents of flexion and extension is often present, but elbow instability is rarely an issue. In such cases, open or arthroscopic debridement (osteocapsular arthroplasty) may significantly improve range of motion and reduce pain at the extremes of motion.[7]

In contract, posttraumatic arthritis may have more severe cartilage loss from the original injury and/or subsequent joint instability that results in incongruent motion and cartilage wear.

Upper Extremity Surgery, Department of Orthopaedic Surgery, Mount Sinai Hospital, 5 East 98th Street, Room 908, New York, NY 10029, USA
* Corresponding author. Mount Sinai Physician Offices, 425 West 59th Street, 5th Floor, New York, NY 10019.
E-mail address: drybalko@gmail.com

Hand Clin 36 (2020) 539–547
https://doi.org/10.1016/j.hcl.2020.07.009
0749-0712/20/

Posterolateral and posteromedial rotatory instabilities can be easily missed and may lead to a painful, arthritic elbow joint if not properly treated. Patients with posttraumatic arthritis often present with pain throughout the entire range of motion because the pathology is often not isolated to the peripheral aspects of the joint, but rather may include the entire joint surface or a large portion of the articular surface. Similarly, patients with inflammatory arthritis typically present with pain throughout the arc of motion. Likewise, radiographic findings reveal pan-articular cartilage loss and narrowing of the entire joint space. These patients also may have attenuation of the ligamentous stabilizers of the elbow joint.

TEA, and specifically semi-constrained TEA, have been shown to have good early results, especially in the low-demand, rheumatoid population.[1,10] However, postoperatively patients are asked to adhere to a permanent lifting restriction of 1 kg for frequent and 5 kg for occasional lifting to avoid excessive forces on the implant.[11] Furthermore, long-term follow-up shows high rates of complications and revision.[1,2,11–13] Consequently, concerns exist with respect to longevity and potentially need for revision, thus limiting its applicability for the young or active patient. Therefore, patients with posttraumatic arthritis, who tend to be younger, are generally poor candidates for this operation.

Less desirable options, such as resection arthroplasty and elbow arthrodesis, are also available. Zarkadas and colleagues[3] reported outcomes of resection arthroplasty in the setting of failed TEA and showed that although the patients benefited from the procedure from the standpoint of pain, their functional performance scores were poor. Similarly, elbow arthrodesis, although an option, may result in a prolonged time to union, has been shown to have numerous complications, and results in substantial limitation in the ability to position the hand in space and is therefore poorly tolerated by patients.[4,14]

In the case of instability due to severe bone loss, bony reconstruction with a vascularized graft, such as a free fibula graft, may be attempted.[15] Alternatively, in cases of non-reconstructible bony deformities of the proximal ulna, the olecranon may be excised and the distal humerus can be associated with the proximal radius with transfer of the triceps to the radial head to maintain some elbow flexion and extension (**Fig. 1**).

For less severe deformities in young, active patients, we prefer interposition arthroplasty, which has been shown to have a high rate of acceptable (but certainly not perfect) results in terms of function and pain relief.[5,16] A number of various resurfacing materials have been proposed for interposition, including fascia, dermis, or tendon.[5,16] The advantage of this procedure is that the bony anatomy is maintained, and ligaments are preserved, repaired, or reconstructed, as necessary. Often, this procedure is combined with temporary joint distraction. Historically, the elbows have been temporarily stabilized with an articulated external fixator.[5,16] However, more recently, an internal joint stabilizer (IJS) device has become an attractive option.[17–19] Finally, TEA remains a viable salvage option at a later time, if the benefits of the interposition arthroplasty deteriorate.

INDICATIONS FOR INTERPOSITION ARTHROPLASTY

Interposition arthroplasty with ligament reconstruction and internal joint stabilization is indicated for patients suffering from severe posttraumatic arthritis or stage II/IIA rheumatoid arthritis in young, high-demand patients[20] (**Fig. 2**). This operation requires adequate bone stock. Although ligament insufficiency may be addressed with ligament reconstruction, instability caused by significant bone loss is a contraindication, unless this can be corrected by way of bone grafting before interposition arthroplasty. Other contraindications include presence of an active infection, open physes, and absence of active elbow flexion.[21]

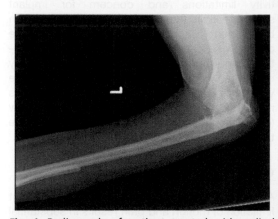

Fig. 1. Radiograph of patient treated with radical resection of proximal ulna for radiation-associated sarcoma and construction of a 1-bone forearm. Distal humerus was placed over the neck of the proximal radius. Biceps tendon was used as an anterior stabilizer, akin to an anterior capsule. Triceps was attached to the radial head with nonabsorbable suture via drill holes. The arm was positioned in neutral rotation. This reconstruction allowed for a reasonably stable, mobile elbow.

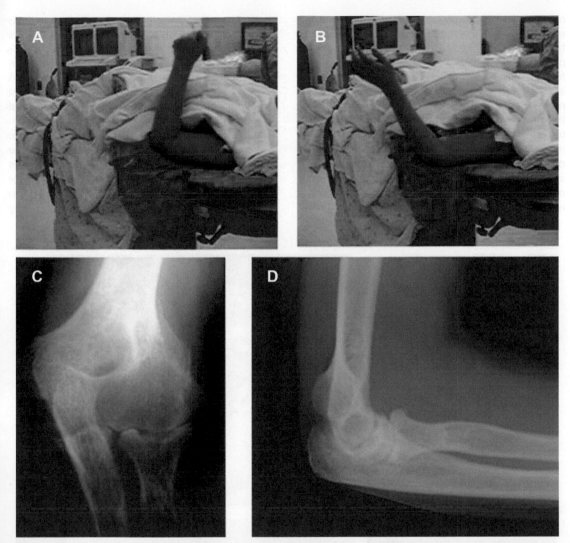

Fig. 2. (*A, B*) A 29-year-old patient presenting with elbow pain and severe range of motion deficit due to rheumatoid arthritis. (*C, D*) Anteroposterior and lateral radiographs of the patient demonstrating Mayo stage II degenerative changes with loss of joint space, but preservation of bony architecture.

TECHNIQUE

These authors prefer the operation to be performed under regional anesthesia with the use of an indwelling interscalene catheter. The patient is placed in the supine position. The authors use an articulated shoulder positioner attached at the forearm to position the forearm above the patient's chest (**Fig. 3**). A sterile tourniquet is applied at the upper arm. The surgeon has an option of a posterior approach or a combination of medial and lateral approaches to the elbow.

Our preference is for a posterior incision, made over the midline of the triceps and is extended distally over the olecranon and the subcutaneous border of the ulna. The length of the incision is

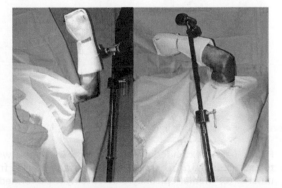

Fig. 3. An articulated shoulder positioner is used to position the arm over the patient's chest.

made such that medial and lateral aspects of the elbow joint may be easily exposed without undue tension on the skin. Full-thickness flaps are raised medially and laterally at the level of triceps and forearm fascia. Medially, care must be taken to identify and protect the ulnar nerve. The ulnar nerve is released from the arcade of Struthers to the flexor carpi ulnaris but does not always need to be circumferentially mobilized (**Fig. 4**). The medial epicondyle is exposed. The flexor tendon origin and medial collateral ligaments are released in 1 of 2 ways. These attachments may either be dissected off subperiosteally or released via a medial epicondyle osteotomy (see **Fig. 4**). The anterior band of the medial collateral ligament attaches onto the anterior-inferior aspect of the medial epicondyle, while the posterior band attaches onto the posterior inferior aspect of the epicondyle and forms the floor of the cubital tunnel. A medial epicondyle osteotomy must be deep and proximal enough to include the medial collateral ligaments and the flexor mass attachments.

Next, the anterior capsule is separated from the brachialis muscle and released. Posteriorly, the posterior capsule is separated from the triceps muscle and is also released. A thorough anterior and posterior release needs to be performed to adequately expose the joint. At this point, it may

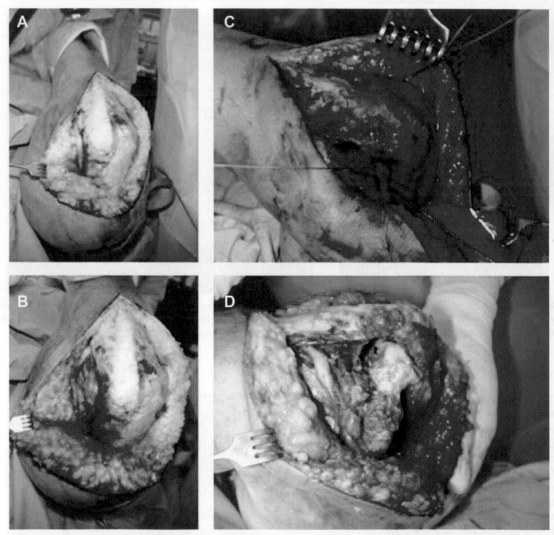

Fig. 4. (*A*) An extended posterior approach is made with thick skin flaps. The ulnar nerve is identified and protected medially. (*B*) The ulnar nerve is decompressed from the arcade of Struthers to the 2 heads of flexor carpi ulnaris. (*C*) Medial epicondyle osteotomy is performed to preserve the medial collateral ligament (MCL) if it is intact. (*D*) The anterior and posterior capsule is fully released, followed by release of the lateral side elbow and the joint is dislocated, exposing the distal humerus.

be possible to hinge the joint open. If the exposure is adequate, the lateral collateral ligament, if intact, may be spared. In the case that the exposure is inadequate, the lateral collateral ligament and the forearm extensor attachments are released subperiosteally from the lateral epicondyle and the elbow can then be dislocated. This may be done from the medial side by hinging the joint open or through the Kocher interval between anconeus and extensor carpi ulnaris.

Patience must be exercised during the elbow dislocation step by following sequential releases as needed. Although the amount of dissection will vary from patient-to-patient, a complete anterior and posterior capsulectomy is always required. It is important to mention that the ulnar nerve needs to be sufficiently visualized and mobilized before dislocation. Failure to do so may impart excessive traction the nerve and result in injury. However, circumferential mobilization should be avoided, if the nerve can be protected while in situ. Finally, if the medial and lateral releases are not adequate to allow safe dislocation or the ulnar nerve cannot be sufficiently mobilized due to scarring, an olecranon osteotomy may be performed to provide excellent exposure. The osteotomy can later be repaired with any number of the available techniques.

Once the distal humerus surface is adequately exposed, the articular surface is evaluated (see Fig. 4). Anterior and posterior synovectomy is performed, and any osteophytes are removed. Finally, the remaining cartilage of the distal humerus is removed with a burr or a curette (**Fig. 5**). Care must be taken not to penetrate or remove subchondral bone, as it provides structural support and helps withstand load. Removal of the subchondral bone may result in late subsidence and if bony resection is excessive can compromise stability of the joint.

Subsequently, the axis pin for application of the IJS (Skeletal Dynamics, Miami, FL) or hinged external fixator is placed. The axis of the pin must coincide with the axis of rotation of the elbow joint. Failure to do so may result in binding, incongruous motion, or accelerated wearing of the graft. The center of rotation of the elbow is located at the center of circles defined by circumference of the trochlea and the capitellum. The pin may be placed freehand, with the use of a guide, or by the radiographic method described previously.[17,19,22,23] Fluoroscopy is used to confirm proper placement of the axis pin (**Fig. 6**).

For the resurfacing portion of the procedure, a number of options are available for choice of graft. Previously described techniques used dermal allograft, fascia lata, allograft fascia, and allograft tendon.[16,21] The authors prefer the use of fascia lata, Achilles tendon allograft, or AlloDerm (BioHorizons, Birmingham, AL). The graft is fashioned

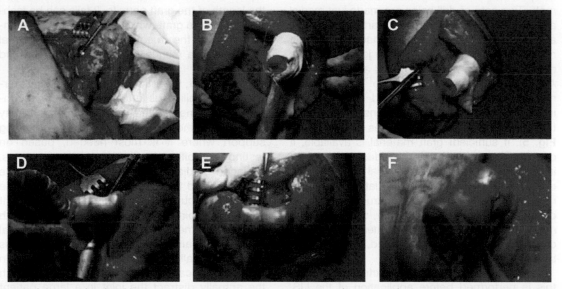

Fig. 5. (*A*) Once the distal humerus is exposed, a rongeur, curette, or burr is used to remove any remaining cartilage. Care is taken not to remove subchondral bone to prevent late subsidence. (*B–F*) The graft is fashioned to the dimensions of the distal humerus. Drill holes are made in the humerus in a mattress fashion. Two sets of drill holes are placed centrally, just medial and just lateral to the center of the distal humerus. A second set of drill holes is made over the medial and lateral aspects of the condyles. A Keith needle is used to pass #2 Kevlar-reinforced sutures in such manner that the graft is well tensioned over the distal humerus to ensure adherence to bone.

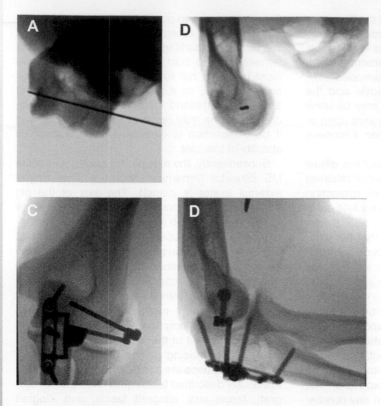

Fig. 6. (*A*, *B*) The axis pin is placed through the center of the axis of rotation of the elbow. This can be done with the guide that comes with the implant set or freehand. Correct placement of this pin is critical to congruent reduction and motion of the elbow. Pin placement must be confirmed by direct and radiographic inspection. (*C*, *D*) Anteroposterior and lateral radiographs showing correct placement of the IJS. This device can be placed either laterally or medially to stabilize the side of the elbow that is most unstable.

to the dimensions of the distal humerus to cover the articular surfaces. Drill holes are made with a Kirshner wire or a small drill in the distal humerus in a proximal-to-distal mattress fashion to created matt. Two sets of drill holes are made just medial and just lateral to the center of articulation. Two additional sets of drill holes are made at the most medial and lateral aspects of the joint. Drill holes need to be large enough to pass a Keith needle. A free Keith needle is used to pass braided, nonabsorbable, Kevlar-reinforced #2 sutures to incorporate the graft. Enough tension is needed to ensure that the graft adheres to bone (see **Fig. 5**). If sufficient graft material is available, it can be folded to provide an additional layer of interposition. Sutures at the medial and lateral aspects of the joint are left long to later be incorporated into the repair/reconstruction of the collateral ligaments. Alternatively, suture anchors may be used for this purpose. When a medial epicondyle osteotomy is performed, it is secured back with 2 screws.

If collateral ligament reconstruction is required, this is performed before application of the IJS. Medial collateral ligament reconstruction is performed using the technique described by Jobe and colleagues,[24] using a palmaris tendon graft. Laterally, several options are available, including reefing of the native capsuloligamentous complex,

reconstruction with a tendon graft as described by O'Driscoll and colleagues,[25] or a technique described by DeLaMora and Hausman[26] using a slip of the lateral triceps tendon. Alternatively, if the length of the graft permits, 2 tails can be fashioned from the graft, which can be used to reconstruct both the medial and lateral collateral ligaments in a manner described by Larson and Morrey.[27]

At this point, the articulated portion of the internal joint stabilizer is attached, and the reconstructed ligaments are tensioned.[19] The IJS may be placed either laterally or medially, providing support where it is most needed, based on testing of stability when tensioning the ligaments. If placed medially, the ulnar nerve needs to be mobilized and transposed out of the way of the IJS. As previously mentioned, proper placement of the axis pin is of utmost importance. With proper placement, the IJS protects the collateral ligament repair, while establishing congruous motion, and allowing early motion. However, in its current incarnation, it is not strong enough the actually distract the joint in a large patient and will eventually fatigue and break along the boom arm. Fluoroscopy is used to confirm final positioning of the IJS and to check for congruent alignment and motion of the elbow joint (see **Fig. 6**).

The detached flexors and extensors are anatomically repaired to their origins at the distal humerus. Skin is closed over a suction drain with a tight closure. A light, loose dressing is applied, and the elbow is splinted.

REHABILITATION

The patient is splinted for approximately 1 week, at which point gentle range of motion is begun under supervision of a therapist. Therapy consists of active and active assisted range of motion exercises, edema control, pain modalities, and home exercise program. Long cycle times of approximately 1 hour are used, and emphasis is placed on obtaining maximum range of motion rather than focusing on the number of cycles. This is done to minimize traction at the incision site and help prevent wound complications. The number of cycles is increased as the wound healing progresses. Continuous passive motion is not used. The IJS is removed at approximately 3 months mark and the patient is allowed to slowly return to usual activities.

DISCUSSION

An unstable, arthritic elbow, particularly in a young, active patient is a challenging problem. Of the treatment options available, none are ideal in this subset of patients. Further, it is important to realize that most geriatric patients eventually must bear weight through their upper limbs and elbows, either with a cane or walker, and they rely heavily on their arms to rise from a seat. For this reason, the "elderly, low-demand patient" may be an oxymoron. Management options for the unstable arthritic elbow include resection arthroplasty, which results in a flail elbow and limited function. Elbow arthrodesis results in substantial functional limitations. Improvements in TEA implants have led to better outcomes; however, patients undergoing TEA are subject to life-long lifting restrictions of no more than 5 kg for occasional and 1 kg for repetitive lifting. Furthermore, durability and longevity of current implant designs, the high rate of revision surgery anticipated in young or active patients, and challenges associated with salvage or revision TEA surgery make this an undesirable option especially for the younger, more active patient.[3,12–14,16] Kwak and colleagues[12] reported a complication and revision rates of 26.5% and 16% in unlinked TEAs, and 19.1% and 13.1% in linked TEAs at 6-year to 8-year follow-up. With multiple revisions, there is risk of significant loss of bone stock or seeding of persistent infection, ultimately precluding

reimplantation and leading to resection arthroplasty. For these reasons, TEA is generally reserved for patients with a limited life expectancy remaining, and should be used with caution.

Interposition arthroplasty has been associated with reasonably satisfactory results particularly in the setting of patients in whom a TEA is undesirable due to young age or high demands. Fernandez-Palazzi and colleagues[28] reported 20-year follow-up results in children and adolescents receiving interposition arthroplasty with 5 of 12 elbows maintaining good to excellent results at last visit. Ljung and colleagues[29] reported no to mild pain in 21 of 28 patients 6 years following interposition arthroplasty. Similarly, Cheng and Morrey[30] demonstrated 69% satisfactory results and 62% excellent results at over 5 months of follow-up. These results were similar in patients with post-traumatic and inflammatory elbow.

Failures of interposition arthroplasty are mostly associated with postoperative elbow instability. Knight and Van Zandt[31] reported 14-year follow-up of interposition arthroplasty results, and noted a 20% failure rate primarily associated with elbow instability. Nolla and colleagues[32] had 2 failures in 13 elbows treated with interposition arthroplasty and temporary hinged external fixation. The elbows developed instability after the external fixator was removed. Reports by Fox and colleagues[33] and Cheng and Morrey[30] showed effective restoration of joint stability and subsequent good outcomes following hardware removal. Therefore, we emphasize the importance of restoring elbow stability, which can be done via ligament reconstruction, bone grafting to restore bony stability, and if necessary, the use of an IJS. Early results of IJS have demonstrated promising results. In a multicenter trial, Orbay and colleagues[18] reported good to excellent results in 23 of 24 patients treated with an IJS for elbow instability, 6 months after removal of the device. The one failure was in a patient with a deficient coronoid. Another report by Sochol and colleagues[19] showed stable elbows following IJS placement in 19 of 20 patients treated for posttraumatic elbow instability. One patient experienced hardware failure, whereas a second patient developed a delayed infection related to the hardware, but was found to have a stable joint at the time of hardware removal.

Interposition arthroplasty in conjunction with ligament reconstruction and an IJS offers a reasonably durable, though imperfect, solution for patients presenting with painful, unstable, arthritic elbows. In the authors' experience, best outcomes for interposition arthroplasty depend on several factors. Most importantly, there must be no substantial loss of bone stock. Patient expectations must be appropriately managed. Patients should understand that they may achieve acceptable, but not complete pain relief and that they will achieve functional but not complete range of motion of the elbow. At the time of surgery, comprehensive joint release must be achieved to maximize exposure and postoperative range of motion. The resurfacing graft should be firmly fixed to the distal humerus to prevent early wear. Elbow stability must be maintained or restored with the use of ligamentous and/or bony reconstruction. The recent availability of an IJS has improved our ability to stabilize select patients and may be used to stabilize the joint and protect the ligament repair/reconstruction. The IJS, however, needs to be placed perfectly at the axis of rotation of the elbow joint to allow for congruent, unobstructed, and painless range of motion, and it should not be used to distract the elbow. Finally, careful postoperative wound management and placement of drains is used to help prevent complications.

Interposition arthroplasty can be an appropriate option for the right patient. Adherence to the principles described will help achieve satisfactory results in this challenging subset of patients.

DISCLOSURE

The authors, their immediate families, and any research foundations with which they are affiliated have not received any financial; payments or other benefits from any commercial entity related to the subject of this article.

REFERENCES

1. Gschwend N, Simmen BR, Matejovsky Z. Late complications in elbow arthroplasty. J Shoulder Elbow Surg 1996;5(2 Pt 1):86–96.
2. Siala M, Laumonerie P, Hedjoudje A, et al. Outcomes of semiconstrained total elbow arthroplasty performed for arthritis in patients under 55 years old. J Shoulder Elbow Surg 2019;1–8. https://doi.org/10.1016/j.jse.2019.08.006.
3. Zarkadas PC, Cass B, Throckmorton T, et al. Long-term outcome of resection arthroplasty for the failed total elbow arthroplasty. J Bone Joint Surg Am 2010;92(15):2576–82.
4. Otto RJ, Mulieri PJ, Cottrell BJ, et al. Arthrodesis for failed total elbow arthroplasty with deep infection. J Shoulder Elbow Surg 2014;23(3):302–7.
5. Chen DD, Forsh DA, Hausman MR. Elbow interposition arthroplasty. Hand Clin 2011;27(2):187–97.
6. Brown TD, Johnston RC, Saltzman CL, et al. Post-traumatic osteoarthritis: a first estimate of incidence,

prevalence, and burden of disease. J Orthop Trauma 2006;20(10):739–44.
7. Biswas D, Wysocki RW, Cohen MS. Primary and posttraumatic arthritis of the elbow. Arthritis 2013;2013. https://doi.org/10.1155/2013/473259.
8. Giannicola G, Bullitta G, Sacchetti FM, et al. Change in quality of life and cost/utility analysis in open stage-related surgical treatment of elbow stiffness. Orthopedics 2013;36(7):923–31.
9. Kauffman JI, Chen AL, Stuchin S, et al. Surgical management of the rheumatoid elbow. J Am Acad Orthop Surg 2003;11(2):100–8.
10. Voloshin I, Schippert DW, Kakar S, et al. Complications of total elbow replacement: a systematic review. J Shoulder Elbow Surg 2011;20(1):158–68.
11. Schoch B, Wong J, Abboud J, et al. Results of total elbow arthroplasty in patients less than 50 years old. J Hand Surg Am 2017;42(10):797–802.
12. Kwak J, Koh K, Jeon I. Total elbow arthroplasty: clinical outcomes, complications, and revision surgery. Clin Orthop Surg 2019;11(4):369.
13. Kaufmann RA, D'Auria JL, Schneppendahl J. Total elbow arthroplasty: elbow biomechanics and failure. J Hand Surg Am 2019;44(8):687–92.
14. Koller H, Kolb K, Assuncao A, et al. The fate of elbow arthrodesis: indications, techniques, and outcome in fourteen patients. J Shoulder Elbow Surg 2008;17(2):293–306.
15. Kouvidis GK, Chalidis BE, Liddington MI, et al. Reconstruction of a severe open distal humerus fracture with complete loss of medial column by using a free fibular osteocutaneous graft. Eplasty 2008;8:e24.
16. Sanchez-Sotelo J. Elbow rheumatoid elbow: surgical treatment options. Curr Rev Musculoskelet Med 2016;9(2):224–31.
17. Orbay JL, Mijares MR. The management of elbow instability using an internal joint stabilizer: Preliminary results. Clin Orthop Relat Res 2014;472(7):2049–60.
18. Orbay JL, Ring D, Kachooei AR, et al. Multicenter trial of an internal joint stabilizer for the elbow. J Shoulder Elbow Surg 2017;26(1):125–32.
19. Sochol KM, Andelman SM, Koehler SM, et al. Treatment of traumatic elbow instability with an internal joint stabilizer. J Hand Surg Am 2019;44(2):161.e1-7.
20. Mansat P. Surgical treatment of the rheumatoid elbow. Joint Bone Spine 2001;68(3):198–210.
21. Morrey BF, Sanchez-Sotelo J, Morrey ME. Chapter 114 - Interposition arthroplasty of the elbow. In: Morrey's the elbow and its disorders. Fifth edition. Philadelphia: Elsevier; 2018.
22. von Knoch F, Marsh JL, Steyers C, et al. A new articulated elbow external fixation technique for difficult elbow trauma. Iowa Orthop J 2001;21:13–9.

23. Bottlang M, O'Rourke MR, Madey SM, et al. Radiographic determinants of the elbow rotation axis: Experimental identification and quantitative validation. J Orthop Res 2000;18(5):821–8.

24. Jobe FW, Stark H, Lombardo SJ. Reconstruction of the ulnar collateral ligament in athletes. J Bone Joint Surg Am 1986;68(8):1158–63.

25. O'Driscoll SW, Bell DF, Morrey BF. Posterolateral rotatory instability of the elbow. J Bone Joint Surg Am 1991;73(3):440–6. Available at: http://www.ncbi. nlm.nih.gov/pubmed/2002081.

26. DeLaMora SN, Hausman M. Lateral ulnar collateral ligament reconstruction using the lateral triceps fascia. Orthopedics 2002;25(9):909–12.

27. Larson AN, Morrey BF. Interposition arthroplasty with an Achilles tendon allograft as a salvage procedure for the elbow. J Bone Joint Surg Am 2008;90(12): 2714–23.

28. Fernandez-Palazzi F, Rodriguez J, Oliver G. Elbow interposition arthroplasty in children and adolescents: long-term follow-up. Int Orthop 2008; 32(2):247–50.

29. Ljung P, Jonsson K, Larsson K, et al. Interposition arthroplasty of the elbow with rheumatoid arthritis. J Shoulder Elbow Surg 1996;5(2 Pt 1):81–5.

30. Cheng SL, Morrey BF. Treatment of the mobile, painful arthritic elbow by distraction interposition arthroplasty. J Bone Joint Surg Br 2000;82(2):233–8.

31. Knight RA, Van Zandt IL. Arthroplasty of the elbow; an end-result study. J Bone Joint Surg Am 1952;24 A(3):610–8. Available at: http://www.ncbi.nlm.nih. gov/pubmed/14946212. Accessed December 15, 2019.

32. Nolla J, Ring D, Lozano-Calderon S, et al. Interposition arthroplasty of the elbow with hinged external fixation for post-traumatic arthritis. J Shoulder Elbow Surg 2008. https://doi.org/10.1016/j.jse.2007.11.008.

33. Fox RJ, Varitimidis SE, Plakseychuk A, et al. The compass elbow hinge: indications and initial results. J Hand Surg Br 2000;25(6):568–72.

1. Publication Title	2. Publication Number	3. Filing Date
HAND CLINICS	000 – 709	9/18/2020

4. Issue Frequency	5. Number of Issues Published Annually	6. Annual Subscription Price
FEB, MAY, AUG, NOV	4	$439.00

7. Complete Mailing Address of Known Office of Publication (Not printer) (Street, city, county, state, and ZIP+4®)

ELSEVIER INC.
230 Park Avenue, Suite 800
New York, NY 10169

Contact Person
Malathi Samayan

Telephone (Include area code)
91-44-4299-4507

8. Complete Mailing Address of Headquarters or General Business Office of Publisher (Not printer)

ELSEVIER INC.
230 Park Avenue, Suite 800
New York, NY 10169

9. Full Names and Complete Mailing Addresses of Publisher, Editor, and Managing Editor (Do not leave blank)

Publisher (Name and complete mailing address)

Dolores Meloni, ELSEVIER INC.
1600 JOHN F KENNEDY BLVD. SUITE 1800
PHILADELPHIA, PA 19103-2899

Editor (Name and complete mailing address)

LAUREN BOYLE, ELSEVIER INC.
1600 JOHN F KENNEDY BLVD. SUITE 1800
PHILADELPHIA, PA 19103-2899

Managing Editor (Name and complete mailing address)

PATRICK MANLEY, ELSEVIER INC.
1600 JOHN F KENNEDY BLVD. SUITE 1800
PHILADELPHIA, PA 19103-2899

10. Owner (Do not leave blank. If the publication is owned by a corporation, give the name and address of the corporation immediately followed by the names and addresses of all stockholders owning or holding 1 percent or more of the total amount of stock. If not owned by a corporation, give the names and addresses of the individual owners. If owned by a partnership or other unincorporated firm, give its name and address as well as those of each individual owner. If the publication is published by a nonprofit organization, give its name and address.)

Full Name	Complete Mailing Address
WHOLLY OWNED SUBSIDIARY OF REED/ELSEVIER, US HOLDINGS	1600 JOHN F KENNEDY BLVD. SUITE 1800 PHILADELPHIA, PA 19103-2899

11. Known Bondholders, Mortgagees, and Other Security Holders Owning or Holding 1 Percent or More of Total Amount of Bonds, Mortgages, or Other Securities. If none, check box ▶ ☐ None

Full Name	Complete Mailing Address
N/A	

12. Tax Status (For completion by nonprofit organizations authorized to mail at nonprofit rates) (Check one)
The purpose, function, and nonprofit status of this organization and the exempt status for federal income tax purposes:
☒ Has Not Changed During Preceding 12 Months
☐ Has Changed During Preceding 12 Months (Publisher must submit explanation of change with this statement)

PS Form **3526**, July 2014 [Page 1 of 4 (see instructions page 4)] PSN 7530-01-000-9931   PRIVACY NOTICE: See our privacy policy on www.usps.com.

13. Publication Title	14. Issue Date for Circulation Data Below
HAND CLINICS	MAY 2020

15. Extent and Nature of Circulation			Average No. Copies Each Issue During Preceding 12 Months	No. Copies of Single Issue Published Nearest to Filing Date
a. Total Number of Copies (Net press run)			304	280
b. Paid Circulation (By Mail and Outside the Mail)	(1)	Mailed Outside-County Paid Subscriptions Stated on PS Form 3541 (Include paid distribution above nominal rate, advertiser's proof copies, and exchange copies)	186	169
	(2)	Mailed In-County Paid Subscriptions Stated on PS Form 3541 (Include paid distribution above nominal rate, advertiser's proof copies, and exchange copies)	0	0
	(3)	Paid Distribution Outside the Mails Including Sales Through Dealers and Carriers, Street Vendors, Counter Sales, and Other Paid Distribution Outside USPS®	88	82
	(4)	Paid Distribution by Other Classes of Mail Through the USPS (e.g., First-Class Mail®)	0	0
c. Total Paid Distribution (Sum of 15b (1), (2), (3), and (4))			274	251
d. Free or Nominal Rate Distribution (By Mail and Outside the Mail)	(1)	Free or Nominal Rate Outside-County Copies included on PS Form 3541	13	12
	(2)	Free or Nominal Rate In-County Copies Included on PS Form 3541	0	0
	(3)	Free or Nominal Rate Copies Mailed at Other Classes Through the USPS (e.g., First-Class Mail)	0	0
	(4)	Free or Nominal Rate Distribution Outside the Mail (Carriers or other means)	13	12
e. Total Free or Nominal Rate Distribution (Sum of 15d (1), (2), (3) and (4))			13	12
f. Total Distribution (Sum of 15c and 15e)			287	263
g. Copies not Distributed (See Instructions to Publishers #4 (page #3))			17	17
h. Total (Sum of 15f and g)			304	280
i. Percent Paid (15c divided by 15f times 100)			95.47%	95.43%

* If you are claiming electronic copies, go to line 16 on page 3. If you are not claiming electronic copies, skip to line 17 on page 3.

16. Electronic Copy Circulation	Average No. Copies Each Issue During Preceding 12 Months	No. Copies of Single Issue Published Nearest to Filing Date
a. Paid Electronic Copies ▶		
b. Total Paid Print Copies (Line 15c) + Paid Electronic Copies (Line 16a) ▶		
c. Total Print Distribution (Line 15f) + Paid Electronic Copies (Line 16a) ▶		
d. Percent Paid (Both Print & Electronic Copies) (16b divided by 16c × 100) ▶		

☒ I certify that 50% of all my distributed copies (electronic and print) are paid above a nominal price.

17. Publication of Statement of Ownership

☒ If the publication is a general publication, publication of this statement is required. Will be printed
in the _____ November 2020 _____ issue of this publication.   ☐ Publication not required.

18. Signature and Title of Editor, Publisher, Business Manager, or Owner

Malathi Samayan - Distribution Controller

Malathi Samayan   Date 9/18/2020

I certify that all information furnished on this form is true and complete. I understand that anyone who furnishes false or misleading information on this form or who omits material or information requested on the form may be subject to criminal sanctions (including fines and imprisonment) and/or civil sanctions (including civil penalties).

PS Form **3526**, July 2014 (Page 3 of 4)   PRIVACY NOTICE: See our privacy policy on www.usps.com.

Moving?

Make sure your subscription moves with you!

To notify us of your new address, find your **Clinics Account Number** (located on your mailing label above your name), and contact customer service at:

Email: journalscustomerservice-usa@elsevier.com

800-654-2452 (subscribers in the U.S. & Canada)
314-447-8871 (subscribers outside of the U.S. & Canada)

Fax number: 314-447-8029

Elsevier Health Sciences Division
Subscription Customer Service
3251 Riverport Lane
Maryland Heights, MO 63043

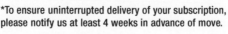

*To ensure uninterrupted delivery of your subscription, please notify us at least 4 weeks in advance of move.

Printed and bound by CPI Group (UK) Ltd, Croydon, CR0 4YY

03/10/2024

01040307-0018